G Proteins,
Receptors,
and
Disease

CONTEMPORARY ENDOCRINOLOGY

P. Michael Conn, SERIES EDITOR

G Proteins, Receptors, and Disease

Edited by

Allen M. Spiegel, MD

Chief, Metabolic Diseases Branch,
National Institute of Diabetes
and Digestive and Kidney Diseases,
National Institutes of Health, Bethesda, MD

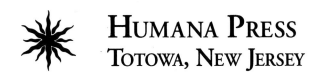

Humana Press
Totowa, New Jersey

G proteins, receptors, and disease/edited by Allen M. Spiegel
    p.   cm.—(Contemporary endocrinology™; 6)
    Includes index.
    ISBN 0-89603-430-5 (alk. paper)
    1. G proteins—Physiological effect. 2. G proteins—Pathophysiology 3. Endocrine glands—Diseases. 4. Cellular signal transduction 5. Pathology, Molecular. I. Spiegel, Allen M. II. Series: Contemporary endocrinology (Totowa, NJ);
    [DNLM: 1. G proteins—physiology. 2. Receptors, Cell Surface—physiology. 3. Endocrine Diseases—genetics. 4. Signal Transduction. QU 55 G1113 1998]
QP552.G16G24 1998
616,4' 071—dc21
DNLM/DLC
for Library of Congress
                                                      97-51985
                                                      CIP

PREFACE

"Theoretically, one should obtain essentially the same clinical picture from failure of an end-organ to respond to a hormone as from a decreased production or absence of said hormone." With these words, Fuller Albright began his now classic paper describing a novel disease, pseudohypoparathyroidism (PHP), and a novel concept, hormone resistance as a cause of disease. Soon, other hormone resistance disorders such as nephrogenic diabetes insipidus (NDI) were recognized, and the concept was extended to resistance to other substances such as calcium ions in familial hypocalciuric hypercalcemia (FHH). Later, diseases characterized by excess rather than deficient hormone action such as McCune-Albright syndrome (MAS) and familial male precocious puberty (FMPP) were recognized to be caused by autonomous endocrine hyperfunction. Although many investigators provided careful and detailed descriptions of the clinical features of these and other related endocrine disorders, an understanding of pathogenesis proved elusive for many years.

In just the past few years, we have gone from clinical description to a molecular understanding of these interesting disorders. This remarkable progress reflects a synthesis of three distinct, but now overlapping, areas of biomedical research: the aforementioned recognition and careful clinical description of specific diseases, the elucidation of the basic mechanisms of signal transduction, and the application of the powerful tools of molecular biology and genetics. Fundamental studies on the mechanisms of hormone action by Rodbell and colleagues at NIH culminated in the discovery of a major signal transduction pathway involving heterotrimeric G proteins. Hundreds of G-protein-coupled receptors (GPCR), over a dozen G proteins, and a comparable number of effectors regulated by G proteins have now been identified and characterized at the molecular and cellular level. Identification and molecular characterization of these signaling proteins and the genes that encode them allowed them to be tested as candidates responsible for diseases of hormone resistance or endocrine hyperfunction. Powerful tools of molecular biology and genetics such as the polymerase chain reaction and gene mapping facilitated testing such hypotheses.

The present volume offers the reader the fruits of the application of molecular biology and genetics to studies of G-protein-coupled signal transduction and disease. Two important and related themes run through each chapter of the book: Many diseases of hormone resistance and of endocrine hyperfunction are caused by loss- and gain-of-function mutations in G proteins or GPCR and the studies of such diseases and the mutations that cause them offer unique insights into the physiologic relevance, structure and function of the involved G protein or GPCR. Many of the chapters include, in addition to discussion of naturally occurring human (or in some instances other mammalian) disorders, a discussion of artificially created disorders using transgenic and gene knockout approaches in mice. The latter also offers powerful insights into G protein and GPCR structure and function, and also suggests new candidate genes for human disorders whose pathogenesis remains unclear.

An introductory chapter provides an overview of G-protein-coupled signal transduction and its relevance to human disease, not only to endocrine disorders, which are the main focus of the book and are covered in detail in the ensuing chapters, but also to other disorders in which G-protein and GPCR mutations play a role, such as retinitis pigmentosa, congenital megacolon, and AIDS. The next section of the book (Chapters 2–6) addresses G proteins, disorders such as PHP and MAS caused by G-protein mutations, and insights gained from G protein mouse gene knockouts. The remainder of the book contains chapters on various GPCR. Chapters 7–9 consider glycoprotein hormone receptors and diseases such as FMPP and hyperthyroidism caused by mutations in these receptors. Chapters 10–15 cover receptors for other peptide hormones such as vasopressin, PTH, ACTH, MSH, as well as the calcium ion receptor. Diseases owing to mutations in these receptors include NDI, FHH, and familial glucocorticoid deficiency. The final section of the book (Chapters 16–18) deals with β-adrenergic and dopamine receptors, including studies on transgenic and knockout mice. Although no single mutation in one of these receptors has clearly been identified as the cause of a human disease, identification of an association between a β3-adrenergic receptor polymorphism and obesity (Chapter 18) highlights the possible contribution of subtle differences in G-protein and GPCR structure to polygenic disorders such as type II diabetes and hypertension.

I hope the reader will share the sense of excitement as leading investigators depict in their respective chapters the discovery of causes for diseases that were mysterious for many years. The impact of these discoveries for disease diagnosis and our appreciation of the structure and function of the involved G proteins and GPCR has been immediate. As has been the case in other parts of the human genetics revolution, the impact on disease prevention and treatment has been less dramatic. A thorough understanding of molecular pathogenesis, nonetheless, should provide the foundation for future efforts directed at prevention and cure of these diseases. With eventual progress in gene therapy and other approaches both old and new, I expect that future versions of these chapters will include expanded sections on the prevention and treatment of their respective diseases.

Allen M. Spiegel, MD

CONTENTS

CONTRIBUTORS

DOMENICO ACCILI, MD, *Developmental Endocrinology Branch, National Institute of Child Health and Human Development, Bethesda, MD*

MEI BAI, PhD, *Endocrine-Hypertension and Renal Divisions, Department of Medicine, Brigham and Women's Hospital, Boston, MA*

DANIEL G. BICHET, MD, *Service de Nephrologie et Centre de Recherche, Hôpital du Sacre-Coeur de Montreal, Quebec, Canada*

LUTZ BIRNBAUMER, PhD, *Department of Anesthesiology, University of California School of Medicine, Los Angeles, CA*

EDWARD M. BROWN, MD, *Endocrine-Hypertension Division, Brigham and Women's Hospital, Boston, MA*

GEORGE P. CHROUSOS, MD, *Developmental Endocrinology Branch, National Institute of Child Health and Human Development, National Institutes of Health, Bethesda, MD*

ROGER D. CONE, PhD, *The Vollum Institute for Advanced Biomedical Research, Oregon Health Sciences University, Portland, OR*

OMAR A. COSO, PhD, *Molecular Signaling Unit, Laboratory of Cellular Development and Oncology, National Institute of Dental Research, National Institutes of Health, Bethesda, MD*

VENITA I. DEALMEIDA, MS, *Department of Biochemistry, Molecular Biology, and Cell Biology, Northwestern University, Evanston, IL*

JOHN DRAGO, MD, PhD, *Neuroscience Laboratory, Department of Anatomy, Monash University, Clayton, Victoria, Australia*

SARA FUCHS, PhD, *Department of Immunology, The Weizmann Institute of Science, Rehovot, Israel*

PATRICIA GALVIN-PARTON, MD, *University Medical Center, State University of New York, Stony Brook, NY*

PAUL A. GODFREY, BS, *Department of Biochemistry, Molecular Biology, and Cell Biology, Northwestern University, Evanston, IL*

JUN HUA GUO, MD, *Departments of Molecular Pharmacology and Pediatrics, University Medical Center, State University of New York, Stony Brook, NY*

J. SILVIO GUTKIND, PhD, *National Institute of Dental Research, National Institutes of Health, Bethesda, MD*

CARRIE HASKELL-LUEVANO, PhD, *The Vollum Institute for Advanced Biomedical Research, Oregon Health Sciences University, Portland, OR*

STEVEN C. HEBERT, MD, *Endocrine-Hypertension and Renal Divisions, Department of Medicine, Brigham and Women's Hospital, Boston, MA*

ILPO T. HUHTANIEMI, MD, PhD, *Department of Physiology, University of Turku, Finland*

HARALD JÜPPNER, MD, *Endocrine Unit, Department of Medicine and Children's Service, Massachusetts General Hospital and Harvard Medical School, Boston, MA*

WALTER J. KOCH, PhD, *Department of Surgery, Howard Hughes Medical Institute, Duke University Medical Center, Durham, NC*

ROBERT J. LEFKOWITZ, MD, *Department of Medicine and Biochemistry, Howard Hughes Medical Institute, Duke University Medical Center, Durham NC*

DONGSI LU, PhD, *The Vollum Institute for Advanced Biomedical Research, Oregon Health Sciences University, Portland, OR*

CRAIG C. MALBON, PhD, *Departments of Molecular Pharmacology and Pediatrics, University Medical Center, State University of New York, Stony Brook, NY*

KELLY E. MAYO, PhD, *Department of Biochemistry, Molecular Biology, and Cell Biology, Northwestern University, Evanston, IL*

CHRISTOPHER M. MOXHAM, PhD, *Department of Molecular Pharmacology and Pediatrics, University Medical Center, State University of New York, Stony Brook, NY*

MARTIN POLLAK, MD, *Endocrine-Hypertension and Renal Divisions, Department of Medicine, Brigham and Women's Hospital, Boston, MA*

UWE RUDOLPH, MD, *Institute of Pharmacology, University of Zurich, Zurich, Switzerland*

ANDREW SHENKER, MD, PhD, *Division of Endocrinology, Department of Pediatrics, Children's Memorial Hospital and Northwestern University Medical School, Chicago, IL*

ALAN R. SHULDINER, MD, *Division of Diabetes, Obesity, and Nutrition, University of Maryland , Baltimore, MD*

KRISTI SILVER, MD, *Division of Endocrinology, Johns Hopkins University School of Medicine, Baltimore, MD*

ALLEN M. SPIEGEL, MD, *Metabolic Diseases Branch, National Institute of Diabetes and Digestive and Kidney Diseases, National Institutes of Health, Bethesda, MD*

CONSTANTINE TSIGOS, MD, PhD, *Department of Experimental Physiology, University of Athens Medical School, Greece*

DAG INGE VAGE, PhD, *Department of Animal Science, Agricultural University of Norway, As, Norway*

GILBERT VASSART, MD, PhD, *Department of Medical Genetics, Institute of Interdisciplinary Research, Universite Libre de Bruxelles, Belgium*

JEREMY WALSTON, MD, *Division of Geriatric Medicine and Gerontology, Johns Hopkins University School of Medicine, Baltimore, MD*

HSIEN-YU WANG, PhD, *Department of Physiology and Biophysics, University Medical Center, State University of New York, Stony Brook, NY*

LEE S. WEINSTEIN, MD, *Metabolic Diseases Branch, National Institute of Diabetes, Digestive, and Kidney Diseases, National Institutes of Health, Bethesda, MD*

KENNETH C. WU, BS, *Department of Biochemistry, Molecular Biology, and Cell Biology, Northwestern University, Evanston, IL*

NINGZHI XU, MD, *Molecular Signaling Unit, Laboratory of Cellular Development and Oncology, National Institute of Dental Research, National Institutes of Health, Bethesda, MD*

1

Introduction to G-Protein-Coupled Signal Transduction and Human Disease

Allen M. Spiegel, MD

CONTENTS

OVERVIEW OF G-PROTEIN-COUPLED SIGNAL TRANSDUCTION

Background

Signal transduction mechanisms can be divided into two major classes, those involving intracellular (cytoplasmic and nuclear) receptors, typified by the thyroid and steroid hormone receptor family, and those involving cell-surface (plasma membrane) receptors. The latter group can be further subdivided according to the effector mechanism employed for receptor signaling. Examples include receptors with intrinsic effector activity, such as tyrosine kinases, serine/threonine kinases, phosphatases, and ligand-gated ion channels, and receptors without intrinsic effector activity typified by the G-protein-coupled receptors (GPCR). Numerous diseases are now known to be caused by defects in signal transduction, and examples exist for each of the major signal transduction mechanisms. This volume focuses on diseases caused by defects in G-protein-coupled signal transduction. This introductory chapter reviews our current understanding of the structure and function of G proteins and the receptors to which they couple, offers some general considerations on how mutations in G proteins and GPCR cause disease, and gives a broad overview of disorders caused by defects in G-protein-coupled signal transduction.

From: *Contemporary Endocrinology: G Proteins, Receptors, and Disease*
Edited by: A. M. Spiegel, Humana Press Inc., Totowa, NJ

Heterotrimeric G Proteins and the Guanosine Triphosphatase (GTPase) Cycle

Heterotrimeric G proteins are members of a gene superfamily encoding proteins that bind guanine nucleotides with high affinity and specificity *(1–3)*. Other members include initiation and elongation factors involved in protein synthesis and "low-mol-wt" GTP-binding proteins in the p21 *ras* oncogene family. The G proteins are heterotrimers consisting of α-, β-, and γ-subunits in decreasing order of molecular weight. It is the α-subunit that binds guanine nucleotides; the β- and γ-subunits form a tightly, but noncovalently associated dimer that functions as a single unit. G proteins act as key intermediates in signal transduction. They couple cell-surface receptors for hormones, neurotransmitters, growth factors, odorants, and photons of light to a diverse set of effector molecules, including ion channels and enzymes that generate second messengers. The very large family of G-protein-coupled receptors shares the common structural motif of seven putative membrane-spanning domains and the common functional feature of agonist-dependent G-protein activation *(4,5)*.

All G proteins share certain common functional features. Chief among these is the GTPase cycle (*see* Fig. 1) that governs G-protein function. G proteins act as timing switches. In the guanosine diphosphate (GDP)-bound conformation, the α-subunit is associated with βγ and is "off" with respect to effector interaction. Agonist-activated receptors act catalytically to release tightly bound GDP from the α-subunit and permit GTP to bind. GTP switches the α-subunit to the "on" conformation, which enables the α-subunit to dissociate from βγ, and interact with and modulate effector activity. βγ-subunits also have been shown to modulate the activity of certain effectors. An intrinsic α-subunit GTPase activity serves as a timing device. By cleaving the terminal phosphate of GTP, GDP is reformed, and the α-subunit resumes its "off" conformation. The heterotrimer reassociates and awaits activated receptor to re-enter another round of the cycle. Some effectors have been shown to speed the α-subunit GTPase activity. This serves as a built-in mechanism to regulate the duration of effector activation by α-subunit. Members of a recently discovered gene family, the (RGS) regulator of G-protein signaling family, have been shown to interact directly with G-protein α-subunits and to stimulate their GTPase activity *(6)*. RGS proteins interact preferentially with a "transition-state" complex between the α-subunit and GTP to facilitate GTP hydrolysis. Specificity in interactions of individual RGS proteins and α-subunits has already been demonstrated, and it is possible that each subset of the α-subunit family has its own corresponding RGS.

GPCR Structure and Function

GENERAL FEATURES

Hydropathy analysis of the primary sequences of all GPCR studied to date shows seven stretches of predominantly hydrophobic amino acids about 20 residues long. These are predicted to form α-helical membrane-spanning domains by extrapolation from the structure of rhodopsin. The seven membrane-spanning domains putatively form a barrel oriented roughly perpendicular to the plane of the membrane, with an extracellular amino-terminus and intracellular carboxy-terminus, three connecting loops located extracellularly (e1–e3) and three located intracellularly (i1–i3). Supporting evidence for this topography comes from studies of susceptibility of specific domains of the receptor to proteolytic cleavage, from immunochemical studies using antibodies against defined epitopes, and from studies of 2-D crystals of purified rhodopsin inserted into lipid bilayers.

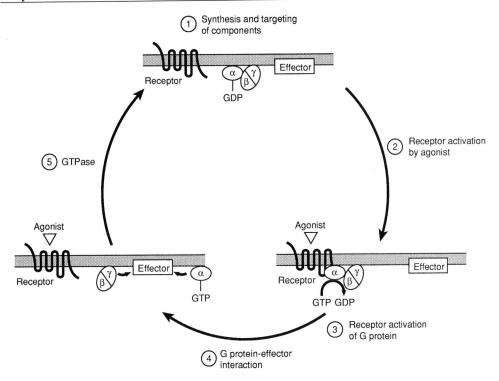

Fig. 1. The G-protein GTPase cycle. Potential sites for disease-causing abnormalities are numbered. In each panel, the stippled region denotes the plasma membrane with extracellular above and intracellular below. In the basal state, the G protein is a heterotrimer with GDP tightly bound to the α-subunit. The agonist-activated receptor catalyzes release of tightly bound GDP, which permits GTP to bind. The GTP-bound α-subunit dissociates from the βγ dimer. Arrows between GTP-bound α subunit and effector and between βγ-dimer and effector indicate regulation of effector activity by the respective subunits. Under physiologic conditions, effector regulation by G-protein subunits is transient and is terminated by the GTPase activity of the α-subunit. The latter converts bound GTP to GDP, thus returning the α-subunit to its inactivated state with high affinity for the βγ-dimer, which reassociates again to form the heterotrimer.

Several posttranslational modifications are found in most GPCR. One or more sites for N-linked glycosylation are present in the amino-terminus (more rarely in one or more of the extracellular loops). Functionally, glycosylation is not critical for ligand binding, but may be important for normal receptor synthesis and membrane insertion.

Most G-protein-coupled receptors have cysteine residues in the e1 and e2 loops that are linked in a disulfide bond. Formation of this disulfide bond appears to be critical for normal folding and subsequent transport from the endoplasmic reticulum. Mutations in rhodopsin, for example, that impair disulfide formation cause receptor to accumulate in the endoplasmic reticulum. This leads to photoreceptor degeneration characteristic of retinitis pigmentosa (*see* Opsins). Most GPCR have one or even two cysteines in the membrane-proximal portion of the carboxy-terminus. This residue has been shown to undergo palmitoylation (reversible thioesterification with a 16-carbon fatty acid). One can speculate that membrane anchoring via the palmitoylated cysteine effectively creates a fourth intracellular loop, but the functional significance of this modification is not completely clear in that mutation of this cysteine to serine does not cause obvious functional alterations in each receptor in which this has been studied. In most GPCR, the carboxy-terminus is rich in serine and threonine residues that are thought to be the sites for phosphorylation by kinases that act to desensitize GPCR (*see* GPCR Regulation). For some GPCR, the sites of phosphorylation are within the i3 loop rather than, or in addition to, the carboxy-terminus.

Superimposed on the common themes outlined above are variations that confer specificity in ligand binding, G-protein coupling, and range of expression of members of the GPCR superfamily. Primary sequence among members of the superfamily may be quite divergent. Only a small number of residues are conserved in virtually all members. Most of these are located in the membrane-spanning domains. The GPCR vary not only in sequence, but also in length of amino- and carboxy-termini and of the various loops most especially the i3 loop. Amino-termini, for example, vary from very short (neurotransmitter receptors) to medium length (members of the parathyroid hormone (PTH)/calcitonin receptor subfamily) to very long (>300 residues) for the glycoprotein hormone receptors and the metabotropic glutamate and calcium-sensing receptors. Variations in posttranslational modifications include number and site of glycosylation, lack of disulfide linking e1 and e2, number and sites of phosphorylation, and number of sites for palmitoylation. The gene structure of members of the GPCR family is highly variable. Rhodopsin, for example, shows typical exon–intron structure, whereas many members of the family have intronless genes or genes with very few introns. Exon–intron borders, where present, often correspond to functional domains (e.g., separate exons for large amino-terminus of glycoprotein hormone receptors vs for seven membrane-spanning domains). Very few GPCR gene promoters have yet been characterized, but these presumably differ significantly and account for major differences in expression range. Some GPCR are restricted in expression to single cell types (e.g., rod and cone opsins), others show a slightly less restricted distribution (glycoprotein hormone receptors), and some are relatively widely distributed (β-adrenergic receptors).

LIGAND BINDING

The first step in signal transduction is binding of ligand to receptor. For GPCR, ligands are very diverse. They range from small molecules, such as biogenic amines and odorants, through small peptides, such as vasopressin, to larger peptides, such as PTH, to much larger proteins, such as the glycoprotein hormones. The best studied GPCR, rhodopsin, actually has its ligand retinal covalently attached. When retinal captures photons of light, it isomerizes and thereby activates rhodopsin. Thus, it depends on photon capture to become an agonist. The ability to couple to and activate G protein is an intrinsic feature of the receptor. A current model of GPCR suggests that the receptor is in a dynamic equilibrium between a state favoring G-protein interaction and one that does not favor G-protein interaction. The role of agonist binding is to favor formation of the activated conformation that promotes G-protein interaction. Antagonists bind specifically to a receptor and can prevent agonists from binding, but they fail to promote the conformation of the receptor capable of activating G proteins. In fact, some antagonists, so-called inverse agonists, actually promote the inactive conformation of the receptor. Rhodopsin binds its ligand, 11-cis retinal, covalently via a protonated Schiff base between the ligand and a lysine residue in the seventh transmembrane domain. The counterion to the protonated Schiff base is a glutamate residue in the third transmembrane domain. The evidence points to a ligand binding pocket within the barrel created by the transmembrane helices. Experimental evidence based on photoaffinity analog labeling, substitution mutagenesis, and chimeric receptors strongly suggests that the ligand binding pocket of GPCR that bind monoamine neurotransmitters is likewise within the transmembrane-spanning helices. In all cases, multiple helices contribute to creation of the ligand binding site. An acidic residue in the third transmembrane domain (comparable to the glutamate in rhodopsin) is characteristic of all biogenic amine binding GPCR. Distinct sites have been identified in several transmembrane domains that affect predominantly antagonist rather than agonist binding. Differences in sequence in the transmembrane domains appear to define specificity of ligand binding. For example, two serines in the fifth transmembrane domain are conserved among all GPCR that bind catecholamines (adrenergic and dopaminergic receptors). Certain serine, threonine, and tyrosine residues within the membrane-spanning domains are characteristic of muscarinic receptors, and appear to be involved in creating the ligand binding pocket. Proline residues in the transmembrane helices may be involved in stabilizing high-affinity agonist binding and in agonist-induced conformational activation of the receptor. A highly conserved aspartate residue in the second transmembrane domain has been shown to confer allosteric regulation (reduction in agonist binding affinity) of GPCR by sodium ions.

The ligand binding site has not been as clearly defined for GPCR with peptide or lipid (e.g., prostaglandins) ligands. Some evidence here too points to the importance of residues in the transmembrane helices. GPCR for larger peptide ligands have larger extracellular amino-termini, which appear to be involved in ligand binding. In the parathyroid hormone/calcitonin receptor subfamily, an approx 100 residue (exclusive of signal sequence) extracellular amino-terminus contains regions shown by deletion analysis to be critical for ligand binding. For the glycoprotein hormone receptors, the comparable region is over 300 residues long and can by itself bind ligand with high affinity. The rest of the receptor, comparable in size to more typical GPCR, is obviously critical for G-protein coupling, but may also contribute to ligand binding. Perhaps the most unique mechanism is found in the thrombin receptor. Here the ligand is a protease. The extracellular amino-terminus of the receptor contains both a ligand-specific anion binding site as well as the specific proteolytic cleavage substrate site. Binding and proteolysis releases an otherwise constrained sequence within the amino-terminus that autoactivates the receptor. The action of thrombin to activate the receptor can be mimicked by small peptides corresponding to the sequence immediately carboxy-terminal to the thrombin cleavage site.

G-PROTEIN COUPLING

Within the GPCR superfamily, subdivisions based on specificity of G-protein coupling can be made (Table 1). These include subfamilies that couple preferentially to G_s, G_i/G_o, and the G_q subfamily, respectively (receptor specificity in coupling to G_{12}/G_{13} has not yet been defined). Detailed study reveals additional levels of complexity in receptor–G-protein coupling. At one extreme, there is evidence for exquisite specificity of coupling within a given subfamily. Certain receptors may show strong preference for individual members of a G-protein subfamily (the C5A receptor prefers G_{16} to other members of the G_q subfamily; the somatostatin and M4 muscarinic receptors couple specifically to the G_{o2} and G_{o1} splice variants, respectively). At the other extreme, certain receptors may normally couple to more than one G-protein

Table 1
Mammalian α-Subunit Diversity

α-Subunit	Toxin Substrate	Expression	Receptor, examples	Effector
G_s	CTX	Ubiquitous	β-Adrenergic, PTH, TSH	↑ Adenylyl cyclase, Ca^{2+} channel
G_{olf}	CTX	Olfactory	Odorant	↑ Adenylyl cyclase
G_{t1}	PTX/CTX	Rod photoreceptors	Rhodopsin	↑ cGMP-phosphodiesterase
G_{t2}	PTX/CTX	Cone photoreceptors	Cone opsins	↑ cGMP-phosphodiesterase
G_{gust}	PTX/CTX?	Taste cells	Taste (?)	?
G_{i1}	PTX	Neural > other	$α_2$-Adrenergic, M2-muscarinic	
G_{i2}	PTX	Ubiquitous		} ↓ Adenylyl cyclase, ↑ K^+ channel
G_{i3}	PTX	Other > neural		
G_o	PTX	Neural, endocrine	Somatostatin	↓ Ca^{2+} channel
G_z	—	Neural, platelets	?	?
G_q	—	Ubiquitous	$α_1$-Adrenergic, M1-muscarinic	
G_{11}	—	Ubiquitous	TRH, V1-vasopressin	} ↑ Phospholipase C-β1
G_{14}	—	Liver, lung, kidney	Interleukin-8	
$G_{15/16}$	—	Blood cells		
G_{12}	—	Ubiquitous	?	?
G_{13}	—	Ubiquitous	?	?

subtype. The thrombin receptor evidently couples to members of both the G_q and G_i subfamilies. The thyroid-stimulating hormone (TSH) receptor can stimulate both cyclic adenosine monophosphate (cAMP) and inositol trisphosphate (IP_3) production, reflecting coupling to both G_s and G_q.

The carboxy-terminus and three intracellular loops are the candidate domains for G-protein interaction, and elucidation of the structural basis for specificity in coupling has focused on these regions. Mutagenesis (insertion, deletion, and substitution), construction of chimeric receptors, receptor antibodies, and synthetic peptides corresponding to these regions have all been used to define the structural determinants for G-protein coupling. The broad picture that emerges from these studies is that no single intracellular domain is solely responsible for G-protein coupling or even for selectivity in G-protein coupling. Lack of data on the 3-D structure of GPCR hampers any attempt to develop a rigorous model of the intracellular receptor domains involved in G-protein coupling, but the data are consistent with the notion that all three intracellular loops and the membrane-proximal portion of the carboxy-terminus contribute to G-protein binding. The regions most important in G-protein coupling may vary among different subsets of the G-protein-coupled receptor superfamily. A variety of experimental approaches provide convincing evidence that the i3 loop is a key determinant of G-protein-coupling specificity. Within the muscarinic receptor subgroup, for example, switching the i3 loop between the M2 and M3 muscarinic receptor subtypes confers G-protein-coupling selectivity of the i3 loop donor. Within the i3 loop, the membrane-proximal (amino- and carboxy-terminal) portions are critical. Much of the i3 loop can be deleted, particularly for receptors with long i3 loops, without altering receptor function. In contrast, changing even limited sequence of the amino-terminal portion of the i3 loop is sufficient to alter G-protein-coupling specificity. Interestingly, such discrete changes may result in a "hybrid" receptor capable of coupling to distinct G-protein classes. Synthetic peptides corresponding to amino- and carboxy-terminal portions of the i3 loop of the β-adrenergic receptor can activate G_s directly. Similar sequences have been identified in the i3 loop of receptors that couple to G_i and G_o. The wasp venom peptide mastoparan also activates G proteins directly, preferentially G_i and G_o. Variations in the i3 loop sequence of a given receptor can occur naturally as a result of alternative splicing. This has been found for the D2-dopamine and pituitary-adenylyl cyclase-activating peptide (PACAP) receptors. For the PACAP receptor, differential G-protein-coupling has been found to result from the alternative splicing.

The i3 loop is not the only determinant of G-protein coupling. Four forms of the prostaglandin E receptor EP3 subtype differing in the carboxy-terminal portion are derived by alternative splicing. These show significant differences in G-protein-coupling specificity. This suggests that the carboxy-terminus may also contribute to defining selectivity in G-protein interaction. The i2 loop likewise plays an important role in G-protein interaction. Certain chimeric receptors (e.g., M1 muscarinic/β-adrenergic) in which the i3 loop is exchanged gain the ability to couple to the G-protein defined by the donor i3 loop, but retain the ability to couple to the G-protein characteristic of the "wild-type" receptor. Determinants in the i2 loop appear responsible for this behavior. The amino acid sequence of the i2 loop is among the most highly conserved among the G-protein-coupled receptor superfamily. The motif DRY (or conservative variants, such as ERW) is characteristic of most G-protein-coupled receptors (the parathyroid hormone receptor subfamily is an exception). Mutation of the R in this motif to H in the V2 vasopressin receptor selectively impairs G-protein coupling. A hydrophobic residue (L, I, V, M, or F) occurs in the middle of this loop in most cloned G-protein-coupled receptors. Substitution of this residue with alanine or with more polar residues severely impairs G-protein coupling without otherwise affecting receptor function. The i2 loop (and this residue in particular) may be a site for interaction with G proteins in general, with other regions, such as the amino-terminal portion of the i3 loop, primarily responsible for selectivity of G-protein coupling.

GPCR REGULATION

GPCR, like other cell-surface receptors, are not static residents of the plasma membrane. They are internalized, and then either degraded or recycled to the plasma membrane in response to various stimuli. Desensitization is a general property of GPCR characterized by loss of responsiveness to prolonged stimulation by agonist. In the homologous form, the receptor is desensitized specifically to the class of agonist to which it has been exposed. In heterologous desensitization, exposure of one receptor to a given agonist may cause loss of responsiveness of other receptor classes to their cognate agonists. Receptor phosphorylation appears to be an early and key event in both types of desensitization. In the heterologous variety, second messenger-activated protein kinases may phosphorylate occupied and unoccupied receptors and cause reduced agonist responsiveness. In homologous desensitization, agonist-occupied receptors are far more susceptible to phosphorylation by a specific class of G-protein-coupled receptor kinases (GRKs). Rhodopsin kinase is a member of this family as is the so-called β-adrenergic receptor kinase (β-ARK). Agonist-occupied receptor activates G protein, presumptively dissociating α- from βγ-subunits (*see* Fig. 1). The latter appears to be critical for membrane and receptor targeting of certain GRKs. The phosphorylated receptor in turn binds a member of a family of soluble proteins termed β-arrestins that compete with G-protein α-subunits for receptor binding, thereby impeding signal transduction. Removal of agonist reverses the process as receptor phosphatases dephosphorylate the desensitized receptors, and GDP-bound α-subunits reassociate with βγ, so that the latter is no longer available for membrane targeting of GRK. The entire mechanism provides a form of negative feedback to blunt the effect of prolonged agonist stimulation. (Desensitization mechanisms are discussed in greater detail in Chapter 16.) Ultimately, however, desensitization mechanisms are unable to prevent inappropriate signaling completely by constitutively activated GPCR (*see* GPCR Gain-of-Function Mutations).

G-Protein Structure and Function

α-SUBUNIT STRUCTURE

All α-subunits (*see* Table 1) are at least 40% identical in amino acid sequence. These regions of identity correspond to five discrete regions ("G boxes") that in the 3-D structure come together to form the guanine nucleotide binding pocket *(7)*. The α-subunits vary in size from 350 to 395 amino acids. The amino- and carboxy-termini as well as the regions inserted between the G boxes show substantial sequence divergence. It is these divergent regions that are believed to confer specificity in G-protein coupling to receptors and effectors. Regions near the carboxy-terminus have been identified as critical for both effector and receptor interactions. The amino-terminus is required for association with the βγ-subunit. The α-subunit is made up of two major domains, a guanine nucleotide binding core very similar in structure to that of other members of the GTPase superfamily, such as *ras*, and an α-helical domain *(7)*. The bound guanine nucleotide is held in a cleft between these two domains. Through yet undefined contacts, activated receptor opens this cleft permitting exhange of GDP for GTP. GTP binding causes a conformational change in certain "switch" regions that is attended by dissociation from $\beta\gamma$ and interaction with effector.

Certain residues have been shown by site-directed mutagenesis to be crucial for α-subunit function. Arginine and glutamine residues (201 and 227, respectively, in the long form of $G\alpha_s$) are conserved in all α-subunits. Mutation of either residue slows GTPase activity and leads to constitutive activation. Cholera toxin modifies the same arginine residue covalently with equivalent effect. The glutamine is identical to that in position 61 of *ras*, a well-known oncogenic "hot spot." Mutation ("H21a") of the adjacent glycine 226 prevents α-subunit activation by GTP by blocking the necessary conformational switch. Mutation ("*unc*") of certain carboxy-terminal residues (e.g., arginine 389 in the long form of $G\alpha_s$) prevents the G protein from coupling to receptor. α-subunits in the G_i/G_o subfamily (Table 1) with a cysteine as the fourth residue from the carboxy-terminus are substrates for covalent modification by pertussis toxin, which likewise causes uncoupling from receptor.

None of the G-protein subunits possesses intrinsic hydrophobic, membrane-spanning domains. However, they behave largely as integral membrane proteins requiring detergent for solubilization from the membrane. A subset (G_i and G_o) of α-subunits undergoes a cotranslational modification in which the 14-carbon fatty acid myristate is attached to amino-terminal glycine. This modification is required for membrane targeting of this subset of α-subunits. It is unclear how other α-subunits, such as $G\alpha_s$ which do not undergo myristoylation, are targeted to the plasma membrane. All α-subunits with the exception of retinal $G\alpha_t$ undergo palmitoylation, a posttranslational modification with this 16-carbon fatty acid. This occurs on one or more cysteine residues near the amino-terminus, and again, this modification is critical for membrane association. Unlike myristoylation, which is a stable modification, palmitoylation is reversible. On α-subunit activation by GTP and dissociation from $\beta\gamma$, palmitate is cleaved; α-subunit hydrolysis of GTP to GDP then promotes repalmitoylation. There is thus a palmitoylation/depalmitoylation cycle stimulated by receptor activation of G protein and superimposed on the basic GTPase cycle. Most α-subunits are associated with the inner surface of the plasma membrane, but some may be localized to other subcellular compartments where their function is not yet clearly elucidated.

βγ-Subunit Structure

β-subunits are about 340 residues long and are highly conserved in sequence. Their 3-D structure has recently been determined both in the $\beta\gamma$ dimer and in the $\alpha\beta\gamma$ heterotrimer *(8)*. β-Subunits consist of an amino-terminal segment that forms a coiled-coil structure with the amino-terminal segment of γ, providing a tight, noncovalent association between the two subunits. The remainder of the β-subunit consists of seven repeats of an approx 40 residue motif (the β-transducin or WD-40 repeat). This element, originally recognized in the β-subunit of the retinal G protein, G_t or transducin, has now been found in a variety of different proteins of disparate subcellular localization and function. The precise functional significance of the WD-40 repeat is as yet unclear, but determination of the 3-D structure reveals that each WD-40 repeat is composed of interlocking β-sheets. The overall β-structure is that of a seven-bladed propeller with each blade composed of four β-sheets. γ-subunits are about 70–80 residues in length and more variable in sequence than β-subunits. The amino-terminal region as noted above is involved in a coiled-coil structure with the corresponding segment of the β-subunit, whereas the carboxy-terminal region forms an α-helix that interacts with one portion of the β-propeller. The carboxy-terminus contains a "CAAX box" motif. This is the site of three sequential posttranslational modifications that are critical for membrane association of the βγ-dimer. The cysteine (C) is the site of isoprenylation, a lipid modification with either a farnesyl or geranyl-geranyl moiety depending on the nature of the amino acid in the X position. Subsequently, a unique protease cleaves the AAX tripeptide. This is followed by methylation of the free carboxyl group of the cysteine. The end result is a very hydrophobic modification of the carboxy-terminus. Mutation of the relevant cysteine does not prevent stable association with the β-subunit, but prevents membrane association of the dimer. The carboxy-terminus of the γ-subunit and the amino-terminus of the α-subunit are thus both modified by addition of hydrophobic lipids, and are thought to be oriented near the inner leaflet of the plasma membrane. Contact between the α-subunit and βγ-dimer is limited to the amino-terminus of α aligned on one side of the β-propeller and certain switch regions of the α-subunit that contact the top surface of the β-propeller only in the GDP-bound conformation of the α-subunit (8).

G-Protein Diversity

The cloning of cDNAs encoding novel G-protein subunits has relied on approaches, such as PCR, using primers for sequences conserved in all members of the gene family. Based on certain common structural features (see α-Subunit Structure), one can reasonably predict that the cDNA encodes, for example, a G-protein α-subunit, but this method does not generally allow prediction of the corresponding function. Thus, for some identified subunits, receptor and effector couplings require further definition. To date, 16 different mammalian α-subunit genes have been cloned (see Table 1). They can be grouped into four subfamilies (G_s, G_i, G_q, and G_{12}) based on amino acid identity and effector regulation. Further diversity is created by alternative splicing of several of these genes. Gene expression varies from highly localized (such as the G proteins involved in visual and odorant transduction) to ubiquitous. At least five mammalian β-subunits and >10 γ-subunits have also been identified. There is evidence for some degree of specificity in which β-subunits will form dimers with which γ-subunits, and for which α-subunits will form heterotrimers with which βγ-dimers. Even with this limitation, there remain a very large number of combinatorial possibilities for which heterotrimers can be formed. The resultant diversity may be important in the specificity of receptor–effector coupling.

Receptor–Effector Coupling Specificity

The diversity of the components of G-protein-mediated signaling pathways (hundreds of receptors, more than a dozen G proteins, and likely more than a dozen effectors) poses the dual questions: how specific is G-protein coupling to receptors and effectors, and what is the basis for specificity? This is not merely an academic question, since in any given cell type, there are multiple receptors, G proteins, and effectors. The effects of drugs targeted to one of these components and the manifestations resulting from dysfunction (e.g., mutation) of one of these components depend on the degree of specificity of the given component's interactions.

Specificity of receptor–effector coupling has been studied experimentally using a variety of approaches. Bacterial toxins have been quite useful (see Table 1). Treatment of intact cells or membranes with cholera toxin leads to constitutive activation of G_s-regulated signaling. Treatment with pertussis toxin blocks signaling through receptors coupled to members of the G_i/G_o subfamily. Certain sets of receptors (e.g., M2 muscarinic, somatostatin) are linked to pertussis toxin-sensitive G-proteins, as are certain effectors (adenylyl cyclase inhibition, potassium channel stimulation). Effector regulation can be both pertussis toxin-sensitive and insensitive. In most cell types, stimulation of phospholipase C (PLC)-β is insensitive, and is mediated by members of the G_q subfamily that are not pertussis toxin substrates. In certain cells (monocyte/macrophages), PLC-β stimulation is blocked by pertussis toxin and is mediated by members of the G_i subfamily. Interestingly, it appears to be the $\beta\gamma$-subunit released from the heterotrimer that stimulates PLC activity in this case. Other approaches to defining specificity of receptor–effector coupling include use of antibodies to the carboxy-terminus of α-subunits, which uncouple specific α-subunits from receptor, reconstitution of receptors and/or effectors with G proteins, and transfection of cDNAs encoding specific receptors, G proteins, or effectors. The picture that emerges from such studies is in general one of relative rather than absolute specificity.

G proteins can be divided into four broad classes. A large number of receptors couple to G_s and thereby stimulate adenylyl cyclase. Another large group couples to members of the G_q subfamily to stimulate PLC. There is overlap in these two receptor groups in that some (e.g., members of the PTH/calcitonin receptor subfamily) appear to stimulate both adenylyl cyclase and PLC possibly by coupling to G_s and G_q. However, another receptor group couples to members of the G_i/G_o subfamily. Finally, the novel G_{12} subfamily likely couples to a different set of receptors and effectors, but this remains to be defined. The importance of the $\beta\gamma$-subunit in receptor–effector coupling has been increasingly appreciated. The γ-subunit may contribute to specificity of receptor–G-protein coupling. The $\beta\gamma$-dimer is directly involved in regulation of certain effectors, including adenylyl cyclase, potassium channels, and PLC-β. Finally, it serves to target GRKs to the plasma membrane and is thus critical for desensitization.

Mutations in G Proteins and GPCR: General Considerations

In theory, mutations in any component of the G-protein-coupled signal transduction pathway could cause disease. Currently, however, the overwhelming majority of identified disease-causing mutations in this pathway involve GPCR and G-protein α-subunits, and they are therefore the focus of this book. With increasing understanding of the structure and function of other components, such as the $\beta\gamma$-dimer, effectors, such as adenylyl cyclase, cyclic GMP phosphodiesterase, and various ion channels, and of proteins that modulate receptor–effector coupling, such as members of the RGS, GRK, and β-arrestin families, additional examples of human diseases caused by mutations in these components are likely to emerge. There are already a few examples of naturally occurring mutations in some of these components in humans (*see 9* and references therein).

There are three principal determinants of the phenotypic expression of mutations in G proteins and GPCR:

1. The range of expression of the mutated gene—mutations in a ubiquitously expressed gene, such as $G\alpha_s$ in general will cause more generalized manifestations than those caused by mutations in a gene, such as a receptor, that is more restricted in expression (*but see 2*);
2. Germline (inherited) vs somatic (postzygotic) mutations—the former potentially cause manifestations in every cell in which the gene is expressed. Somatic mutation of even a

ubiquitously expressed gene, in contrast, would still lead to manifestations that are local-ized to the cells derived from the progenitor in which the original somatic mutation occurred; and

3. Nature of the mutation—mutations can be broadly divided into those causing gain vs loss of function.

Loss of function mutations block normal mRNA and/or protein synthesis, prevent the synthesized protein from reaching its normal subcellular location, the plasma membrane in the case of GPCR and G proteins (*see* #1 in Fig. 1), or impair function despite synthesis and normal targeting of the protein. Many GPCR mutations, including missense muta-tions, will cause abnormal folding of the protein with retention in the endoplasmic reticu-lum. GPCR mutations compatible with normal protein synthesis and trafficking may nonetheless cause loss of function by impairing agonist binding to or activation of recep-tor (#2 in Fig. 1), or by impairing receptor coupling to and activation of G protein (#3 in Fig. 1). G protein loss of function mutations, in addition to impairing normal protein syn-thesis or trafficking, may block receptor coupling or activation by GTP (#3 in Fig. 1) or impair effector interaction (#4 in Fig. 1).

Gain of function mutations cause inappropriate or constitutive activation. A constitu-tively activated GPCR presumptively assumes the conformation that leads to G-protein activation, even without binding of the hormone that normally activates the receptor. Likewise, a constitutively activated G protein signals its effector despite the lack of nor-mal "upstream" signals from a hormone-activated GPCR. Such mutations could either accelerate release of GDP and lead to receptor-independent G-protein activation (#3 in Fig. 1) or block the GTPase reaction that terminates G-protein activation (#5 in Fig. 1). Gain of function mutations are by definition dominant, and thus, heterozygotes for germline mutations will be clinically affected. For loss of function mutations, the situa-tion is more complex. Pure loss of function mutations may cause no overt clinical dys-function in heterozygotes. For many GPCR, there is sufficient signal sensitivity and amplification such that a 50% reduction in receptor number does not lead to clinically apparent disease.

Loss-of-function mutations are generally associated with inherited disorders, whereas gain of function mutations may occur in the germline in inherited disorders or as somatic events in sporadic disorders. In the latter case, a gain-of-function mutation confers a proliferative advantage on the cell in which the somatic event occurs, leading to a clonal neoplasm and eventually clinically evident disease. Germline mutations of certain GPCR and G proteins may never be detected simply because they would be incompatible with life. This could be true of both heterozygous gain of function muta-tions or of homozygous null mutations in which inappropriate signal activation or total lack of signaling, respectively, would be lethal. When such germline mutations are com-patible with life, the timing of onset of clinical disease may be quite variable, even though the mutation is already present at birth. For gain of function mutations, the timing of disease onset may reflect several factors, including the degree of constitutive activation of the particular mutation, critical developmental events, such as cell prolif-eration necessary for a response to signal activation, and the eventual failure of mecha-nisms attempting to compensate for inappropriate signal activation.

Mere identification of sequence variation in a GPCR or G-protein gene does not constitute proof of a disease-causing mutation. Some sequence differences may simply be polymorphisms of no pathophysiologic consequence (*but see* GPCR and G-Protein

Polymorphisms and Disease for possible role of polymorphisms in predisposing to disease). Identification of mutations only in affected members of a kindred and not in un-affected members or in "normal control" subjects is suggestive of pathophysiologic relevance. Also, certain mutations may be predicted to be functionally significant, e.g., those causing truncation of a GPCR, based on available information on GPCR and G-protein structure and function. More rigorous proof that a mutation identified is responsible for the disease being studied requires mutagenesis of the normal gene and appropriate functional studies of the expressed gene product. Mutations in certain GPCR or G proteins cause predictable effects, e.g., loss-of-function mutation of a hormone receptor causes resistance to the action of the corresponding hormone. In some cases, the consequences of a particular mutation are surprising and not readily predictable based on the presumptive function of the involved gene product, e.g., loss of function mutation of the endothelin-B receptor causes congenital megacolon (Hirschsprung disease).

Many, but by no means all, diseases caused by G protein and GPCR mutations are endocrine diseases. Most endocrine diseases can be classified into those involving either hypo- or hypersecretion of a given hormone or hormones. G protein and GPCR mutations can cause diseases of either type. In general, loss-of-function mutations lead to hyposecretion, and gain of function mutations lead to hypersecretion of the hormone regulated by the involved GPCR or G protein. For example, loss-of-function mutations of the TSH receptor would cause hypothyroidism, and gain of function mutations, hyperthyroidism. If, however, an activated GPCR or G protein normally inhibits hormone secretion (e.g., inhibition of PTH secretion by activated calcium receptor or inhibition of prolactin secretion by activated G_i/G_o), the effect of loss or gain of function mutations will be hyper- or hyposecretion, respectively. Loss-of-function mutations of a given GPCR or of the G protein to which it is coupled will cause hormone resistance with a clinical phenotype closely resembling that caused by deficiency of the hormone normally activating the corresponding receptor or receptors. Hormone resistance caused by GPCR or G-protein loss-of-function mutations is characterized by increased circulating concentration of the corresponding hormone agonist. Gain of function mutations will lead to a state resembling hypersecretion of the hormone normally activating the involved GPCR, but circulating concentrations of the involved hormone will actually be suppressed, reflecting autonomous hyperfunction of the target gland.

DISEASES CAUSED BY GPCR MUTATIONS

GPCR Loss-of-Function Mutations (Table 2)

Mutations that disrupt GPCR function at any of several steps in the activation cycle (Fig. 1) can cause disease. Nonsense and frameshift mutations that truncate the protein anywhere up to and including the membrane-proximal portion of the carboxy-terminus generally cause complete loss of function. A variety of missense mutations located in almost any portion of a GPCR can also disrupt normal function in a variety of ways. Expression and study of such naturally occurring mutations provide valuable clues to the normal structure and function of the involved GPCR. Specific examples are given below with those not covered elsewhere in this volume described in greater detail.

Table 2
Diseases Caused by GPCR Loss-of-Function Mutations

Receptor	Disease	Inheritance
Cone opsins	Color-blindness	X-linked; aut. rec.
Rhodopsin	RP	Aut. dom.; aut. rec.
V2 vasopressin	Nephrogenic diabetes insipidus	X-linked
ACTH	Familial ACTH resistance	Aut. rec.
LH	Male-pseudohermaphroditism	Aut. rec.
TSH	Familial hypothyroidism	Aut. rec.
CaR	Familial hypocalciuric Hypercalcemia/neonatal	Aut. dom.
	Severe primary Hyperparathyroidism	Aut. rec.
Thromboxane A2	Congenital bleeding	Aut. dom.
Endothelin-B	Hirschsprung disease	Aut. rec.
FSH	Hypergonadotropic Ovarian failure	Aut. rec.
TRH	Central hypothyroidism	Aut. rec.
GHRH	GH deficiency	Aut. rec.

OPSINS

The four visual pigments in humans, rhodopsin (the rod photoreceptor pigment) and the blue, green, and red cone opsins, are prototypical GPCR with a core structure consisting of seven membrane-spanning helices with a retinal covalently bound to a lysine (296 in rhodopsin) in the seventh transmembrane domain *(10)*. As discussed above, photon capture in rhodopsin converts a bound antagonist to an agonist by causing isomerization of 11-cis retinal to all-trans. This leads to a shift in protonation to glutamate 134 at the cytoplasmic base of the third transmembrane domain, and a likely conformational change in the cytoplasmic loops that promotes G-protein activation. The discovery that the β-adrenergic receptor shares with rhodopsin the core seven membrane-spanning domain structure led to the eventual identification of the many other members of this superfamily *(4,10)*. Disease-causing mutations of GPCR were also first discovered in the opsin family. Mutations in each of the visual pigments lead to a number of disorders in humans. These have been reviewed extensively, including a full listing of the specific mutations *(5,11–13)*. Common forms of color-blindness are owing to loss-of-function mutations in either the red or green cone opsin genes *(14)*. The red and green pigment genes are arranged in tandem on the X chromosome and are relatively frequently subject to unequal recombination events, resulting in gain/loss of entire genes or formation of red–green hydrid genes with altered absorption properties. A number of heterozygous point mutations in the blue pigment gene on chromosome 7 cause autosomal-dominant forms of deficient blue spectral sensitivity. A common polymorphism, serine vs alanine at position 180, in the red pigment gene accounts for genetic variation in sensitivity to long-wavelength light *(14)*.

Retinitis pigmentosa (RP) is characterized by progressive photoreceptor degeneration and blindness. The disorder shows extensive phenotypic and genetic heterogeneity, with

X-linked, autosomal-recessive and dominant forms. About 30% of the latter form is owing to >60 different mutations in the rhodopsin gene on chromosome 3 *(5,11–14)*. These are not simple loss-of-function mutations, but rather act dominantly, in ways not completely clarified, to cause photoreceptor degeneration. The majority are thought to cause abnormal protein folding with retention in the endoplasmic reticulum and eventual cell destruction. Missense mutations in the amino-terminus, transmembrane domains, and first and second extracellular loops are most often involved. In autosomal-recessive forms of RP, pure loss-of-function mutations of both alleles of the rhodopsin gene have been found *(15,16)*.

OTHER GPCR

Since the discovery that opsin loss-of-function mutations could cause human disease, numerous examples of other human diseases caused by GPCR loss-of-function mutations have been identified (Table 2). Several are described in detail in separate chapters of this volume: hypothyroidism resulting from TSH receptor mutations (Chapter 7), pseudo-hermaphroditism caused by LH receptor mutations (Chapter 8), hypergonadotropic ovarian failure caused by FSH receptor mutations (Chapter 9), nephrogenic diabetes insipidus owing to V2 vasopressin receptor mutations (Chapter 10), familial hypocalciuric hypercalcemia caused by calcium receptor mutations (Chapter 11), GH-deficient dwarfism owing to GHRH receptor mutations (Chapter 13), and familial ACTH resistance owing to ACTH receptor mutations (Chapter 15).

Hirschsprung disease (congenital megacolon) is a multigenic disorder characterized by failure of innervation of the gastrointestinal tract. One form of the disease appears to be the result of loss-of-function mutation in the endothelin-B receptor *(17)*. Homozygotes for the mutation have a substantially greater risk of developing the disease than do heterozygotes. Exactly how this mutation leads to the phenotype is unclear, since the physiologic effects of endothelin receptor agonists were thought to be limited to vasopressor actions. Based on the association between loss-of-function mutations in the receptor and the disease phenotype, an essential role for this receptor in development of certain neural crest-derived cells has been suggested *(18)*. The phenotypic consequences of LH receptor (Chapter 8) and FSH receptor (Chapter 9) loss-of-function mutations provide additional examples of a developmental role for GPCR. In the first endothelin-B receptor mutation to be identified, cysteine is substituted for trytophan276, a highly conserved residue in the fifth transmembrane domain *(17)*. Subsequently, additional loss-of-function mutations of the endothelin B receptor have been identified in other kindreds with the disease *(18)*.

An arginine60leucine mutation in the first intracellular loop of the thromboxane A_2 receptor has been identified in platelets from affected members of two unrelated families with a dominantly inherited bleeding disorder *(19)*. The mutation does not affect binding, but impairs second messenger production specifically in response to thromboxane A_2 receptor agonists, but not other platelet agonists, such as thrombin. Even subjects with the mutation in heterozygous form showed impaired platelet response, suggesting that the mutation could act as a "dominant-negative" perhaps by binding agonist and then failing to activate G protein. Loss-of-function mutations in the TRH receptor have recently been identified in a family with autosomal-recessive central hypothyroidism. This presumptively causes resistance to TRH, deficiency of TSH, and resultant hypothyroidism *(20)*.

Table 3
Diseases Caused by GPCR Gain-of-Function Mutations

Receptor	Disease	Inheritance
Rhodopsin	Cong. night blindness	Aut. dom.
LH	Familial male precocious puberty	Aut. dom.
TSH	Sporadic hyperfunctional thyroid nodules	Somatic
TSH	Familial nonautoimmune hyperthyroidism	Aut. dom.
CaR	Familial hypoparathyroidism	Aut. dom.
PTH/PTHrP	Jansen metaphyseal chondrodysplasia	Aut. dom.
FSH	Gonadotropin-independent spermatog.	Aut. dom.

MOUSE MODELS OF GPCR LOSS OF FUNCTION

Mouse models of human disease, both naturally occurring and artificially created, that involve GPCR loss-of-function mutations have also been described. Hypothyroid mice caused by TSH receptor mutation (Chapter 7), dwarf mice owing to GHRH receptor mutation (Chapter 13), and pigment deficiency owing to melanocortin receptor mutations (Chapter 14) are examples of naturally occurring mouse models. In addition to naturally occurring mutations, mouse gene targeting methodology has provided the opportunity to disrupt any gene and to create artificial loss-of-function mutations in genes encoding any GPCR. With targeted disruption of mouse genes ("knockout" mouse) becoming almost routine, not surprisingly a very large number of GPCR genes have been knocked out in mice to study the phenotypic consequences, and gain insight into physiologic functions and possible functional redundancy of receptor subtypes. The sheer number of these knockouts, with new ones reported almost weekly, precludes comprehensive coverage here, but a few instructive examples will be cited. The mouse calcium receptor gene knockout provides a useful model of the naturally occurring human disease (Chapter 11). Heterozygous mutant mice have mild calcium insensitivity as seen in some kindreds with familial hypocalciuric hypercalcemia, whereas homozygotes are lethal early postnatally as with the human counterpart, severe neonatal hyperparathyroidism. Knockout of genes for dopamine receptor subtypes (Chapter 17) has provided valuable information on the distinct functions of members of the subfamily. Targeted disruption of the endothelin-B receptor gene in mice leads to a similar phenotype (congenital megacolon) as that seen in a naturally occurring mutant mouse (piebald-lethal) with a deletion of the receptor gene *(21)*. Both the naturally occurring and artifically created mouse models bolster the case that mutations in this receptor identified in humans with congenital megacolon are indeed responsible for the observed phenotype.

GPCR Gain-of-Function Mutations (Table 3)

Artificial site-directed mutagenesis of adrenergic receptors showed that missense mutations of critical residues at the junction of the sixth transmembrane domain and third intracellular loop cause constitutive (agonist-independent) G-protein activation *(22)*. This observation provided the theoretical basis for identification of naturally occurring gain-of-function mutations in GPCR that cause constitutive activation and disease. Examples for several different GPCR have now been found (Table 3).

Interestingly, such mutations have been identified not only in the residues corresponding to those originally shown to cause constitutive activation of adrenergic receptors, but also at various other locations depending on the GPCR involved. For some GPCR, such as that for TSH, almost every part of the receptor may be involved, possibly indicative of a greater inherent tendency for this receptor to assume the activated conformation (*see* Chapter 7). Activating mutations lend support to a dynamic model of GPCR function involving an equilibrium between active and inactive conformations. The mutations presumptively eliminate or diminish inhibitory constraints preventing activation that under physiologic conditions are relieved by agonist binding. Mutation location provides clues to the mechanism of GPCR activation. Specific examples are given below; details are provided only for rhodopsin, which is not covered elsewhere in the volume.

Congenital stationary night blindness is an autosomal-dominant disorder considered distinct from RP. Affected individuals do not show progressive photoreceptor degeneration, but show night blindness from earliest childhood. The disease shows genetic heterogeneity with dominant mutations in rhodopsin, cyclic GMP phosphodiesterase, and the α-subunit of rod transducin (*see* G-Protein α-Subunit Gain-of-Function Mutations), and recessive mutations in arrestin (the rod photoreceptor-specific member of the β-arrestin family) and rhodopsin kinase (the rod photoreceptor-specific member of the GRK family) *(9)*. Heterozygous rhodopsin mutations identified in this disorder include glycine90aspartate (second transmembrane domain) and alanine292glutamate (seventh transmembrane domain) *(14)*. Either mutant adds negative charge to the retinal binding pocket that may weaken the normal salt bridge between lysine296 and glutamate113. Although the mutants still bind retinal and are thus not always constitutively activated a small percentage of unliganded opsins postulated to occur at steady state would, if mutant, be activated. The resultant background "noise" would diminish low-light sensitivity, yielding the night blindness phenotype. Lack of photoreceptor degeneration may reflect the mild degree of rhodopsin activation.

Other disorders caused by GPCR gain-of-function mutations include inherited and sporadic forms of thyroid hyperfunction owing to germline and somatic mutations, respectively, in the TSH receptor (Chapter 7), familial male precocious puberty (LH receptor; Chapter 8), familial hypoparathyroidism (calcium receptor; Chapter 11), and Jansen's metaphyseal chondrodysplasia (PTH/PTHrP receptor; Chapter 12). An activating mutation of the FSH receptor has been suggested to be a cause of gonadotropin-independent spermatogenesis *(23)*. Several viruses contain open reading frames encoding putative GPCR in the chemokine receptor subfamily. The Kaposi's sarcoma-associated herpesvirus contains such a receptor gene, which in in vitro expression studies caused constitutive activation of phospholipase C and stimulation of cell proliferation *(24)*. This may represent an example of a constitutively activated GPCR acting as a viral oncogene.

Mouse models provide additional examples; naturally occurring hyperpigmentation phenotypes in mice and other mammals have been shown to be caused by activating mutations of the melanocortin type 1 receptor (Chapter 14). Transgenic overexpression of even wild-type β-adrenergic receptors in hearts of mice causes agonist-independent activation equal to maximal stimulation by agonist in normal controls (Chapter 16). This result is consistent with the dynamic model of GPCR function: each GPCR is in equilibrium between an active and inactive conformation with agonist and activating mutations

Table 4
Human Diseases Caused by G-Protein α-Subunit Mutations

G-protein α-subunit	Disease	Mutation type
α_s	Pseudohypoparathyroidism (PHP) type Ia	Loss
α_s	PHP Ia with precocious puberty	Loss/gain
α_s	Acromegaly, hyperfunctional thyroid nodules, McCune-Albright syndrome	Gain
α_{i2}	Ovarian and adrenalcortical tumors (?)	Gain
α_{t1}	Congenital stationary night blindness (Nougaret type)	Gain (?)

driving the equilibrium toward the active state. With sufficiently high levels of expression, the small fraction of total receptor spontaneously reaching the active conformation is capable of fully activating "downstream" components. Spontaneous activation achieved by receptor overexpression and constitutive activation caused by gain-of-function GPCR mutations can be inhibited by so-called inverse agonists. Such compounds bind to receptor and drive the equilibrium toward the inactive conformation. Examples of inverse agonists for the PTH/PTHrP receptor (Chapter 12), melanocortin receptors (Chapter 14), and β-adrenergic receptors (Chapter 16) are given in this volume. Such agents may eventually prove therapeutically useful. The melanocortin receptors also provide a unique paradigm: the agouti protein, a naturally occurring antagonist of a GPCR. Not only is it involved in physiologic regulation of mammalian skin and hair color, but its ectopic expression also causes obesity through inhibition of the melanocortin type 4 receptor in a naturally occurring mouse mutant (Chapter 14).

DISEASES CAUSED BY G-PROTEIN α-SUBUNIT MUTATIONS

G-Protein α-Subunit Loss-of-Function Mutations

Heterozygous germline, loss-of-function mutations of $G\alpha_s$ cause generalized hormone resistance (pseudohypoparathyroidism type Ia; PHP Ia) and other phenotypic features of Albright hereditary osteodystrophy (Table 4). The complexities of the human disease and of a mouse $G\alpha_s$ gene knockout model are discussed in Chapter 2. As yet, naturally occurring human or mouse diseases caused by loss-of-function mutations in other G-protein α-subunits have not been described. Such mutations have been sought and excluded in a number of diseases, including hypertension (25), Usher syndrome (26), and bipolar disorder (27). Quantitative and/or qualitative G-protein abnormalities have been reported in several disorders, including alcoholism (28), opiate dependence (29), hypertension (30, 31), cardiac diseases (32) (see also Chapter 16), and aging (30), but the functional significance and molecular basis for such alterations remain unclear.

Knockouts of mouse genes encoding other G-protein α-subunits have been reported, and these provide interesting insights into function. Germline knockout of the $G\alpha_{i2}$ gene causes ulcerative colitis, an unanticipated phenotype that may be owing to critical functions of this protein in lymphocytes (Chapter 4). Both these results and the effects of tissue-selective $G\alpha_{i2}$ gene knockout using antisense technology (Chapter 5) suggest nonredundant functions of $G\alpha_i$ subtypes. $G\alpha_{13}$ gene knockout causes embryonic lethality in the homozygous state owing to abnormal blood vessel development *(33)*. Further study of this model may provide insight into the normal role of this protein in receptor–effector coupling. Germline knockout of the $G\alpha_o$ gene causes no gross disruption of the nervous system despite the fact that this protein makes up about 0.5% of neuronal membrane protein *(34)*. Homozygous null mice show tremor and reduced survival for reasons not yet clear. A defect in cardiac calcium channel regulation in these mice defines a specific function for $G\alpha_o$ that cannot be compensated by other $G\alpha_i$ subtypes.

G-Protein α-Subunit Gain-of-Function Mutations

Heterozygous somatic, activating mutations in the $G\alpha_s$ gene cause acromegaly, thyroid adenomas, fibrous dysplasia, or McCune-Albright syndrome (Table 4), depending on the site and timing of the mutation (Chapter 3). These mutations involve highly conserved residues responsible for normal GTPase activity. A unique $G\alpha_s$ gene mutation causing both loss of function associated with PHP Ia and gain of function in testicular Leydig cells associated with precocious puberty is also discussed in Chapter 3. Activating somatic mutations of the $G\alpha_{i2}$ gene were intially identified in ovarian and adrenocortical tumors *(35)*. Several subsequent studies have failed to confirm this observation, casting doubt on the role of such mutations in causing tumors of these or other tissues *(36–38)*. A heterozygous germline missense mutation, glycine 38 to aspartate, in the rod photoreceptor transducin α-subunit gene has been identified in a dominantly inherited form of congenital stationary night blindness (Nougaret type) *(39)*. The residue equivalent to glycine 38 is highly conserved not only in all heterotrimeric G-protein α-subunits, but also in more distantly related members of the GTPase superfamily, such as *ras*. Missense mutations in this residue in *ras* are oncogenic, because they reduce GTPase activity. This suggests that the glycine38 mutation in the transducin α-subunit gene is likewise an activating mutation owing to reduction in GTPase activity. This suggestion is consistent with the dominant inheritance pattern and with the ability of activating mutations of other phototransduction components, such as rhodopsin and cGMP phosphodiesterase, to give the same phenotype (*see* GPCR Gain-of-Function Mutations).

Naturally occurring mutations in other α-subunits have not been identified to date. Transfection of cell lines with constitutively activated mutant forms of either $G\alpha_{12}$ or $G\alpha_{13}$ leads to cell transformation (Chapter 6). This suggests that such mutant α-subunits could act as oncogenes and should be sought in various neoplasms.

GPCR AND G-PROTEIN POLYMORPHISMS AND DISEASE

The loss- and gain-of-function mutations described thus far are all associated in a clear way with a disease phenotype, and in several cases, cause-and-effect relationships have been demonstrated. As with many other genes, however, a variety of polymorphisms in the genes encoding GPCR and G-protein α-subunits have been identified. Even when these cause no change in coding sequence, they may be useful in linkage and other studies attempting to identify asociated diseases. In several instances, DNA sequence variations that change amino acid sequence have been identified. The functional significance of such sequence differences and their possible role in predisposing to disease is a subject of current study, particularly in complex disorders likely to involve polygenic inheritance. Chapter 18 details such studies of a coding polymorphism in the β3-adrenergic receptor in relation to type II diabetes and obesity. Chapter 14 discusses allelic variation in the melanocortin type 1 receptor in relation to variations in skin and hair color. Susceptibility to development of type II diabetes has been associated with a glucagon receptor polymorphism *(40)*, a correlation between nocturnal asthma and a β2-adrenergic receptor polymorphism observed *(41)*, and an association between risk-taking behavior and a particular D4-dopamine receptor polymorphism identified *(42)* (*see also* Chapter 17).

One of the most striking examples of a polymorphism associated with altered disease susceptibility concerns the identification of a critical role for GPCR in the chemokine receptor subfamily as coreceptors with CD4 in entry of HIV-1 into target cells. The chemokine receptor termed CCR-5 allows infection by macrophage-tropic strains of HIV-1. A 32-bp deletion in the coding region of the CCR-5 gene causing a frameshift, and loss of function was identified in population studies. Individuals homozygous for the null allele appear to be resistant to viral infection; heterozygotes may display partial resistance *(43,44)*. As yet, no deleterious consequences of homozygous loss of function have been identified. This apparently beneficial phenotype conferred by a GPCR loss-of-function mutation has spurred efforts to develop pharmacologic agents to block CCR-5 function in individuals with normal alleles.

These are but a few examples of what surely will eventually be a large number of correlations between particular structural variants of components of the G-protein-coupled signal transduction pathway and particular phenotypes, such as disease susceptibility. Each chapter that follows offers insights into examples of human diseases already well studied at the molecular level, and provides glimpses of future prospects in this rapidly developing field at the interface of molecular and clinical science.

REFERENCES

1. Spiegel AM, Jones TLZ, Simonds WF, Weinstein LS. G-Proteins. R.G. Landes, Austin, TX, 1994.
2. Neer EJ. Heterotrimeric G proteins: organizers of transmembrane signals. Cell 1995;80:249–257.
3. Dessauer CW, Posner BA, Gilman AG. Visualizing signal transduction: receptors, G-proteins, and adenylate cyclases. Clin Sci 1996;91:527–537.
4. Strader CD, Fong TM, Tota MR, Underwood D. Structure and function of G-protein-coupled receptors. Annu Rev Biochem 1994;63:101–132.
5. Iismaa TP, Biden TJ, Shine J. *G-Protein-Coupled Receptors*. R.G. Landes, Austin, TX, 1995.
6. Berman DM, Wilkie TM, Gilman AG. GAIP and RGS4 are GTPase-activating proteins for the G_i subfamily of G-protein α subunits. Cell 1996;86:445–452.
7. Coleman DE, Berghuis AM, Lee E, Linder ME, Gilman AG, Sprang SR. Structures of active conformations of G_{ia1} and the mechanism of GTP hydrolysis. Science 1994;265:1405–1412.
8. Wall MA, Coleman DE, Lee E, Iñiguez-Lluhi JA, Posner BA, Gilman AG, Sprang SR. The structure of the G-protein heterotrimer $G_{ia1}\beta_1\gamma_2$. Cell 1995;83:1047–1058.
9. Yamamoto S, Sippel KC, Berson EL, Dryja TP. Defects in the rhodopsin kinase gene in the Oguchi form of stationary night blindness. Nat Genet 1997;15:175–178.
10. Baldwin JM. Structure and function of receptors coupled to G proteins. Curr Opinion Cell Biol 1994;6:180–190.
11. Min KC, Zvygaga TA, Cypress AM, Sakmar TP. Characterization of mutant rhodopsins responsible for autosomal dominant retinitis pigmentosa: mutations on the cytoplasmic surface affect transducin activation. J Biol Chem 1993;268:9400–9404.
12. Sung C-H, Davenport CM, Nathans J. Rhodopsin mutations responsible for autosomal dominant retinitis pigmentosa: clustering of functional classes along the polypeptide chain. J Biol Chem 1993;268: 26,645–26,649.
13. Macke JP, Davenport CM, Jacobson SG, Hennessey JC, Gonzalez-Fernandez F, Conway BP, Heckenlively J, Palmer R, Maumenee IH, Sieving P, Gouras P, Good W, Nathans J. Identification of novel rhodopsin mutations responsible for retinitis pigmentosa: implications for the structure and function of rhodopsin. Am J Hum Genet 1993;53:80–89.

14. Nathans J. In the eye of the beholder: visual pigments and inherited variation in human vision. Cell 1994;78:357–360.

15. Rosenfeld PJ, Cowley GS, McGee TL, Sandberg MA, Berson EL, Dryja TP. A *Null* mutation in the rhodopsin gene causes rod photoreceptor dysfunction and autosomal recessive retinitis pigmentosa. Nature Genetics 1992;1:209–213.

16. Kumaramanickavel G, Maw M, Denton MJ, John S, Srikumari CRS, Orth U, Oehlmann R, Gal A. Missense rhodopsin mutation in a family with recessive RP. Nature Genet 1994;8:10,11.

17. Puffenberger EG, Hosoda K, Washington SS, Nakao K, DeWit D, Yanagisawa M, Chakravarti A. A missense mutation of the endothelin-B receptor gene in multigenic Hirschsprung's disease. Cell 1994;79:1257–1266.

18. Chakravarti A. Endothelin receptor-mediated signaling in Hirschsprung disease. Hum Mol Genet 1996;5:303–307.

19. Hirata T, Kakizuka A, Ushikubi F, Fuse I, Okuma M, Narumiya S. Arg[60] to Leu mutation of the human thromboxane A_2 receptor in a dominantly inherited bleeding disorder. J Clin Invest 1994;94:1662–1667.

20. Collu R, Tang JQ, Castagne J, Lagace G, Masson N, Deal C, Huot C, Van Vliet G. Isolated central hypothyroidism caused by inactivating mutations in the thyrotropin-releasing hormone receptor gene. Horm Res 1997;46:1 (Abstract).

21. Hosoda K, Hammer RE, Richardson JA, Baynash AG, Cheung JC, Giaid A, Yanagisawa M. Targeted and natural (piebald-lethal) mutations of endothelin-B receptor gene produce megacolon associated with spotted coat color in mice. Cell 1994;79:1267–1276.

22. Lefkowitz RJ, Cotecchia S, Samama P, Costa T. Constitutive activity of receptors coupled to guanine nucleotide regulatory proteins. Trends Pharmacol Sci 1994;14:303–307.

23. Gromoll J, Simoni M, Nieschlag E. An activating mutation of the follicle-stimulating hormone receptor autonomously sustains spermatogenesis in a hypophysectomized man. J Clin Endocrinol Metab 1996;81:1367–1370.

24. Arvanitakis L, Geras-Raaka E, Varma A, Gershengorn MC, Cesarman E. Human herpesvirus KSHV encodes a constitutively active G-protein-coupled receptor linked to cell proliferation. Nature 1997;385:347–350.

25. Gurich RW, Beach RE, Caflisch CR. Cloning of the α-subunit of G_s protein from spontaneously hypertensive rats. Hypertension 1994;24:595–599.

26. Magovcevic I, Berson EL, Morton CC. Detection of cone alpha transducin mRNA in human fetal cochlea: negative mutation analysis in Usher syndrome. Hear Res 1996;99:7–12.

27. Ram A, Guedj F, Cravchik A, Weinstein L, Cao QH, Badner JA, Goldin LR, Grisaru N, Manji HK, Belmaker RH, Gershon ES, Gejman PV. No abnormality in the gene for the G-protein stimulatory α subunit in patients with bipolar disorder. Arch Gen Psychiatry 1997;54:44–48.

28. Wand GS, Waltman C, Martin CS, McCaul ME, Levine MA, Wolfgang D. Differential expression of guanosine triphosphate binding proteins in men at high and low risk for the future development of alcoholism. J Clin Invest 1994;94:1004–1011.

29. Manji HK, Chen G, Potter W, Kosten TR. Guanine nucleotide binding proteins in opioid-dependent patients. Biol Psychiatry 1997;41:130–134.

30. Feldman RD, Tan CM, Chorazyczewski J. G-protein alterations in hypertension and aging. Hypertension 1995;26:725–732.

31. Siffert W. Genetically fixed enhanced G-protein activation in essential hypertension. Renal Physiol Biochem 1996;19:172–173.

32. Schnabel P, Böhm M. Heterotrimeric G proteins in heart disease. Cell Signal 1996;8:413–423.

33. Offermanns S, Mancino V, Revel JP, Simon MI. Vascular system defects and impaired cell chemokinesis as a result of Galpha13 deficiency. Science 1997;275:533–536.

34. Valenzuela D, Han X, Mende U, Fankhauser C, Mashimo H, Huang P, Pfeffer J, Neer EJ, Fishman MC. G-alpha-o is necessary for muscarinic regulation of Ca^{2+} channels in mouse heart. Proc Natl Acad Sci USA 1997;94:1727–1732.

35. Lyons J, Landis CA, Harsh G, Vallar L, Grünewald K, Feichtinger H, Duh Q-Y, Clark OH, Kawasaki E, Bourne HR, McCormick F. Two G-protein oncogenes in human endocrine tumors. Science 1990;249:655–659.

36. Reincke M, Karl M, Travis W, Chrousos GP. No evidence for oncogenic mutations in guanine nucleotide-binding proteins of human adrenocortical neoplasms. J Clin Endocrinol Metab 1993;77:1419–1422.

2

Albright Hereditary Osteodystrophy, Pseudohypoparathyroidism, and G$_s$ Deficiency

Lee S. Weinstein, MD

CONTENTS

OVERVIEW

Pseudohypoparathyroidism (PHP) is a term that refers to a heterogeneous group of metabolic disorders in which resistance to parathyroid hormone (PTH), characterized by hypocalcemia, hyperphosphatemia, and elevation of serum PTH in the setting of normal renal function, is the major clinical feature. In the original report by Fuller Albright, PHP patients showed reduced calcemic and phosphaturic responses to injected bovine parathyroid extract compared to patients with primary hypoparathyroidism *(1)*. This observation led to the speculation that PHP is caused by a defect in PTH action within its target tissues, and was the first description of a hormone resistance syndrome. Subsequent studies describing parathyroid hyperplasia and elevation of immunoreactive serum PTH in untreated PHP patients confirmed that PTH resistance was the underlying defect *(2,3)*.

From: *Contemporary Endocrinology: G Proteins, Receptors, and Disease*
Edited by: A. M. Spiegel, Humana Press Inc., Totowa, NJ

In Albright's original report, PHP patients were noted to have several distinct physical features, including short stature, centripetal obesity, short neck, and brachydactyly. This constellation of findings is referred to as Albright hereditary osteodystrophy (AHO), and has subsequently been shown to also include subcutaneous ossification and mental dysfunction in some cases *(4,5)*. The relationship of AHO to PTH resistance was unclear until Albright described a patient with the physical features of AHO, but without PTH resistance *(6)*. He termed this entity pseudopseudohypoparathyroidism (PPHP). The occurrence of AHO in the absence of PTH resistance suggests that AHO is not the consequence of abnormal calcium metabolism.

The defect in PHP was further defined when it was determined that PTH stimulates formation of intracellular cAMP in its target organs, and that in most PHP patients, the renal cAMP response to exogenous bovine PTH (as reflected in urinary excretion of cAMP) is markedly reduced when compared to normal subjects or patients with primary hypoparathyroidism *(7)*. Many patients with a blunted urinary cAMP response (termed PHP type I) were shown to have deficient activity of a guanine nucleotide binding protein G_s that couples receptors for hormones and other extracellular signals to the stimulation of cAMP formation (PHP type Ia) *(8,9)*. The molecular defect in these patients has been shown to reside in the gene encoding the $G\alpha_s$-subunit (GNAS1) *(10,11)*. These patients have PTH resistance in association with AHO and resistance to other hormones (eg., TSH, gonadotropins) whose receptors couple to G_s. Other PHP type I patients present with multiple hormone resistance, AHO, and a blunted urinary cAMP response to PTH, but with no evidence of G_s deficiency (PHP type Ic) *(12–14)*, whereas others have PTH resistance in isolation without AHO or G_s deficiency (PHP type Ib) *(13,15)*. Rare patients with PHP have been shown to have normal urinary cAMP response, but a deficient phosphaturic response to PTH, which indicates a defect distal to cAMP generation (PHP type II) *(16)*. This chapter will review all forms of PHP with emphasis on the pathogenesis of the G_s-deficient forms (PHP Ia and PPHP). Preliminary observations of $G\alpha_s$ knockout mice, recently generated in our laboratory, will be presented and implications of these observations on the regulation of the $G\alpha_s$ gene and the pathogenesis of PHP Ia and PPHP will be discussed.

PHYSIOLOGY OF CALCIUM AND PHOSPHATE METABOLISM

The serum ionized calcium and phosphate concentrations are maintained within narrow limits through the actions of PTH and vitamin D. PTH is synthesized in the parathyroid glands as a 115 amino acid polypeptide, preproPTH, and secreted as the mature 84 amino acid peptide hormone *(17)*. A decrease in serum ionized calcium stimulates secretion of PTH. PTH raises the extracellular fluid calcium concentration through its direct actions on kidney and bone and indirect actions (via vitamin D) on the gastrointestinal tract.

PTH has three major effects on the kidney:

1. Increased renal calcium reabsorption through an action on sites in the distal tubule, resulting in decreased net urinary calcium excretion for a given filtered load of calcium *(18)*;
2. Increased renal phosphate clearance through actions primarily in the proximal tubule, resulting in lower serum phosphate concentrations *(18)*; and
3. Increased formation of 1,25-dihydroxyvitamin D.

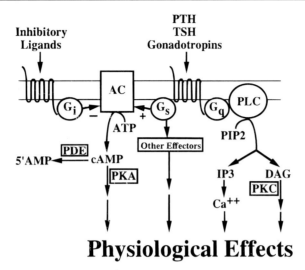

Physiological Effects

Fig. 1. Signal pathways for PTH. PTH and other hormones bind to specific receptors, which leads to activation of G_s and $G_{q/11}$. G_s stimulates adenylyl cyclase (AC), which catalyzes the formation of cAMP from ATP. Inhibitory hormones bind to their specific receptors, which inhibit AC activity through activation of various inhibitory G proteins (G_i). cAMP stimulates PKA, which phosphorylates cell-specific substrates. cAMP is degraded by various PDEs. G_s can also modulate other effectors, such as calcium channels. Activation of $G_{q/11}$ stimulates PLC. PLC catalyzes the hydrolysis of the phosphoinositide PIP2 to inositol triphosphate (IP_3), which increases intracellular calcium, and diacylglycerol (DAG), which activates PKC. These proximal signals modulate downstream pathways, which result in specific physiological effects.

Vitamin D is either synthesized in skin after exposure to uv light (cholecalciferol) or ingested as a plant sterol (ergocalciferol). In the liver, these forms of vitamin D are hydroxylated in the 25 position in a constitutive manner to form 25-hydroxyvitamin D. 1,25-Dihydroxyvitamin D, the active metabolite, is formed by the action of 25-hydroxycholecalciferol 1α hydroxylase, a highly regulated microsomal enzyme present in the kidney. PTH directly (and indirectly, through the lowering of serum phosphate concentrations) increases the activity of 1α hydroxylase. Increased serum levels of 1,25-dihydroxyvitamin D results in increased intestinal calcium absorption. 1,25-Dihydroxyvitamin D is also required for release of calcium from bone in response to PTH.

PTH has two major actions on bone, an acute calcemic effect through mobilization of calcium from bone to the extracellular fluid, presumably through effects of PTH on osteocytes (18), and a chronic skeletal remodeling effect owing to stimulation of osteoclast-mediated bone resorption. The remodeling effect is most likely the result of the direct actions of PTH on osteoblasts, which alters osteoblast function and stimulates release of factors which increase osteoclast resorption (19,20). 1,25-Dihydroxyvitamin D is required for the acute calcemic response of bone to PTH, but is not required for the remodeling effect.

MECHANISM OF PTH ACTION

PTH binds to specific receptors on the surface of its target cells, resulting in the generation of intracellular second messengers (18) (see Fig. 1). Activated receptors interact with one or more members of a family of heterotrimeric guanine nucleotide binding proteins (G proteins) *(21–24)*. G proteins in their inactive state are heterotrimers composed of α-, β- and γ-subunits. The α-subunits bind guanine nucleotide and interact with receptors and effectors. β- and γ-subunits form stable noncovalent heterodimers, which are tightly associated with cell membranes. In its inactive state, an α-subunit is associated with a βγ complex and has GDP bound to its guanine nucleotide binding site. On activation by ligand-bound receptor, the G-protein α-subunit exchanges bound GDP for GTP and dissociates from βγ. The free GTP-bound α-subunit directly interacts with and modulates its appropriate effector or effectors (usually intracellular enzymes or ion channels). βγ also appears to modulate certain effectors directly, such as some isoforms of adenylyl cyclase *(25)* and phospholipase C (PLC) *(26,27)*. Inactivation occurs via an intrinsic GTPase activity of the α-subunit, which converts bound GTP to GDP by the hydrolysis of the γ phosphate and results in reassociation with the βγ complex.

PTH stimulates the formation of intracellular cAMP by adenylyl cyclase *(7,18)* and the breakdown of phosphoinositides by PLC, resulting in the generation of inositol 1,4,5 triphosphate, diacylglycerol, and increased cytosolic calcium *(28–33)*. The stimulation of adenylyl cyclase is mediated through G_s, whereas stimulation of PLC is presumed to be mediated through one or more members of the $G_{q/11}$ family *(34)*. G_s is also capable of modulating Ca^{2+} channels *(35)*. Although cAMP is the most well-studied second messenger generated by PTH and is important for PTH action, it is likely that other effector pathways also have a significant role in PTH action.

Administration of exogenous PTH increases both urinary *(7,18)* and plasma *(36)* cAMP. These result from PTH action on the renal proximal tubule and are useful clinically as tests of renal responsiveness to PTH *(7,36)*. G_s activation leads to stimulation of adenylyl cyclase, the enzyme that catalyzes formation of cAMP from ATP and Mg^{2+}. cAMP stimulates a specific cAMP-dependent protein kinase (protein kinase A or PKA) that, in turn, regulates the function of key substrates through phosphorylation. One set of substrates for PKA is the cAMP-responsive element binding (CREB) proteins, a family of transcription factors whose activity is regulated by phosphorylation. cAMP is degraded by cyclic nucleotide phosphodiesterases (PDEs).

Both the increase in phosphate clearance *(37,38)* and the stimulation of 25-hydroxy-cholecalciferol-1α-hydroxylase *(39,40)* observed after administration of PTH are probably mediated by cAMP. It is still unclear whether cAMP is important in the anticalciuric effect of PTH *(41,42)*. In bone, the role of cAMP-dependent pathways in PTH action is less clear *(19,43,44)*, although PTH stimulates cAMP formation in osteoblast cells *(19)*. It appears that cAMP may play a role regulating the differentiation pathway of osteoblasts, and that cAMP stimulates proliferation and inhibits differentiation of osteoprogenitor cells *(45–47)*.

COMPONENTS OF THE SIGNAL TRANSDUCTION PATHWAY

The components of G_s signaling pathways include receptors (in this case the PTH/PTHrP receptor), G_s, adenylyl cyclase, PKA, PDEs, and specific cellular substrates for PKA *(48)*. Defects of specific receptors or cell-specific substrates downstream of PKA would be predicted to lead to resistance to a specific hormone. There are many examples of isolated hormone resistance resulting from defects in specific receptors, and several are discussed in detail in other chapters of this book. Since G_s is a component common to virtually all signaling pathways that stimulate cAMP formation, G_s

defects would be predicted to result in multihormone resistance and pleiotropic manifestations. Although adenylyl cyclase and cAMP phosphodiesterase are common components in the pathway, each exists as multiple subtypes with differences in their regulation and tissue-specific expression *(25,49–51)*. Defects in these components might therefore result in relatively isolated abnormalities. Some forms of adenylyl cyclase are also negatively regulated by distinct inhibitory hormones that bind to their specific receptors and activate one or more G_i (i for inhibitory) proteins (*see* Fig. 1).

Receptors

Several cDNAs isolated from different species encode a single receptor that binds with PTH and the related protein PTHrP with equal affinity and that is expressed in bone and kidney (as well as other tisssues) *(52–54)*. The cDNA encodes a protein with a predicted overall topography similar to that of other members of the G-protein-coupled receptor family, with seven potential membrane-spanning domains. Binding of either PTH or PTHrP to the expressed receptor stimulates adenylyl cyclase and PLC *(52,53)*, making it likely that receptor activation leads to interaction with both G_s and one or more members of the $G_{q/11}$ family. A second receptor that binds only PTH has been cloned, but its expression appears to be limited to the central nervous system *(55)* and therefore is not likely to be defective in PHP. The existence of multiple PTH receptors within bone and kidney has been suggested by pharmacological studies *(56–58)*. However, photoaffinity labeling experiments with PTH identifies a single protein of 70 kDa in bone and kidney *(59)*, and a second receptor in either bone or kidney has yet to be identified. Activating mutations of the PTH/PTHrP receptor have been identified in Jansen's metaphyseal chondrodysplasia *(60)*. The PTH/PTHrP receptor is discussed in more detail in Chapter 12.

G_s

G_s couples many receptors, including the PTH/PTHrP receptor, to the stimulation of adenylyl cyclase. It also can increase the opening of specific calcium channels *(35)*. Like other G proteins, G_s consists of three subunits, α, β, and γ, each the product of a separate gene. The α-subunit ($G\alpha_s$) directly interacts with and stimulates all forms of adenylyl cyclase, whereas $\beta\gamma$-dimers inhibit or stimulate only specific isoforms of adenylyl cyclase *(25,51)*. $G\alpha_s$ binds guanine nucleotide and confers specificity for receptor and effector coupling.

Many biochemical studies and the more recent crystal structures of both α-subunits *(61–64)* and $\alpha\beta\gamma$-heterotrimers *(65,66)* have increased our understanding of G protein structure and function. The 3-D structure consists of a GTPase domain, containing five domains (G1–G5), which converge to form the guanine nucleotide binding pocket, and a helical domain, which is unique for each α-subunit. Both the amino- and carboxy-terminis are important for receptor interactions. On activation, three discrete regions (switch regions 1–3) within the GTPase domain undergo a conformational shift. In the inactive GDP-bound state, the switch 2 region directly interacts with $\beta\gamma$. GTP binding causes the switch 2 region to move inward toward the switch 3 region, and this presumably results in dissociation from $\beta\gamma$. Specific residues within the GTPase domain of $G\alpha_s$ that interact with adenylyl cyclase have been identified *(67)*.

The human gene encoding $G\alpha_s$ (GNAS1) is a complex gene spanning about 20 kb and composed of 13 exons *(68)*. Analysis of the mouse gene (Gnas) shows its organization to be similar to that of the human (L. S. W., unpublished data). The conserved G1–G5 regions are in exons 2, 8, 9, 11, and 13, respectively. The 5′-flanking regions of the human and mouse genes have a high G + C content and multiple "GC" boxes (potential binding sites for transcriptional factor Sp1), and lack canonical "TATA" boxes (ref. *68* and L. S. W., unpublished data). These features are found in the promoters of other "housekeeping" genes, which, like GNAS1, are ubiquitously expressed. The GNAS1 (human) gene has been mapped to 20q13 *(69)*, whereas Gnas (mouse) has been mapped to the distal arm of chromosome 2 *(70)* in a region syntenic with 20q13 in humans. Gnas maps within a region that is implicated as having one or more imprinted genes *(71,72)*.

Four major species of human $G\alpha_s$ cDNA have been identified and appear to result from alternative splicing of a single gene *(68,73)*. Two long and two short forms are the result of the splicing in or out of exon 3, respectively, and correspond to the long and short forms of $G\alpha_s$ identified on immunoblots. Further heterogeneity is produced by the use of 2 alternative 3′ splice sites for intron 3, resulting in the presence or absence of an extra CAG codon at the junction of the exon 3 and 4 coding sequences. There is little evidence to suggest that these four forms are functionally different *(35,74)*, although they are differentially expressed in different tissues *(75)*. Another alternatively spliced form of $G\alpha_s$ cDNA has been identified and shown to be present within intracellular compartments in secretory cells *(76)*. This form, referred to as $XL\alpha s$ because it encodes a very large amino-terminal extension to the $G\alpha_s$ protein, appears to result from the use of an alternative first exon of the GNAS1 gene. However, the existence of this sequence as an independent exon within the gene has yet to be established. Several reports have documented the presence of other alternatively spliced forms of $G\alpha_s$, including the use of a still different alternative exon 1 and the splicing out of other internal exons *(77,78)*. The extent to which these forms are expressed as protein and their physiological significance is still largely unknown.

Mutations of $G\alpha_s$ have been identified in vitro and in vivo. $G\alpha_s$ mutations in mouse S49 lymphoma cells can lead to total deficiency of $G\alpha_s$ expression (cyc–), uncoupling from receptors (unc) or failure to undergo activation by GTP (H21a) *(79)*. Substitutions of residues Arg^{201} or Gln^{227} inhibit the intrinsic GTPase "turn off" mechanism and therefore lead to constitutive activation. These mutations have been identified in sporadic endocrine tumors, fibrous dysplasia of bone, and the McCune-Albright syndrome (MAS) (*see* Chapter 3). Cholera toxin catalyzes the ADP ribosylation of residue Arg^{201} and this covalent modification leads to constitutive activation of $G\alpha_s$, which clinically manifests itself as severe diarrhea in patients with intestinal cholera. Residue Gln^{227} is analogous to residue Gln^{61} in the related Ras protein, which when mutated leads to inhibition of the GTPase and constitutive activation.

Adenylyl Cyclase

At least eight subtypes of adenylyl cylase encoded by independent genes have been identified *(51)*. The encoded proteins are large with multiple membrane-spanning domains and have a predicted topography similar to that for ATP binding transport proteins. However, there is no evidence that adenylyl cyclase has any transporter function. The tissue distribution varies widely with some restricted to the central nervous system (types 1 and 3) and others more ubiquitously expressed (e.g., type 4). Although all adenylyl cyclases are stimulated by $G\alpha_s$, their regulation otherwise varies widely *(51,80)*. Some are stimulated by calcium and calmodulin (type 1), whereas others are inhibited by calcium (types 5 and 6). βγ inhibits adenylyl cyclase type 1, but stimulates adenylyl cyclase types 2 and 4 *(81)*. Some subtypes are also phosphorylated by PKA or PKC. Defects in calmodulin-sensitive adenylyl cyclase have been associated with learning defects in drosophila *(82)* and mice *(83)*. The physiological significance of the molecular diversity of adenylyl cyclase is still poorly understood.

Downstream Components

Multiple forms of cyclic nucleotide phosphodiesterase, differing in substrate (cAMP vs cGMP) specificity, hormonal regulation, and tissue distribution, have been identified *(49,50,84)*. Mutations resulting in deficient *(85)* and excess *(86)* cAMP phospho-diesterase activity have been described. PKA is a tetramer, consisting of two regulatory (cAMP binding) and two catalytic subunits. Binding of cAMP promotes regulatory sub-unit dissociation and activation of catalytic subunits. Defects in regulatory subunits can lead to constitutive activation *(87)*, whereas defects in catalytic subunits have been associated with decreased PKA activity *(79)*. CREB is a common substrate for PKA, and in bone leads to increased Fos expression *(88)*. Further substrates for PKA in both bone and kidney are poorly defined.

PATHOPHYSIOLOGY OF PHP

Common to all forms of PHP is a defect in the renal response to PTH. The majority of patients with PHP show a markedly diminished rise in urinary cAMP excretion in response to PTH infusion when compared to normal controls or patients with PTH-deficient forms of hypoparathyroidism *(7)*. Patients with blunted cAMP response, who presumably have a defect proximal to cAMP generation, are classified as PHP type I. In these patients, the phosphaturic response to PTH is also diminished, and this is likely to be a direct consequence of the lack of cAMP response *(37)*, since administration of dibu-tyryl cAMP in these patients produces a normal phosphaturic response *(38)*. Decreased phosphate clearance leads to hyperphosphatemia. Hyperphosphatemia and renal resistance to PTH both lead to diminished formation of 1,25-dihydroxyvitamin D *(38,40,89–92)*. It is likely that cAMP also mediates this effect *(91)*. 1,25 Dihydroxyvitamin D deficiency con-tributes to hypocalcemia through a decrease in both gastrointestinal absorption of calcium and calcium mobilization from bone in response to PTH *(93–95)*. Rarely, patients with PHP show a normal urinary cAMP response, but a decreased phosphaturic response to infused PTH, indicating a defect located distal to cAMP generation (PHP type II) *(16)*.

Although the response of renal phosphate clearance and 1α-hydroxylase to PTH is diminished in PHP, the anticalciuric action of PTH appears to remain intact *(42)*. There are several possible explanations for why renal handling of calcium is unaffected. One possibility is that a small rise in intracellular cAMP is sufficient to stimulate the maximal anticalciuric response. It is equally likely that other effector pathways (e.g., phos-phoinositide pathway), which remain intact in PHP type I, mediate the anticalciuric response to PTH. The site of action of the anticalciuric effect of PTH (distal tubule) is dis-tinct from the site of PTH action leading to phosphaturia and increased vitamin D metab-olism (proximal tubule). The severity of the primary signaling defect may vary between different cell types, so that the defect in the proximal tubule may be more severe than in the distal tubule. The physiologic response to vasopressin, a hormone that raises cAMP in the distal tubule, has been shown to be normal in patients with PHP type I *(96,97)*.

Although the diminished renal responsiveness to PTH is well established, the extent to which PTH signaling in bone is defective is less clear. The calcemic response to PTH (presumed to be secondary to mobilization of calcium of bone) is diminished in many PHP patients. However, correction of 1,25-dihydroxyvitamin D deficiency restores the calcemic response *(93–95)*. This suggests that the diminished calcemic response to PTH and resultant hypocalcemia are not secondary to primary skeletal resistance to PTH, but rather to 1,25-dihydroxyvitamin D deficiency resulting from renal resistance to PTH *(38,40,89–92)*. In one unusual case, selective deficiency of 1,25-dihydroxyvitamin D was invoked as the cause of isolated skeletal resistance to PTH *(98)*. Patients with PHP occasionally show evidence of rickets *(99,100)* or osteomalacia *(95)* secondary to 1,25-dihydroxyvitamin D deficiency.

The bone remodeling response to PTH, which does not require normal levels of 1,25-dihydroxyvitamin D, is intact to a greater or lesser extent in patients with PHP. The clinical manifestations are variable and range from decreased bone density *(101)* to overt osteitis fibrosa cystica *(102–104)*. Whether the variable manifestations are a result of differences in skeletal resistance to PTH or to differences in circulating levels of PTH or 1,25-dihydroxyvitamin is unclear. Overt hyperparathyroid bone disease is rare in PHP type Ia *(103)*, but is seen in patients with PHP type Ib. The possibility that PHP with osteitis fibrosa cystica is a distinct entity is discussed in the section on PHP type Ib. Consistent with the notion that skeletal resistance to PTH is normal in PHP type I, bone cells derived from two PHP type I patients demonstrated normal responsiveness to PTH in vitro *(104,105)*.

PTH antagonists, such as abnormal forms of PTH or other unrelated molecules that block PTH binding to its receptor, could theoretically result in PHP. An abnormal form of PTH may lack biological activity and result in hypoparathyroidism, but should not result in the resistance to normal exogenous PTH, which is characteristic of PTH. There is no evidence that either abnormal forms of PTH, which may be present in some hypoparathyroid patients *(106–108)*, or PTH analogs synthesized in vitro *(58)* can function as potent PTH antagonists in vivo. Molecular genetic analysis of the PTH gene suggests that the secretion of mutated forms of PTH is probably a rare event *(109,110)*. One group has reported a dissociation between PTH biologic activity and immunoreactivity in patients with PHP type I using ultrasensitive renal and metatarsal cytochemical assays for PTH *(111,112)*. Whereas immunoreactivity was supranormal, biologic activity was in the normal range. Plasma from these patients was also shown to be able to block the activity of normal PTH in these assays *(113)*, suggesting the existence of a circulating inhibitor of PTH action in patients with PHP type I. Another group reported similar findings in patients treated for nutritional vitamin D deficiency using the same assay *(114)*. The improvement in PTH responsiveness observed in PHP patients after correction of hypocalcemia with vitamin D treatment *(115)* or after parathyroidectomy *(113)* prompted speculation that secretion of an abnormal form of PTH or another inhibitor of PTH by the parathyroid glands could lead to PTH resistance. Consistent with this possibility, Mitchell and Goltzman demonstrated the presence of abnormal forms of immunoreactive PTH in some PHP patients *(116)*. However, there is no evidence that vitamin D treatment or parathyroidectomy restores a normal urinary cAMP response to PTH *(7)*. It is likely that the elevated levels of PTH present in untreated PHP patients may lead to decreased PTH sensitivity secondary to downregulation of the PTH/PTHrP receptor, and that hypocalcemia or vitamin D deficiency may inhibit steps in PTH action that are distal to the generation of cAMP *(see* PHP Type II). The hypothesis that PHP is

Table 1
Classification of AHO and PHP

	AHO	Hormone resistance	PTH infusion	G_s defect	Comments
PHP Ia	Yes	Multiple	cAMP-↓ phosphaturia-↓	Yes	
PPHP	Yes	None	Normal response	Yes	Within PHP Ia kindreds
PHP Ib	No	PTH only	cAMP-↓ phosphaturia-↓	No	? PTH receptor defect
PHP Ic	Yes	Multiple	cAMP-↓ phosphaturia-↓	No	? AC defect
PHP II	No	PTH only	cAMP-normal phosphaturia-↓	No	Usually reverses with treatment
AHO-like syndrome	Yes[a]	None	Normal response	No	Deletion at 2q37

[a] Brachydactyly and mental retardation.

primarily the result of inhibitors of PTH action is not proven and could certainly not explain the generalized hormone resistance and multiple somatic, neurological, and sensory defects present in PHP type Ia, PPHP, and PHP type Ic.

CLASSIFICATION OF PHP AND AHO

In the sections that follow, PHP is classified according to the presumed locus of the defect causing PTH resistance. PHP is divided into type I (defect proximal to cAMP production) and type II (defect distal to cAMP generation). PHP type I may be further subdivided into Ia (generalized hormone resistance, AHO, and G_s deficiency), Ib (resistance limited to PTH, no AHO or G_s deficiency) and Ic (generalized hormone resistance and AHO without G_s deficiency). PPHP is the term applied to individuals with G_s deficiency and AHO, but without hormone resistance. Some distinct genetic syndromes that present with features of AHO are discussed briefly. The classification is summarized in Table 1.

PHP Type Ia and PPHP

PATHOPHYSIOLOGY

The majority of patients with PHP have, in addition to PTH resistance, resistance to other hormones (e.g., TSH, gonadotropins) which raise intracellular cAMP in their target tissues and a constellation of somatic features referred to as AHO (1,13). The features of AHO include short stature, centripetal obesity, round face, brachydactyly, subcutaneous ossifications, and mental retardation. The diminished urinary cAMP response to exogenous PTH, which is observed in these patients (7,117), and the presence of multihormone resistance would lead to the prediction that a general component of the signal transduction pathway proximal to the generation of cAMP (e.g., G_s or adenylyl cyclase) is defective in these patients. In most PHP subjects with AHO and generalized hormone resistance, an approx 50% deficiency of G_s function is found in the membranes of various cell types (e.g., erythrocytes, fibroblasts, platelets, transformed lymphoblasts, renal tissue) examined by the cyc– functional complementation assay *(8,9,117–126)*. In this assay, cell membranes prepared from patients or normal subjects are reconstituted with membranes from mutant S49 mouse lymphoma cells (cyc–), which have receptors and adenylyl cyclase, but totally lack G_s, and the adenylyl cyclase response to the β-adrenergic stimulator isoproterenol is determined. Stimulation is proportional to the amount of functional G_s in the test membranes. In some of these studies, levels of G_s were also examined by measuring the extent of cholera toxin-catalyzed incorporation of radioactive ADP ribose into $G\alpha_s$. Patients with multihormone resistance, AHO, and G_s deficiency are diagnosed as having PHP type Ia. The formation of the high affinity ternary complex among ligand, β-adrenergic receptor, and G_s was shown to be significantly decreased in erythrocyte membranes from some PHP type Ia patients *(127)*. More recently real-time metabolic responses to a β-adrenergic agonist were shown to be decreased in cultured fibroblasts of affected patients *(128)*. In contrast to G_s, the expression of G_i has been shown to be normal in several PHP type Ia patients *(129,130)*.

After the initial description of PHP, Albright *(6)* reported a patient with the physical features of AHO, but without evidence of PTH resistance and termed this condition PPHP. The genetic linkage between PHP and PPHP was recognized early *(3)* and re-emphasized more recently *(131)*. Subsequently, it has been shown that patients with PPHP show no evidence of resistance to any hormone and, in contrast to patients with PHP type Ia, show a perfectly normal urinary cAMP response to exogenous PTH *(117)*. However, similar to PHP type Ia patients, patients with PPHP also have an approx 50% deficiency in functional G_s in cell membranes *(117,132)*. AHO can be considered a specific genetic disorder associated with G_s deficiency with two variants defined by the presence (PHP type Ia) or absence (PPHP) of multihormone resistance. Since many of the features of AHO are nonspecific (obesity, short stature) or may be found in other disorders, the term PPHP is best restricted to relatives of patients with PHP Ia who show phenotypic features of Albright osteodystrophy and a normal rise in urinary cAMP excretion in response to PTH *(7,117)*.

Initially, PHP type Ia was proposed to be transmitted in an X-linked-dominant *(3)* or autosomal-recessive *(133)* manner. A report of father-to-son transmission of G_s deficiency made X-linked inheritance unlikely *(134)*, and subsequent reports were more consistent with an autosomal-dominant mode of inheritance *(119,131,135,136)*. The functional G_s deficiency present in PHP type Ia and PPHP is most often accompanied by a similar deficiency in amounts of $G\alpha_s$ steady-state mRNA *(126,137,138)* and/or $G\alpha_s$ protein *(139,140)*. The genetic defect in patients with PHP Ia and PPHP has been confirmed by the identification of multiple heterozygous loss-of-function mutations within the GNAS1 gene (*see* Table 2). The mapping of this gene to 20q13 *(69)* also confirms that the disease is transmitted in an autosomal-dominant manner.

With one exception (*see below*), each GNAS1 mutation associated with PHP Ia has been identified in a single kindred. In many cases, the mutations result in abnormal RNA processing and lack of expression of the mutant allele (i.e., base substitution at a splice junction site, coding frameshift mutations, large deletion) *(11,138,140–148;* L.S.W., unpublished data). One specific 4-bp deletion within exon 7 of GNAS1 has been identified in affected members from eight unrelated PHP Ia kindreds (*see* Fig. 2) *(138,145–148)*. A previously defined consensus sequence for arrest of DNA polymerase α has been found to be prone to sporadic deletion mutations *(149)*. The GNAS1 exon 7 deletion site coincides with this consensus sequence (*see* Fig. 2). The presence of CT dinucleotide repeats

Table 2
G$_s\alpha$ Mutations in PHP Type Ia and PPHP

	Mutation	Type	mRNA	Protein	Comments	Ref.
Exon 1	A→G	Missense M1V	N1[a]	Abnormal 70K form; N1 form ↓	Cyc–assay ↓	10
Intron 3	A→G	Acceptor splice junction	ND[b]	ND		141
Exon 4	43-bp deletion		ND	ND		143
Exon 4	2-bp deletion	Frameshift	↓	ND		130, Unpublished (L. S. W.)
Exon 4	3-bp deletion	Missense ΔN99	ND	ND		Unpublished (L. S. W.)
Exon 4	T→C	Missense L99P	ND	↓		140
Exon 5	1-bp deletion	Frameshift	ND	ND	Cyc–assay ↓	142
Exon 5	C→T	Missense P115S	ND	ND		146
Intron 5	G→A	Donor splice junction	ND	ND		144
Exon 6	C→T	Missense R165C	NI	↓		140
Exon 7	4-bp deletion	Frameshift	↓	ND	Present in several kindreds; Cyc–assay ↓	138, 145–148
Exon 7	T→G	Missense Y190D	ND	ND		141

(continued)

Table 2 (*continued*)

	Mutation	Type	mRNA	Protein	Comments	Ref.
Exon 8	4-bp deletion	Frameshift	NI	↓		140
Exon 9	G → A	Missense R231H	ND	ND	Defective receptor-dependent signaling	155
Exon 10	C → G	Missense S250R	NI	↓	Cyc–assay ↓	Unpublished (L. S. W.)
Exon 10	C → T	Missense R258W	NI	↓	Cyc–assay ↓	Unpublished (L. S. W.)
Exon 10	A → G	Missense E259V	ND	ND		146
Exon 10	1-bp insertion	Frameshift	ND	ND	Cyc–assay ↓	142
Exon 10	1-bp deletion	Frameshift	ND	ND		11
Intron 10	G → C	Donor splice junction	↓	ND		11
Exon 13	G → T	Missense A366S	ND	ND	PHP Ia and testotoxicosis; Cyc–assay ↓ at 37°C; rapid GDP release and activation at low temp.	154
Exon 13	3-bp deletion	Missense ΔI383	ND	ND		141
Exon 13	G → A	Missense R385H	ND	Moderate ↓	Cyc–assay ↓; uncoupled from receptor	150

[a] NI, normal.
[b] ND, not determined or not available.

Normal Allele

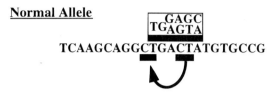

TCAAGCAGGCTGACTATGTGCCG

Mutant Allele

TCAAGCAGGCTATGTGCCG

Fig. 2. GNAS1 deletion hot-spot. A stretch of the normal coding sequence of GNAS1 exon 7 *(68)* is shown on top and the 4-bp deletion mutation is shown below *(147)*. CT dinucleotide repeats in the vicinity and within the deletion are underlined. A consensus sequence that has been derived from comparison of deletion hot-spot sites in other genes *(149)* is shown in a box aligned above the normal GNAS1 sequence. The mutation is presumed to be secondary to pausing of DNA polymerase, and single-strand mispairing and slippage during replication (shown with arrow).

flanking the deletion is consistent with slipped strand mispairing of a CT repeat during replication and excision of the resulting 4-base single-stranded loop *(149)*. Therefore, this mutation appears to be a deletion hot spot likely to be a result of arrest of polymerization and slipped strand mispairing during DNA replication *(147)*.

A number of missense mutations in GNAS1 have also been identified. In some cases, the encoded amino acid substitution (L99P and R165C; ref. *140*; S250R, D. Warner, L. S. W., unpublished data) appears to alter globally the tertiary structure, interaction with βγ, or intracellular trafficking, since in each case, the level of Gα$_s$ mRNA is normal, but the level of membrane Gα$_s$ protein is decreased. In one kindred, a mutation at the translational start site codon is associated with the expression of an abnormally large form of Gα$_s$ protein, which is presumed to be functionally deficient (10). For several missense mutations (ΔN99, P115S, Y190D, E259V, ΔI383), the biochemical defect remains to be determined *(141,146*; and L. S. W., unpublished data).

In several cases, missense mutations within GNAS1 encode Gα$_s$ proteins with a specific biochemical abnormality that may further our understanding of the molecular mechanisms of G protein activation, guanine nucleotide binding, or interactions with βγ and receptor. One missense mutation (R385H) identified in the carboxy-terminal region, known to be a region important for receptor interaction, results in a specific defect in receptor coupling *(150)*. This is nearby the unc mutation (R389P), which was identified in S49 mouse lymphoma cells and shown to disrupt receptor coupling *(151,152)*. A missense mutation (A366S) within the highly conserved G5 region of Gα$_s$ was recently identified in two unrelated males who presented with AHO, PTH resistance, and gonadotropin-independent precocious puberty *(153)*. This mutation was shown to decrease the protein's affinity for GDP *(154)*. Increased release of GDP has two functional consequences: (1) an increased time that the protein is unbound to guanine nucleotide leading to instability of the protein, and (2) an increased activation of G$_s$ pathways, since GDP release is normally the rate-limiting step in G protein activation. At internal body temperature (37°C), the former effect is predominant, leading to decreased expression of Gα$_s$ protein and the clinical expression of AHO and hormone resistance. At the slightly lower temperatures (the ambient temperature of the testes), the latter effect predominates, leading to G_s activation, increased intracellular cAMP, and gonadotropin-independent precocious puberty.

Missense mutations which encode amino acid substitutions within regions that undergo major conformational shifts on receptor activation (switch regions) have also been identified. A mutation (R231H) within the switch 2 region, the major site of βγ interaction, was shown to result in a specific defect in receptor-dependent activation *(155)*. Further studies should give a better understanding of how this mutation would lead to this specific defect. Two mutations have been identified in the switch 3. One mutation (E259V) has not been studied biochemically *(146)*, but since this acidic residue interacts with basic residues within the switch 2 region on activation, it would be predicted that this mutation would not allow the protein to switch to the active conformation. We have recently identified a mutation (R258W) in the switch 3 region that is somewhat unstable at 37°C owing to a marked decrease affinity for GDP, but that at lower temperatures demonstrates a specific defect in receptor-dependent activation (Warner D., L. S. W., unpublished data).

Consistent with the equivalent functional G_s deficiency present in both forms of AHO, identical GNAS1 mutations were identified in both PHP type Ia and PPHP patients within several kindred *(10,11,140,145*; for example, *see* Fig. 3). The presence of GNAS1 mutations with subtle *(11)* or absent *(140)* clinical findings suggests that these mutations are associated with a wide spectrum of clinical severity. The mechanism by which an identical GNAS1 mutation can lead to such a variable phenotype is discussed in more detail at the end of the chapter. In contrast to PHP type Ia, in which inactivating GNAS1 mutations are associated with generalized hormone resistance, in the McCune Albright syndrome, activating GNAS1 mutations are associated with hormone-independent activation, leading to gonadotropin-independent precocious puberty, hyperthyroidism, hypercortisolism, and growth hormone excess *(156,157*; and Chapter 3).

CLINICAL FEATURES

Generalized Resistance to Hormones and Sensory Stimuli. Resistance to PTH is the most commonly recognized hormonal abnormality, although it is not necessarily the first to appear in patients with PHP type Ia. The classical clinical picture is hypocalcemia and hyperphosphatemia with elevation of circulating PTH. Hypocalcemia is not present from birth in patients with PHP Ia. PTH resistance usually slowly develops over the first several years, initially presenting with hyperphosphatemia and elevated serum PTH before the development of overt or subclinical hypocalcemia *(158–160)*. An infant had normal serum calcium and PTH levels and a normal cAMP response to exogenous PTH, but by age 2.5 yr had developed overt PTH resistance with no significant cAMP response to PTH *(160)*. This suggests that PTH responsiveness is initially normal and decreases after birth. Whether this is secondary to a progressive decrease in G_s in renal tubules after birth or to changes in other factors in early childhood is unclear. Some patients with clear-cut PTH resistance (elevated serum PTH, blunted urinary cAMP response to PTH) remain normocalcemic *(94,161)* or fluctuate between low and normal calcium concentrations *(162)*. It is likely that the variability in the serum calcium concentration among patients with PHP is at least partially owing to differences in the concentrations of 1,25-dihydroxyvitamin D, which alters the intestinal absorption of calcium and the ability of PTH to stimulate calcium release from skeletal stores *(93,94)*. Estrogens and placental synthesis of 1,25-dihydroxyvitamin D (which is not regulated by PTH) may alter the serum calcium concentration and decrease requirements for vitamin D supplementation in PHP patients during pregnancy *(163,164)*.

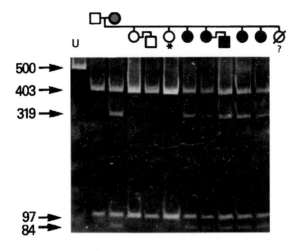

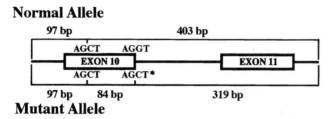

Fig. 3. An identical GNAS1 mutation is present in both PHP type Ia and PPHP. In the upper panel, the pedigree of an AHO kindred is shown. Pedigree members with PHP type Ia are blackened, and that for the member with PPHP is stippled. The asterisk denotes an unaffected member with four unaffected sons who were not analyzed. One subject who died in infancy and whose disease status is unknown is listed with a question mark. Genomic DNA was isolated from each family member and a 500-bp genomic fragment, including GNAS1 exons 10 and 11, was amplified using the polymerase chain reaction. The fragments were digested with the restriction endonuclease *Alu*I, and the digests were electrophoresed in a nondenaturing 5% acrylamide gel. The size of the restriction fragments is depicted on the left with the 500-bp undigested fragment shown in lane U. Unaffected members show 403- and 97-bp fragments, whereas affected subjects show two additional fragments of 319- and 84-bp. A schematic of the GNAS1 genomic fragment with the *Alu*I restriction sites is shown below. The 500-bp genomic fragment contains an *Alu*I restriction site 97 bp from the 5′-end within the normal sequence of exon 10, predicting 97- and 403-bp fragments in the normal allele as shown above the diagram. A G to C base substitution at the donor splice junction site of intron 10 (which was defined by direct sequencing) creates a new *Alu*I restriction site, predicting 319-, 97-, and 84-bp fragments. Therefore, all affected members within the kindred, both with PHP type Ia and PPHP, were heterozygous for this mutation. The mother with PPHP had very mild signs of AHO, including only unilateral brachydactyly of a distal thumb and pinpoint subcutaneous calcifications detected only on X-ray (from Weinstein et al. *[11]*).

Clinical studies of patients with PHP type Ia provide evidence for resistance to hormones other than PTH, which is presumed to be secondary to G_s deficiency within multiple endocrine glands. Primary thyroid resistance to TSH appears to be extremely common, if not universal, in patients with PHP type Ia *(13,165)*. Defective adenylyl cyclase stimulation by GTP and TSH in thyroid membranes obtained from a patient with

PHP type Ia provides direct evidence for thyroid resistance to TSH in this disease (166). In contrast to patients with more common forms of primary hypothyroidism, no goiter is present in PHP type Ia, since TSH resistance would lead to decreased thyroid growth and hormone secretion. There is generally no evidence of autoimmune thyroid disease. The serum TSH levels are mildly to moderately elevated, and usually the thyroid hormone levels are slightly low or low normal. Several cases of PHP type Ia initially came to medical attention owing to elevated TSH levels detected in neonatal screening (167–169).

Clinical evidence of hypogonadism is common in patients, particularly in females, and is manifested as primary or secondary amenorrhea, oligomenorrhea, or infertility (13,170–172). Although endocrine studies of the reproductive axis are often normal, there are some patients in whom gonadotropin-resistance is evident on basal measurements or after stimulation with gonadotropins or gonadotropin-releasing hormone (97,125,170). Prolactin deficiency has also been reported in many (but not all) PHP type Ia patients (13,97,130,173–175). The cause of this abnormality has not been elucidated. In anecdotal case reports, some PHP type Ia patients have shown evidence of growth hormone deficiency (172,176), whereas others have not (97,177).

For some hormones, such as glucagon (13,178), and isoproterenol (179), the cAMP response in PHP type Ia patients is reduced when compared to control subjects, but the downstream responses (increase in serum glucose) remain relatively intact. It appears that either plasma cAMP measurements are too crude to distinguish the cAMP response in specific cells or that the cAMP response is sufficient to stimulate maximally the physiologic response. One study with only two PHP type Ia patients reported a normal rise in serum-free fatty acids in response to isoproterenol (180), but a subsequent study reported blunted free fatty acid responses to isoproterenol (181).

Patients with PHP type Ia do not show resistance to all hormones that activate G_s coupled pathways. There is no evidence of resistance to vasopressin (96,97) or ACTH (13,97). Whether or not the cAMP responses to either hormone are normal has not been studied. A single patient with PTH and ACTH resistance and prolactin deficiency, but without AHO has been reported (182), but it is unclear whether the patient has PHP type Ia or another PHP variant.

An early study of PHP patients reported decreased sensitivity to gustatory and olfactory stimuli, which was not corrected after treatment of hypocalcemia (183). Subsequent studies demonstrated decreased olfactory function in PHP type Ia patients, but not in PHP type Ib patients (normal G_s) (184,185). Recently, olfaction was shown to be abnormal in PHP type Ia, but normal in PPHP (186). It is unclear if the difference in olfaction between PHP type Ia and PPHP is related to differences in extracellular calcium concentrations, hormonal status, or G_s expression within critical central nervous system pathways. It is unlikely that G_s deficiency has a direct effect on the initial signaling from odorant or taste receptors, since distinct G proteins, G_{olf} (187) and gustducin (188), are responsible for transduction of primary odorant and gustatory stimuli, respectively. It is more likely that G_s deficiency may lead to defects in higher-level processing of sensory signals in the central nervous system. Sensorineural hearing loss has also been reported in PHP Ia (189). In interpreting studies of sensory perception in patients in PHP type Ia, it is important to remember that many of these patients have mild mental retardation (5), which may affect the ability of these patients to perform a given task properly.

Albright Hereditary Osteodystrophy. The phenotypic features that characterize AHO include short stature, obesity, rounded face, mental retardation, subcutaneous

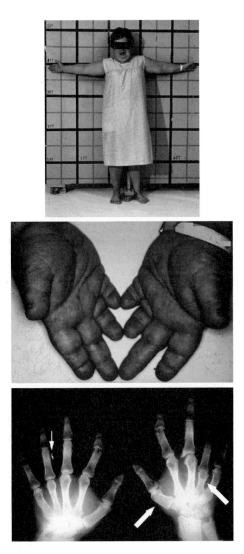

Fig. 4. Features of AHO. Top: Patient with AHO showing the features of short stature, obesity and rounded face with depressed nasal bridge. Center: Severe brachydactyly particularly of the first, second, fourth and fifth digits bilaterally. Notice the shortening and widening of the distal thumbs. Bottom: Hand radiograph showing evidence of subcutaneous ossification (thin arrow) and brachydactyly (thick arrows).

ossification, and characteristic shortening and widening of long bones in the hands and feet (brachydactyly) (Fig. 4). Many patients also show characteristic facial features, including depressed nasal bridge and hypertelorism. The pathogenesis of AHO in patients with PHP type Ia and PPHP is less well understood than the pathogenesis of generalized hormone resistance. The severity of the AHO phenotype varies greatly between patients with G_s deficiency, with some patients showing few *(11)* or no *(140)* somatic features. Although G_s deficiency is presumed to have a major role in the pathogenesis of AHO, the role of downstream pathways (abnormal cAMP generation vs other G_s-coupled effector pathways) is poorly established.

The most characterisitic feature of AHO is brachydactyly, which involves the phalanges of the hands and feet in either a symmetric or asymmetric manner. Shortening and widening of the distal phalanx of the thumb is the most common abnormality, followed by shortening of the third through fifth metacarpals *(190–192)*. This pattern of involvement is somewhat specific for AHO when compared to other disorders in which brachydactyly is a feature *(190,191)*. Brachydactyly becomes clinically evident within the first decade and is associated with premature closure of the epiphyseal growth plate *(193)*. Generalized short stature is also commonly present in AHO *(193)*. Other skeletal abnormalities that have been reported in association with AHO include thickening of the calvarium, spinal cord compression, and bowing or shortening of the axial long bones *(131,190,194–196)*. Subcutaneous heterotopic ossifications (osteoma cutis) are also present in a significant number of AHO patients *(4,158,197,198)*. They may be large and palpable or pinpoint and only detectable by radiological examination *(11)*, and can present in a migratory fashion *(158,197)*.

The absence of the skeletal features of AHO in patients with primary hypoparathyroidism or PHP type Ib and the presence of these features in patients with normal calcium metabolism (i.e., PPHP) strongly suggest that the skeletal abnormalities are not related to hypocalcemia, hyperphosphatemia, or elevated PTH *per se*. PTH/PTHrP receptors are present within proliferative chondrocytes in the endochondral growth plates of long bones, and PTHrP acts in a paracrine manner through G_s-coupled pathways to inhibit the transition from proliferative to hypertrophic chondrocytes *(199)*. As predicted, mice with disruption of the PTHrP *(200)* or PTH/PTHrP receptor *(201)* genes had narrow growth plates with evidence of acceleration of the endochondral process and abnormal bone growth. Similar histological findings have been found in some mice with a knockout of the $G\alpha_s$ gene *(see below)*. It is likely that growth plates within long bones affected with brachydactyly have a similar histologic appearance and that brachdactyly at least in part is owing to G_s deficiency within growth plates, which results in abnormal endochondral ossification. The factors that influence the specific pattern of brachydactyly are unknown. The effect of growth hormone deficiency, which is present in some PHP type Ia patients *(see above)*, on the severity of short stature and brachydactyly has not been examined.

Several lines of evidence suggest that G_s activation inhibits the differentiation of osteoprogenitor cells to mature osteoblasts in a cAMP-dependent manner and, conversely, that decreased G_s expression leads to increased osteoblast differentiation. Treatment of osteoprogenitor cells with either PTH *(46)* or forskolin *(45)*, a direct stimulator of adenylyl cyclase, inhibited differentiation to an osteoblast phenotype in vitro. In patients with MAS, activating $G\alpha_s$ mutations are found in lesions of polyostotic fibrous dysplasia, which histologically are composed of poorly differentiated mesenchymal precursor cells *(47)*. cAMP likely mediates this effect by the activation of PKA, which phosphorylates CREB, a family of cAMP-responsive transcription factors. Phosphorylated CREB then promotes the expression of Fos, another transcription factor that, in combination with other transcription factors, promotes the expression of growth-related genes and suppresses the expression of osteoblast-specific genes (e.g., osteocalcin) *(88)*. In support of this model, Fos has been shown to be expressed at high levels within lesions of fibrous dysplasia *(202)* and overexpression of Fos in transgenic mice resulted in fibrous bone lesions *(203)*. Treatment of cells cultured from rat calvaria with oligonucleotides antisense to $G\alpha_s$ promoted their differentiation to an osteoblast phenotype *(204)*. It is reasonable to speculate that in patients with PHP type Ia, G_s deficiency in pluripotential cells might promote the formation of bone in heterotopic locations and lead to subcutaneous ossifications.

There are several potential mechanisms by which general G_s deficiency may lead to obesity. Similar to the reported effects of G_s deficiency on osteoblast differentiation, treatment of 3T3-L1 preadipocytes with oligonucleotides antisense to $G\alpha_s$ promoted their differentiation to adipocytes (205). However, for these cells, the effect was assumed to be mediated by a cAMP-independent mechanism, since coincubation with a cAMP analog did not block the effect of antisense oligonucleotides. In mature adipocytes, agents that stimulate lipolysis, such as β-adrenergic agonists, do so through the activation of G_s and elevation of intracellular cAMP. Isoproterenol-stimulated adenylyl cyclase activity was demonstrated to be low in adipocyte plasma membranes isolated from four obese patients with PHP type Ia (181). Serum free fatty acid concentrations were also low in these patients, consistent with decreased lipolytic activity in vivo. In brown adipose tissue, β-adrenergic agents induce the expression of uncoupling protein and increase the rate of thermogenesis. It is therefore plausible, but unproven, that G_s deficiency in brown adipose tissue could lead to decreased energy expenditure and result in obesity (206). Untreated hypothyroidism could also potentially increase the severity of obesity in PHP type Ia patients.

Mental retardation or developmental delay is seen in a significant number of AHO patients (5). The mechanisms involved are not defined, but abnormalities in cAMP metabolism are associated with learning defects in invertebrate model systems (82,125) and in transgenic mice (83). However, behavioral testing of $G\alpha_s$ knockout mice (see below) has not revealed any significant abnormalities (Paylor R., Crawley J., unpublished data). The role, if any, of associated hormonal abnormalities in the development of mental retardation is not well studied, but is probably not very significant. Mental retardation has been associated with brachydactyly in a genetically distinct disorder (207,208).

PHP Type Ib

Patients with PHP type Ib have PTH resistance but no evidence of AHO, decreased G_s activity, or generalized hormone resistance (13,15,209). In these patients, as in PHP type Ia, the urinary cAMP response to exogenous bovine parathyroid extract is diminished, suggesting the defect of PTH action in the kidney lies in a component that is proximal to cAMP generation (PTH/PTHrP receptor, G_s, or adenylyl cyclase) (13). Since only the PTH-stimulated pathway is abnormal (15), a defect in the PTH/PTHrP receptor, which would result in specific resistance to PTH, could explain the hormone resistance present in these patients. However, screening of many patients failed to reveal mutations in the structural portion of the gene encoding the PTH/PTHrP receptor (210,211). This may not be totally surprising, since defects in the PTH/PTHrP receptor gene might be expected to lead to developmental bone abnormalities similar to those present in AHO as well as PTH resistance. In vitro fibroblast cultures derived from some PHP type Ib patients had decreased levels of PTH/PTHrP receptor mRNA, and both the cAMP response to PTH and the levels of PTH/PTHrP receptor mRNA were normalized after treatment of cells with dexamethasone (212,213). Although these results suggest that defects in regulation of expression of the PTH/PTHrP receptor may be the cause of PHP type Ib, in vivo studies in affected patients will be required to confirm this possibility. The PTH/PTHrP receptor and potential defects in PHP are covered more fully in Chapter 12.

There is evidence that PHP type Ib itself is a heterogeneous group of disorders. Although PHP type Ib is most often sporadic *(15,210)*, it has also been reported to be familial *(173,210,214)*. Although most patients do not display evidence of overt hyperparathyroid bone disease, a subset have elevation in alkaline phosphatase or osteitis fibrosa cystica *(102–104)*. Those with overt bone disease may represent one end of a wide spectrum of clinical presentations of the same underlying defect *(103)*. Although cultured skin fibroblasts from most PHP type Ib patients showed selective PTH resistance, this was not found in all cases *(15)*. It is interesting that one PHP type Ib patient with normal PTH responsiveness in cultured fibroblasts *(15)* as well as another patient with normal PTH responsiveness in cultured bone cells *(104)* showed evidence of osteitis fibrosa cystica. This suggests that those patients with PHP type Ib and overt skeletal disease may represent a subset with a distinct molecular defect. Prolactin deficiency has been reported in some, but not all patients with PHP type Ib *(13,173–175)*. The mechanism for this is unclear.

PHP Type Ic

PHP type Ic refers to a small number of patients with generalized hormone resistance and AHO that have been reported to have normal G_s activity *(12–14)*. In one family, hypothyroidism, rather than PTH resistance, was the most significant hormonal abnormality *(215)*. The molecular defect in this form of PHP has not been established. A single PHP type Ic patient has been reported in whom in vitro biochemical data were most compatible with a defect in the catalytic subunit of adenylyl cyclase *(14)*. Multiple isoforms of adenylyl cyclase encoded by separate genes have been identified *(51)*. A potential candidate for molecular defects in PHP type Ic would be a subtype of adenylyl cyclase, which is widely expressed, particularly in bone, kidney, and endocrine glands. Subtle defects in G_s or defects in other components of the cAMP pathway (G_i, cAMP phosphodiesterases) may also be present in patients with PHP type Ic. Levels of $G\alpha_i$-subunits, determined by pertussis toxin-catalyzed ADP-ribosylation assays, have been shown to be normal in three patients with PHP type Ic *(129)*. In one kindred, AHO and PTH resistance was present in a mother and daughter with a deletion of a proximal portion of the long arm of chromosome 15 *(216)*.

PHP Type II

PHP type II refers to rare patients with unequivocal clinical evidence of PTH resistance in which the urinary cAMP response to exogenous PTH is normal, but the phosphaturic response is reduced *(16)*. It therefore appears to involve a defect distal to PTH-stimulated cAMP production. Patients with PHP type II have no evidence of AHO or generalized hormone resistance. The inability of cAMP to generate a normal physiological response could theoretically be a result of a defect at any point along the pathway from PKA to the renal sodium-phosphate transporter. At present, there is no direct evidence for a specific defect.

In most or perhaps all cases, PHP type II may be an acquired rather than inherited genetic defect *(217)*. Patients with vitamin D deficiency can also have findings similar to PHP type II with normal urinary cAMP, but decreased phosphaturic response to exogenous PTH *(217,218)*. Calcium infusion or vitamin D treatment can normalize the phosphaturic response to PTH in patients diagnosed with PHP type II or vitamin D deficiency *(217–219)*. This implies that calcium and perhaps unidentified effects of vitamin D on the renal tubule are important in the mechanism by which cAMP stimulates the phosphaturic response. In one case, PHP type II was associated with Sjögren syndrome and the presence of antirenal tubular plasma membrane autoantibodies *(220)*.

Other AHO Syndromes

As discussed above, AHO is characteristic of patients with PHP type Ia and Ic and PPHP. However, other familial forms of AHO have been recognized. One form, characterized primarily by brachydactyly and mental retardation, has been associated with deletions at 2q37 and therefore is clearly genetically distinct from PHP type Ia and PPHP *(207,208)*. Another familial syndrome, acrodysostosis, has many features in common with AHO, and it has been questioned whether it is in fact a distinct entity or a variant of AHO *(221)*.

DIAGNOSIS

Hypocalcemia, hyperphosphatemia, and elevated immunoreactive PTH in the setting of normal renal function generally establishe the diagnosis of PHP. Patients may occasionally be normocalcemic even with evidence of PTH resistance (elevated PTH and phosphate) *(94,61)*. Although patients could theoretically have elevated immunoreactive PTH resulting from the presence of bioinactive forms of PTH rather than PTH resistance, this occurs rarely *(106–108)*. In some cases when the clinical picture is unclear, measurement of serum ionized calcium may prove useful. If necessary, the diagnosis of PHP can be confirmed by measuring the response of urinary cAMP and phosphate excretion to exogenous PTH. Initially, bovine parathyroid extract was used *(7)*, but more recently the PTH (1–34) synthetic peptide analog is available for diagnostic testing *(222)*. In patients with PHP type I, both the urinary cAMP and phosphaturic responses to PTH are low. In patients with PHP type II, the urinary cAMP response is normal, but the phosphaturic response is low. In PTH-deficient states, both responses are normal. The response of plasma cAMP to exogenous PTH is also a useful discriminator between PHP type I and other types of hypoparathyroidism, and may be especially useful in young children *(160,223)*. The plasma cAMP response in normal infants is not as great as in older subjects *(223)*. Basal nephrogenous cAMP measurements (total urinary cAMP excreted filtered load of cAMP per deciliter of glomerular filtrate) may be useful in discriminating between PHP types I and II *(224)*. The normal rise in plasma 1,25-dihydroxyvitamin D levels in response to PTH in normals and patients with primary hypoparathyroidism is absent in patients with PHP type I *(40)*.

The presence of manifestations of AHO and/or evidence of generalized hormone resistance helps to distinguish PHP type Ia and Ic from PHP type Ib. Sometimes patients with PHP type Ia or Ic come to initial medical attention for the evaluation of one or more features of AHO *(197)* or after the detection of hypothyroidism *(167–169)*. In order to distinguish PHP type Ia from PHP type Ib or Ic, a functional or genetic G_s defect needs to be identified by either G_s biochemical assay *(8)*, $G\alpha_s$ quantitation by immunoblot *(139)*, or genetic screening of the GNAS1 gene *(225)*. These assays are cumbersome and are presently only performed in a few research laboratories.

Many features of AHO are quite nonspecific (short stature, obesity) or are present in other disorders (brachydactyly). Therefore, the diagnosis of PPHP should only be made in those patients with characteristic features of AHO who either are in PHP type Ia kindreds or in whom a G_s defect has been demonstrated by laboratory testing. The isolated finding of brachydactyly is relatively nonspecific and insufficient to make the diagnosis of PPHP *(226)*. Brachydactyly is a feature of a number of other genetic diseases, including Turner's syndrome *(190)*, acrodysostosis *(221)*, and a recently defined inherited syndrome that is associated with deletions at 2q37 *(207,208)*. The coexistence of brachydactyly and subcutaneous ossification probably increases the likelihood that PPHP is the correct diagnosis.

TREATMENT

The long-term treatment of hypocalcemia in patients with PHP is similar to treatment of other forms of hypoparathyroidism *(18)*. Treatment with vitamin D (ergocalciferol) or one of its more active metabolites (in many patients with oral calcium supplementation) should be given at doses that are adequate to maintain normocalcemia and relieve hypocalcemic symptoms. Since there is evidence that excess PTH may lead to skeletal demineralization in PHP *(227)*, it is probably most beneficial to treat aggressively in order to normalize the serum PTH, which can usually be accomplished. In contrast to PTH-deficient forms of hypoparathyroidism, correction of hypocalcemia in patients with PHP type Ia does not typically lead to hypercalciuria *(227–229)*. Patients receiving vitamin D treatment must be closely monitored (including measurement of urinary calcium excretion) to avoid under- or overtreatment. In patients with PHP Ia or Ic, treatment of associated endocrinopathies, in particular hypothyroidism and hypogonadism, may be indicated. There are no specific treatments for the various manifestations of AHO. Rarely subcutaneous ossifications are surgically excised if they are particularly large or bothersome. Whether growth hormone therapy may be useful in the management of AHO has not been studied.

GENERATION AND CHARACTERIZATION OF Gα$_S$ KNOCKOUT MICE

Based on the pattern of inheritance of PHP type Ia and PPHP in humans and the localization of the mouse gene encoding Gα$_s$ (Gnas) to an "imprinted" region on chromosome 2, it has been speculated that GNAS1 is an imprinted gene. Mice with a genetic knockout of Gnas were generated in our laboratory (Yu S., Yu D., Lee E., Westphal H. L. S. W., unpublished data) in order to characterize the resulting phenotype and to deter-mine whether genomic imprinting of Gnas leads to the observed phenotypic variability, particularly in the expression of generalized hormone resistance (PHP type Ia vs PPHP). A genomic clone including exons 1–3 of Gnas was isolated from a genomic library, and a DNA "cassette" encoding the expression of a neomycin resistance gene was spliced into the second exon, disrupting the Gnas coding sequence. The DNA targeting construct was transfected into pluripotential embryonic stem (ES) cells, and chimeras containing the Gα$_s$ knockout (GsKO) were generated by standard gene knockout technology. Mating of chimeras with wild-type (wt) CD1 mice resulted in successful germline transmission of GsKO. Preliminary characterization of GsKO mice suggests that Gnas is an imprinted gene.

VARIABLE PHENOTYPE IN G$_S$ DEFICIENCY: PHP IA VS PPHP

One of the basic questions that remains unanswered is how apparently equivalent G$_s$ deficiency and identical GNAS1 mutations can lead to such variable phenotypic expression,

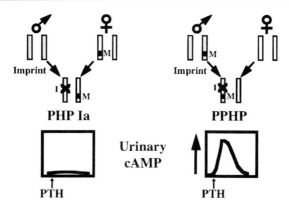

Fig. 5. Imprinting model of PHP type Ia and PPHP. According to the imprinting model, the GNAS1 gene is imprinted in specific tissues, such as the site of PTH action (the renal proximal tubule). In these tissues, the allele derived from the father (paternal allele, shown as hatched) is normally not expressed because of an imprint (I) that is placed on the gene during some point of spermatogenesis. Inheritance of a loss-of-function mutation (M) from the mother (shown on the left) would result in loss of expression in both alleles (owing to an imprint on the paternal allele and a mutation of the maternal allele). This should result in severe or total G_s deficiency and hormone resistance, represented below by a totally blunted urinary cAMP response to PTH. In contrast, inheritance of a mutation from the father (shown on right) should have no consequences, since the mutation is present in the paternal allele, which owing to imprinting is not expressed anyway. G_s expression and hormone responsiveness should therefore be normal, as shown below.

particularly in terms of the presence (PHP type Ia) or absence (PPHP) of generalized hormone resistance. Although the stoichiometric concentration of $G\alpha_s$ relative to other signaling components is not exactly defined, it is generally expressed at significantly higher concentrations than receptors, so it is not clear how 50% deficiency would result in so many physiological abnormalities. Another unexplained feature is that there is resistance to some (e.g., PTH, TSH, and gonadotropins), but not all hormones (e.g., vasopressin, ACTH) that activate G_s-coupled pathways. At least for some hormones (e.g., glucagon, β-adrenergic), it appears that a partial cAMP response is sufficient to evoke a full physiologic response.

Genomic imprinting of the GNAS1 gene was recently proposed as a potential mechanism to explain the occurrence of PHP type Ia and PPHP in patients with GNAS1 mutations, based on the observation that when the disease is maternally transmitted, all offspring have PHP type Ia, whereas paternal transmission leads to PPHP *(232)*. This has been confirmed in a sporadic case of PPHP in which an inactivating mutation was demonstrated to be present on the paternal allele based on segregation of a silent polymorphism *(144)*. According to this model (*see* Fig. 5), the paternal GNAS1 allele is normally not expressed in specific tissues, such as the proximal renal tubule, owing to an imprinting mechanism. If a loss-of-function mutation is present within the maternal allele (because of inheritance from the mother), neither allele is expressed (secondary to imprinting of the paternal allele and mutation within the maternal allele) and severe or total G_s deficiency within the target tissue should lead to hormone resistance. In contrast, inheritance of a loss-of-function mutation within the paternal allele would disrupt an allele that is normally not expressed owing to imprinting, so that the mutation should have no effect on G_s expression or hormone action. This is consistent with the observed response of urinary cAMP to exogenous PTH, which is almost fully blunted in PHP type Ia, but totally normal in PPHP *(117)*.

According to this model, imprinting of GNAS1 would be presumed to be tissue-specific, limited mainly to tissues in which there is parent-of-origin specific differences in hormone responsiveness, such as the renal proximal tubule and thyroid. In most tissues, there would be no imprinting, resulting in a 50% decrease in G_s activity regardless of the parent-of-origin of the mutation, as has been shown in erythrocyte membranes *(117)*. One possible explanation for the lack of resistance to hormones, such as vasopressin and ACTH, is that GNAS1 is not imprinted within their targets of action (collecting ducts, adrenal cortex). The resulting G_s deficiency would be partial and not severe enough to result in hormone resistance. This possibility remains to be proven.

The mouse gene (Gnas) maps within a defined "imprinted" region in the distal portion of chromosome 2 *(70–72)*. Preliminary observations in G_sKO mice are consistent with the imprinting model. However, despite strong genetic evidence for imprinting of the human GNAS1 gene, this has not as yet been proven with molecular studies. One study that examined multiple human fetal tissues showed no evidence for monoalleleic expression of GNAS1, although specific targets of hormone action were not tested *(233)*. A single case report describes the apparent expression of PHP type Ia in an infant in which G_s deficiency was inherited from his father *(234)*. The diagnosis was based on a blunted cAMP response to exogenous PTH. However, baseline calcium, phosphorus, and PTH, as well as thyroid function tests, were all normal, making the diagnosis of PHP type Ia somewhat equivocal. Other mechanisms may also contribute to the variable phenotypic expression of G_s deficiency, including genetic variability in other components of the signal transduction system (e.g., adenylyl cyclases, phosphodiesterases), which themselves have multiple isoforms with unique patterns of tissue-specific expression.

REFERENCES

1. Albright F, Burnett CH, Smith PH, Parson W. Pseudohypoparathyroidism: an example of "Seabright-Bantam syndrome." Endocrinology 1942;30:922–932.
2. Tashjian AH, Jr., Frantz AG, Lee JB. Pseudohypoparathyroidism: assays of parathyroid hormone and thyrocalcitonin. Proc Natl Acad Sci USA 1966;56:1138–1142.
3. Mann JB, Alterman S, Hills AG. Albright's hereditary osteodystrophy comprising pseudo-hypoparathyroidism and pseudopseudohypoparathyroidism with a report of two cases representing the complete syndrome occurring in successive generations. Ann Intern Med 1962;56:315–342.
4. Eyre WG, Reed WB. Albright's hereditary osteodystrophy with cutaneous bone formation. Arch Dermatol 1971;104:634–642.
5. Farfel Z, Friedman E. Mental deficiency in pseudohypoparathyroidism type I is associated with Ns-protein deficiency. Ann Intern Med 1986;105:197–199.
6. Albright F, Forbes AP, Henneman PH. Pseudopseudohypoparathyroidism. Trans Assoc Am Physicians 1952;65:337–350.
7. Chase LR, Melson GL, Aurbach GD. Pseudohypoparathyroidism: defective excretion of 3′,5′-AMP in response to parathyroid hormone. J Clin Invest 1969;48:1832–1844.
8. Levine MA, Downs RW Jr, Singer M, Marx SJ, Aurbach GD, Spiegel AM. Deficient activity of guanine nucleotide regulatory protein in erythrocytes from patients with pseudohypoparathyroidism. Biochem Biophys Res Commun 1980;94:1319–1324.
9. Farfel Z, Brickman AS, Kaslow HR, Brothers VM, Bourne HR. Defect of receptor-cyclase coupling protein in pseudohypoparathyroidism. N Engl J Med 1980;303:237–242.
10. Patten JL, Johns DR, Valle D, et al. Mutation in the gene encoding the stimulatory G protein of adenylate cyclase in Albright's hereditary osteodystrophy. N Engl J Med 1990;322:1412–1419.
11. Weinstein LS, Gejman PV, Friedman E, et al. Mutations of the G_s α-subunit gene in Albright hereditary osteodystrophy detected by denaturing gradient gel electrophoresis. Proc Natl Acad Sci USA 1990;87:8287–8290.

12. Radeke HH, Auf'mkolk B, Jüppner H, Krohn HP, Keck E, Hesch RD. Multiple pre- and postreceptor defects in pseudohypoparathyroidism (a multicenter study with twenty four patients). J Clin Endocrinol Metab 1986;62:393–402.

13. Levine MA, Downs RW Jr, Moses AM, et al. Resistance to multiple hormones in patients with pseudohypoparathyroidism. Association with deficient activity of guanine nucleotide regulatory protein. Am J Med 1983;74:545–556.

14. Barrett D, Breslau NA, Wax MB, Molinoff PB, Downs RW Jr. New form of pseudohypoparathyroidism with abnormal catalytic adenylate cyclase. Am J Physiol 1989;257:E277–E283.

15. Silve C, Santora A, Breslau N, Moses A, Spiegel A. Selective resistance to parathyroid hormone in cultured skin fibroblasts from patients with pseudohypoparathyroidism type Ib. J Clin Endocrinol Metab 1986;62:640–644.

16. Drezner M, Neelon FA, Lebovitz HE. Pseudohypoparathyroidism type II: a possible defect in the reception of the cyclic AMP signal. N Engl J Med 1973;289:1056–1060.

17. Vasicek TJ, McDevitt BE, Freeman MW, et al. Nucleotide sequence of the human parathyroid hormone gene. Proc Natl Acad Sci USA 1983;80:2127–2131.

18. Aurbach GD, Marx SJ, Spiegel AM. Parathyroid Hormone, Calcitonin, and the Calciferols. In: Wilson JD, Foster DW, eds. Williams Textbook of Endocrinology, 8th ed. Saunders, Philadelphia, 1992, pp. 1397–1476.

19. Rodan GA, Rodan SB. Hormone-adenylate cyclase coupling in osteosarcoma clonal cell lines. Adv Cyclic Nucleotide Protein Phosphorylation Res 1984;17:127–134.

20. Jilka RL. Are osteoblastic cells required for the control of osteoclast activity by parathyroid hormone. Bone Miner 1986;1:261–266.

21. Spiegel AM, Shenker A, Weinstein LS. Receptor-effector coupling by G proteins: Implications for normal and abnormal signal transduction. Endocr Rev 1992;13:536–565.

22. Bourne HR, Sanders DA, McCormick F. The GTPase superfamily: a conserved switch for diverse cell functions. Nature 1990;348:125–132.

23. Kaziro Y, Itoh H, Kozasa T, Nakafuku M, Satoh T. Structure and function of signal-transducing GTP-binding proteins. Annu Rev Biochem 1991;60:349–400.

24. Birnbaumer L, Abramowitz J, Brown AM. Receptor-effector coupling by G proteins. Biochim Biophys Acta Rev Biomembr 1990;1031:163–224.

25. Tang W-J, Gilman AG. Type-specific regulation of adenylyl cyclase by G protein $\beta\gamma$ subunits. Science 1991;254:1500–1503.

26. Camps M, Hou C, Sidiropoulos D, Stock JB, Jakobs KH, Gierschik P. Stimulation of phospholipase C by guanine-nucleotide-binding protein beta gamma subunits. Eur J Biochem 1992;206:821–831.

27. Blank JL, Brattain KA, Exton JH. Activation of cytosolic phosphoinositide phospholipase C by G-protein $\beta\gamma$ subunits. J Biol Chem 1992;267:23069–23075.

28. Reid IR, Civitelli R, Halstead LR, Avioli LV, Hruska KA. Parathyroid hormone acutely elevates intracellular calcium in osteoblastlike cells. Am J Physiol 1987;253:E45–E51.

29. Civitelli R, Reid IR, Westbrook S, Avioli LV, Hruska KA. PTH elevates inositol polyphosphates and diacylglycerol in a rat osteoblast-like cell line. Am J Physiol 1988;255:E660–E667.

30. Cosman F, Morrow B, Kopal M, Bilezikian JP. Stimulation of inositol phosphate formation in ROS 17/2.8 cell membranes by guanine nucleotide, calcium, and parathyroid hormone. J Bone Miner Res 1989;4:413–420.

31. Dunlay R, Hruska K. PTH receptor coupling to phospholipase C is an alternate pathway of signal transduction in bone and kidney. Am J Physiol 1990;258:F223–F231.

32. Gupta A, Martin KJ, Miyauchi A, Hruska KA. Regulation of cytosolic calcium by parathyroid hormone and oscillations of cytosolic calcium in fibroblasts from normal and pseudohypoparathyroid patients. Endocrinology 1991;128:2825–2836.

33. Bringhurst FR, Juppner H, Guo J, et al. Cloned, stably expressed parathyroid hormone (PTH)/PTH-related peptide receptors activate multiple messenger signals and biological responses in LLC-PK$_1$ kidney cells. Endocrinology 1993;132:2090–2098.

34. Gutowski S, Smrcka A, Nowak L, Wu D, Simon M, Sternweis PC. Antibodies to the α_q subfamily of guanine nucleotide-binding regulatory protein α subunits attenuate activation of phosphatidylinositol 4,5-bisphosphate hydrolysis by hormones. J Biol Chem 1991;266:20519–20524.

35. Mattera R, Graziano MP, Yatani A, et al. Splice variants of the alpha subunit of the G protein G$_s$ activate both adenylyl cyclase and calcium channels. Science 1989;243:804–807.

36. Lewin IG, Papapoulos SE, Tomlinson S, Hendy GN, O'Riordan JL. Studies of hypoparathyroidism and pseudohypoparathyroidism. Q J Med 1978;47:533–548.

37. Caverzasio J, Rizzoli R, Bonjour JP. Sodium-dependent phosphate transport inhibited by parathyroid hormone and cyclic AMP stimulation in an opossum kidney cell line. J Biol Chem 1986;261: 3233–3237.

38. Bell NH, Avery S, Sinha T, Clark CM, Jr, Allen DO, Johnston C, Jr. Effects of dibutyryl cyclic adenosine 3′,5′-monophosphate and parathyroid extract on calcium and phosphorus metabolism in hypoparathyroidism and pseudohypoparathyroidism. J Clin Invest 1972;51:816–823.

39. Shigematsu T, Horiuchi N, Ogura Y, Miyahara T, Suda T. Human parathyroid hormone inhibits renal 24-hydroxylase activity of 25-hydroxyvitamin D3 by a mechanism involving adenosine 3′,5′-monophosphate in rats. Endocrinology 1986;118:1583–1589.

40. Miura R, Yumita S, Yoshinaga K, Furukawa Y. Response of plasma 1,25-dihydroxyvitamin D in the human PTH(1-34) infusion test: an improved index for the diagnosis of idiopathic hypoparathyroidism and pseudohypoparathyroidism. Calcif Tissue Int 1990;46:309–313.

41. Puschett JB. Are all of the renal tubular actions of parathyroid hormone mediated by the adenylate cyclase system. Miner Electrolyte Metab 1982;7:281–284.

42. Stone MD, Hosking DJ, Garcia-Himmelstine C, White DA, Rosenblum D, Worth HG. The renal response to exogenous parathyroid hormone in treated pseudohypoparathyroidism. Bone 1993;14: 727–735.

43. Löwik CWGM, van Leeuwen JPTM, van der Meer JM, van Zeeland JK, Scheven BAA, Herrmann-Erlee MPM. A two-receptor model for the action of parathyroid hormone on osteoblasts: a role for intracellular free calcium and cAMP. Cell Calcium 1985;6:311–326.

44. Peck WA. Cyclic AMP as a second messenger in the skeletal actions of parathyroid hormone: a decade-old hypothesis. Calcif Tissue Int 1979;29:1–4.

45. Turksen K, Grigoriadis AE, Heersche JNM, Aubin JE. Forskolin has biphasic effects on osteoprogenitor cell differentiation in vitro. J Cell Physiol 1990;142:61–69.

46. Bellows CG, Ishida H, Aubin JE, Heersche JNM. Parathyroid hormone reversibly suppresses the differentiation of osteoprogenitor cells into functional osteoblasts. Endocrinology 1990;127:3111–3116.

47. Shenker A, Weinstein LS, Sweet DE, Spiegel AM. An activating $G_s\alpha$ mutation is present in fibrous dysplasia of bone in the McCune-Albright syndrome. J Clin Endocrinol Metab 1994;79:750–755.

48. Spiegel AM, Gierschik P, Levine MA, Downs RW, Jr. Clinical implications of guanine nucleotide-binding proteins as receptor-effector couplers. N Engl J Med 1985;312:26–33.

49. Nicholson CD, Chaliss RAJ, Shahid M. Differential modulation of tissue function and therapeutic potential of selective inhibitors of cyclic nucleotide phosphodiesterase isoenzymes. Trends Pharmacol Sci 1991;12:19–27.

50. Conti M, Jin S-LC, Monaco L, Repaske DR, Swinnen JV. Hormonal regulation of cyclic nucleotide phosphodiesterases. Endocr Rev 1991;12:218–234.

51. Iyengar R. Molecular and functional diversity of mammalian G_s-stimulated adenylyl cyclases. FASEB J 1993;7:768–775.

52. Jüppner H, Abou-Samra A-B, Freeman M, et al. A G protein-linked receptor for parathyroid hormone and parathyroid hormone-related peptide. Science 1991;254:1024–1026.

53. Abou-Samra A-B, Jüppner H, Force T, et al. Expression cloning of a common receptor for parathyroid hormone and parathyroid hormone-related peptide from rat osteoblast-like cells: a single receptor stimulates intracellular accumulation of both cAMP and inositol trisphosphates and increases intracellular free calcium. Proc Natl Acad Sci USA 1992;89:2732–2736.

54. Schipani E, Karga H, Karaplis AC, et al. Identical complementary deoxyribonucleic acids encode a human renal and bone parathyroid hormone (PTH)/PTH-related peptide receptor. Endocrinology 1993;132:2157–2165.

55. Usdin TB, Gruber C, Bonner TI. Identification and functional expression of a receptor selectively recognizing parathyroid hormone, the PTH2 receptor. J Biol Chem 1995;270:15,455–15,458.

56. Demay M, Mitchell J, Goltzman D. Comparison of renal and osseous binding of parathyroid hormone and hormonal fragments. Am J Physiol 1985;249:E437–E446.

57. Martin KJ, Bellorin-Font E, Morrissey JJ, Jilka RL, MacGregor RR, Cohn DV. Relative sensitivity of kidney and bone to the amino-terminal fragment b-PTH (1-30) of native bovine parathyroid hormone: implications for assessment of bioactivity of parathyroid hormone fragments in vivo and in vitro. Calcif Tissue Int 1983;35:520–525.

58. Horiuchi N, Rosenblatt M, Keutmann HT, Potts JT, Jr, Holick MF. A multiresponse parathyroid hormone assay: an inhibitor has agonist properties in vivo. Am J Physiol 1983;244:E589–E595.

59. Goldring SR, Tyler GA, Krane SM, Potts JT, Jr, Rosenblatt M. Photoaffinity labeling of parathyroid hormone receptors: comparison of receptors across species and target tissues and after desensitization to hormone. Biochemistry 1984;23:498–502.

60. Schipani E, Kruse K, Juppner H. A constitutively active mutant PTH-PTHrP receptor in Jansen-type metaphyseal chondrodysplasia. Science 1995;268:98–100.

61. Coleman DE, Berghuis AM, Lee E, Linder ME, Gilman AG, Sprang SR. Structures of active conformations of $G_{i\alpha1}$ and the mechanism of GTP hydrolysis. Science 1994;265:1405–1412.

62. Sondek J, Lambright DG, Noel JP, Hamm HE, Sigler PB. GTPase mechanism of G proteins from the 1.7-Å crystal structure of transducin α-GDP-AlF$_4^-$. Nature 1994;372:276–279.

63. Noel JP, Hamm HE, Sigler PB. The 2.2 Å crystal structure of transducin-α complexed with GTPγS. Nature. 1993;366:654–663.

64. Lambright DG, Noel JP, Hamm HE, Sigler PB. Structural determinants for activation of the α-subunit of a heterotrimeric G protein. Nature 1994;369:621–628.

65. Wall MA, Coleman DE, Lee E, et al. The structure of the G protein heterotrimer $G_{i\alpha1\beta1\gamma2}$. Cell 1995;83:1047–1058.

66. Lambright DG, Sondek J, Bohm A, Skiba NP, Hamm HE, Sigler PB. The 2.0A crystal structure of a heterotrimeric G protein. Nature 1996;379:297–299.

67. Berlot CH, Bourne HR. Identification of effector-activating residues of $G_{s\alpha}$. Cell 1992;68:911–922.

68. Kozasa T, Itoh H, Tsukamoto T, Kaziro Y. Isolation and characterization of the human Gs alpha gene. Proc Natl Acad Sci USA 1988;85:2081–2085.

69. Gejman PV, Weinstein LS, Martinez M, et al. Genetic mapping of the Gs-α subunit gene (GNAS1) to the distal long arm of chromosome 20 using a polymorphism detected by denaturing gradient gel electrophoresis. Genomics 1991;9:782–783.

70. Wilkie TM, Gilbert DJ, Olsen AS, et al. Evolution of the mammalian G protein α subunit multigene family. Nature Genetics 1992;1:85–91.

71. Peters J, Beechey CV, Ball ST, Evans EP. Mapping studies of the distal imprinting region of mouse Chromosome 2. Genet Res 1994;63:169–174.

72. Cattanach BM, Kirk M. Differential activity of maternally and paternally derived chromosome regions in mice. Nature 1985;315:496–498.

73. Bray P, Carter A, Simons C, et al. Human cDNA clones for four species of Gαs signal transduction protein. Proc Natl Acad Sci USA 1986;83:8893–8897.

74. O'Donnell JK, Sweet RW, Stadel JM. Expression and characterization of the long and short splice variants of Gsα in S49 cyc–cells. Mol Pharmacol 1991;39:702–710.

75. Cooper DMF, Boyajian CL, Goldsmith PK, Unson CG, Spiegel A. Differential expression of low molecular weight form of G_s-α in neostriatum and cerebellum: correlation with expression of calmodulin-independent adenylyl cyclase. Brain Res 1990;523:143–146.

76. Kehlenbach RH, Matthey J, Huttner WB. XLαs is a new type of G protein. Nature 1994;372:804–809.

77. Swaroop A, Agarwal N, Gruen JR, Bick D, Weissman SM. Differential expression of novel Gsα signal transduction protein cDNA species. Nucleic Acids Res 1991;19:4725–4729.

78. Ali IU, Reinhold W, Salvador C, Aguanno S. Aberrant splicing of Gsα transcript in transformed human astroglial and glioblastoma cell lines. Nucleic Acids Res 1992;20:4263–4267.

79. Farfel Z, Salomon MR, Bourne HR. Genetic investigation of adenylate cyclase: mutations in mouse and man. Annu Rev Pharmacol Toxicol 1981;21:251–264.

80. Taussig R, Tang WJ, Hepler Jr., Gilman AG. Distinct patterns of bidirectional regulation of mammalian adenylylcyclases. J Biol Chem 1994;269:6093–6100.

81. Tang WJ, Gilman AG. Type-specific regulation of adenylyl cyclase by G protein $\beta\gamma$ subunits. Science 1991;254:1500–1503.

82. Levin LR, Han P-L, Hwang PM, Feinstein PG, Davis RL, Reed RR. The Drosophila learning and memory gene *rutabaga* encodes a Ca^{2+}/calmodulin-responsive adenylyl cyclase. Cell 1992;68:479–489.

83. Wu ZL, Thomas SA, Villacres EC, et al. Altered behavior and long-term potentiation in type I adenylyl cyclase mutant mice. Proc Natl Acad Sci USA 1995;92:220–224.

84. Charbonneau H, Beier N, Walsh KA, Beavo JA. Identification of a conserved domain among cyclic nucleotide phosphodiesterases from diverse species. Proc Natl Acad Sci USA 1986;83:9308–9312.

85. Chen CN, Denome S, Davis RL. Molecular analysis of cDNA clones and the corresponding genomic coding sequences of the Drosophila dunce+ gene, the structural gene for cAMP phosphodiesterase. Proc Natl Acad Sci USA 1986;83:9313–9317.

86. Brothers VM, Walker N, Bourne HR. Increased cyclic nucleotide phosphodiesterase activity in a mutant S49 lymphoma cell. Characterization and comparison with wild type enzyme activity. J Biol Chem 1982;257:9349–9355.

87. Matsumoto K, Uno I, Oshima Y, Ishikawa T. Isolation and characterization of yeast mutants deficient in adenylate cyclase and cAMP-dependent protein kinase. Proc Natl Acad Sci USA 1982;79: 2355–2359.

88. Stein GS, Lian JB. Molecular mechanisms mediating proliferation/differentiation interrelationships during progressive development of the osteoblast phenotype. Endocr Rev 1993;14:424–442.

89. Lambert PW, Hollis BW, Bell NH, Epstein S. Demonstration of a lack of change in serum 1α, 25-dihydroxyvitamin D in response to parathyroid extract in pseudohypoparathyroidism. J Clin Invest 1980;66:782–791.

90. Braun JJ, Birkenhäger JC, Visser TJ, Juttmann JR. Lack of response of 1,25-dihydroxycholecalciferol to exogenous parathyroid hormone in a patient with treated pseudohypoparathyroidism. Clin Endocrinol (Oxford) 1981;14:403–407.

91. Yamaoka K, Seino Y, Ishida M, et al. Effect of dibutyryl adenosine 3′,5′-monophosphate administration on plasma concentrations of 1,25-dihydroxyvitamin D in pseudohypoparathyroidism type I. J Clin Endocrinol Metab 1981;53:1096–1100.

92. Breslau NA, Weinstock RS. Regulation of 1,25 (OH)2D synthesis in hypoparathyroidism and pseudohypoparathyroidism. Am J Physiol 1988;255:E730-E736.

93. Drezner MK, Neelon FA, Haussler M, McPherson HT, Lebovitz HE. 1,25-dihydroxycholecalciferol deficiency: the probable cause of hypocalcemia and metabolic bone disease in pseudohypoparathyroidism. J Clin Endocrinol Metab 1976;42:621–628.

94. Drezner MK, Haussler MR. Normocalcemic pseudohypoparathyroidism. Association with normal D3 metabolism. Am J Med 1979;66:503–508.

95. Epstein S, Meunier PJ, Lambert PW, Stern PH, Bell NH. 1α,25-dihydroxyvitamin D3 corrects osteomalacia in hypoparathyroidism and pseudohypoparathyroidism. Acta Endocrinol (Copenh) 1983;103: 241–247.

96. Moses AM, Weinstock RS, Levine MA, Breslau NA. Evidence for normal antidiuretic responses to endogenous and exogenous arginine vasopressin in patients with guanine nucleotide-binding stimulatory protein-deficient pseudohypoparathyroidism. J Clin Endocrinol Metab 1986;62:221–224.

97. Faull CM, Welbury RR, Paul B, Kendall-Taylor P. Pseudohypoparathyroidism: its phenotypic variability and associated disorders in a large family. Q J Med 1991;78:251–264.

98. Metz SA, Baylink DJ, Hughes MR, Haussler MR, Robertson RP. Selective deficiency of 1,25-dihydroxycholecalciferol. A cause of isolated skeletal resistance to parathyroid hormone. N Engl J Med 1977;297:1084–1090.

99. Wilson JD, Hadden DR. Pseudohypoparathyroidism presenting with rickets. J Clin Endocrinol Metab 1980;51:1184–1189.

100. Dabbagh S, Chesney RW, Langer LO, DeLuca HF, Gilbert EF, DeWeerd JH, Jr. Renal-nonresponsive, bone-responsive pseudohypoparathyroidism. A case with normal vitamin D metabolite levels and clinical features of rickets. Am J Dis Child 1984;138:1030–1033.

101. Breslau NA, Moses AM, Pak CY. Evidence for bone remodeling but lack of calcium mobilization response to parathyroid hormone in pseudohypoparathyroidism. J Clin Endocrinol Metab 1983;57:638–644.

102. Frame B, Hanson CA, Frost HM, Block M, Arnstein AR. Renal resistance to parathyroid hormone with osteitis fibrosa: "pseudohypohyperparathyroidism." Am J Med 1972;52:311–321.

103. Kidd GS, Schaaf M, Adler RA, Lassman MN, Wray HL. Skeletal responsiveness in pseudohypoparathyroidism. A spectrum of clinical disease. Am J Med 1980;68:772–781.

104. Murray TM, Rao LG, Wong M-M, et al. Pseudohypoparathyroidism with osteitis fibrosa cystica: direct demonstration of skeletal responsiveness to parathyroid hormone in cells cultured from bone. J Bone Miner Res 1993;8:83–91.

105. Ish-Shalom S, Rao LG, Levine MA, et al. Normal parathyroid hormone responsiveness of bone-derived cells from a patient with pseudohypoparathyroidism. J Bone Miner Res 1996;11:8–14.

106. Nusynowitz ML, Klein MH. Pseudoidiopathic hypoparathyroidism. Hypoparathyroidism with ineffective parathyroid hormone. Am J Med 1973;55:677–686.

107. Connors MH, Irias JJ, Golabi M. Hypo-hyperparathyroidism: evidence for a defective parathyroid hormone. Pediatrics 1977;60:343–348.

108. McElduff A, Wilkinson M, Lackmann M, et al. Familial hypoparathyroidism due to an abnormal parathyroid hormone molecule. Aust N Z J Med 1989;19:22–30.

109. Ahn TG, Antonarakis SE, Kronenberg HM, Igarashi T, Levine MA. Familial isolated hypopara-thyroidism: a molecular genetic analysis of 8 families with 23 affected persons. Medicine (Baltimore) 1986;65:73–81.

110. Arnold A, Horst SA, Gardella TJ, Baba H, Levine MA, Kronenberg HM. Mutation of the signal peptide-encoding region of the preproparathyroid hormone gene in familial isolated hypopara-thyroidism. J Clin Invest 1990;86:1084–1087.

111. de Deuxchaisnes CN, Fischer JA, Dambacher MA, et al. Dissociation of parathyroid hormone bio-activity and immunoreactivity in pseudohypoparathyroidism type I. J Clin Endocrinol Metab 1981;53: 1105–1109.

112. Bradbeer JN, Dunham J, Fischer JA, de Deuxchaisnes CN, Loveridge N. The metatarsal cyto-chemical bioassay of parathyroid hormone: validation, specificity, and application to the study of pseudohypoparathyroidism type I. J Clin Endocrinol Metab 1988;67:1237–1243.

113. Loveridge N, Fischer JA, Nagant De Deuxchaisnes C, et al. Inhibition of cytochemical bioactivity of parathyroid hormone by plasma in pseudohypoparathyroidism type I. J Clin Endocrinol Metab 1982;54:1274–1275.

114. Allgrove J, Chayen J, Jayaweera P, O'Riordan JL. An investigation of the biological activity of parathyroid hormone in pseudohypoparathyroidism: comparison with vitamin D deficiency. Clin Endocrinol (Oxford) 1984;20:503–514.

115. Stögmann W, Fischer JA. Pseudohypoparathyroidism. Disappearance of the resistance to parathyroid extract during treatment with vitamin D. Am J Med 1975;59:140–144.

116. Mitchell J, Goltzman D. Examination of circulating parathyroid hormone in pseudohypopara-thyroidism. J Clin Endocrinol Metab 1985;61:328–334.

117. Levine MA, Jap TS, Mauseth RS, Downs RW, Spiegel AM. Activity of the stimulatory guanine nucleotide-binding protein is reduced in erythrocytes from patients with pseudohypoparathyroidism and pseudopseudohypoparathyroidism: biochemical, endocrine, and genetic analysis of Albright's hereditary osteodystrophy in six kindreds. J Clin Endocrinol Metab 1986;62:497–502.

118. Farfel Z, Bourne HR. Deficient activity of receptor-cyclase coupling protein in platelets of patients with pseudohypoparathyroidism. J Clin Endocrinol Metab 1980;51:1202–1204.

119. Farfel Z, Brothers VM, Brickman AS, Conte F, Neer R, Bourne HR. Pseudohypoparathyroidism: inheritance of deficient receptor-cyclase coupling activity. Proc Natl Acad Sci USA 1981;78:3098–3102.

120. Bourne HR, Kaslow HR, Brickman AS, Farfel Z. Fibroblast defect in pseudohypoparathyroidism, type I: reduced activity of receptor-cyclase coupling protein. J Clin Endocrinol Metab 1981;53: 636–640.

121. Spiegel AM, Levine MA, Aurbach GD, et al. Deficiency of hormone receptor-adenylate cyclase coupling protein: basis for hormone resistance in pseudohypoparathyroidism. Am J Physiol 1982;243:E37–E42.

122. Motulsky HJ, Hughes RJ, Brickman AS, Farfel Z, Bourne HR, Insel PA. Platelets of pseudo-hypoparathyroid patients: evidence that distinct receptor-cyclase coupling proteins mediate stimula-tion and inhibition of adenylate cyclase. Proc Natl Acad Sci USA 1982;79:4193–4197.

123. Farfel Z, Abood ME, Brickman AS, Bourne HR. Deficient activity of receptor-cyclase coupling pro-tein in transformed lymphoblasts of patients with pseudohypoparathyroidism type I. J Clin Endocrinol Metab 1982;55:113–117.

124. Levine MA, Eil C, Downs RW, Jr., Spiegel AM. Deficient guanine nucleotide regulatory unit activity in cultured fibroblast membranes from patients with pseudohypoparathyroidism type I. A cause of impaired synthesis of 3',5'-cyclic AMP by intact and broken cells. J Clin Invest 1983;72:316–324.

125. Downs RW, Jr., Levine MA, Drezner MK, Burch WM, Jr, Spiegel AM. Deficient adenylate cyclase regulatory protein in renal membranes from a patient with pseudohypoparathyroidism. J Clin Invest 1983;71:231–235.

126. Levine MA, Ahn TG, Klupt SF, et al. Genetic deficiency of the α-subunit of the guanine nucleotide-binding protein Gs as the molecular basis for Albright hereditary osteodystrophy. Proc Natl Acad Sci USA 1988;85:617–621.

127. Heinsimer JA, Davies AO, Downs RW, et al. Impaired formation of beta-adrenergic receptor-nucleotide regulatory protein complexes in pseudohypoparathyroidism. J Clin Invest 1984;73:1335–1343.

128. Ong OC, Van Dop C, Fung BKK. Real-time monitoring of reduced β-adrenergic response in fibro-blasts from patients with pseudohypoparathyroidism. Anal Biochem 1996;238:76–81.

129. Downs RW, Sekura RD, Levine MA, Spiegel AM. The inhibitory adenylate cyclase coupling protein in pseudohypoparathyroidism. J Clin Endocrinol Metab 1985;61:351–354.

130. Schuster V, Eschenhagen T, Kruse K, Gierschik P, Kreth HW. Endocrine and molecular biological studies in a German family with Albright hereditary osteodystrophy. Eur J Pediatr 1993;152:185–189.

131. Fitch N. Albright's hereditary osteodystrophy: a review. Am J Med Genet 1982;11:11–29.

132. Fischer JA, Bourne HR, Dambacher MA, et al. Pseudohypoparathyroidism: inheritance and expression of deficient receptor-cyclase coupling protein activity. Clin Endocrinol (Oxford) 1983;19: 747–754.

133. Cedarbaum SD, Lippe BM. Probable autosomal recessive inheritance in a family with Albright's hereditary and evaluation of the genetics of the disorder. Am J Hum Genet 1973;25:638–645.

134. Van Dop C, Bourne HR, Neer RM. Father to son transmission of decreased Ns activity in pseudo-hypoparathyroidism type Ia. J Clin Endocrinol Metab 1984;59:825–828.

135. Weinberg AG, Stone RT. Autosomal dominant inheritance in Albright's hereditary osteodystrophy. J Pediatr 1971;79:996–999.

136. Van Dop C, Bourne HR. Pseudohypoparathyroidism. Annu Rev Med 1983;34:259–266.

137. Carter A, Bardin C, Collins R, Simons C, Bray P, Spiegel A. Reduced expression of multiple forms of the α subunit of the stimulatory GTP-binding protein in pseudohypoparathyroidism type Ia. Proc Natl Acad Sci USA 1987;84:7266–7269.

138. Weinstein LS, Gejman PV, De Mazancourt P, American N, Spiegel AM. A heterozygous 4-bp deletion mutation in the $G_s\alpha$ gene (GNAS1) in a patient with Albright hereditary osteodystrophy. Genomics 1992;13:1319–1321.

139. Patten JL, Levine MA. Immunochemical analysis of the α-subunit of the stimulatory G protein of adenylyl cyclase in patients with Albright's hereditary osteodystrophy. J Clin Endocrinol Metab 1990;71:1208–1214.

140. Miric A, Vechio JD, Levine MA. Heterogeneous mutations in the gene encoding the α subunit of the stimulatory G protein of adenylyl cyclase in Albright hereditary osteodystrophy. J Clin Endocrinol Metab 1993;76:1560–1568.

141. Ringel MD, Schwindinger WF, Levine MA. Clinical implications of genetic defects in G proteins. The molecular basis of McCune-Albright syndrome and Albright hereditary osteodystrophy. Medicine (Baltimore) 1996;75:171–184.

142. Shapira H, Mouallem M, Shapiro MS, Weisman Y, Farfel Z. Pseudohypoparathyroidism type Ia: two new heterozygous frameshift mutations in exons 5 and 10 of the Gs alpha gene. Hum Genet 1996;97:73–75.

143. Luttikhuis MEMO, Wilson LC, Leonard JV, Trembath RC. Characterization of a *de novo* 43-bp deletion of the Gsα gene (GNAS1) in Albright hereditary osteodystrophy. Genomics 1994;21:455–457.

144. Wilson LC, Oude Luttikhuis ME, Clayton PT, Fraser WD, Trembath RC. Parental origin of Gs α gene mutations in Albright's hereditary osteodystrophy. J Med Genet 1994;31:835–839.

145. Nakamoto JM, Hakakha MJ, Englund AT, Brickman AS, Van Dop C. Variable parathyroid hormone resistance in a family with a G_s protein mutation and Albright hereditary osteodystrophy. Clin Res 1992;40:95A (Abstract).

146. Dixon PH, Ahmed SF, Bonthron DT, Barr DGO, Kelnar CJH, Thakkar RV. Mutational analysis of the GNAS1 gene in pseudohypoparathyroidism. J Bone Miner Res 1996;11(Supp 1):S494 (Abstract).

147. Yu SH, Yu D, Hainline BE, et al. A deletion hot-spot in exon 7 of the $G_s\alpha$ gene (GNAS1) in patients with Albright hereditary osteodystrophy. Hum Mol Genet 1995;4:2001–2002.

148. Yokoyama M, Takeda K, Iyota K, Okabayashi T, Hashimoto K. A 4-base pair deletion mutation of Gs alpha gene in a Japanese patient with pseudohypoparathyroidism. J Endocrinol Invest 1996;19: 236–241.

149. Krawczak M, Cooper DN. Gene deletions causing human genetic disease: mechanisms of mutagenesis and the role of the local DNA sequence environment. Hum Genet 1991;86:425–441.

150. Schwindinger WF, Miric A, Zimmerman D, Levine MA. A novel $G_s\alpha$ mutant in a patient with Albright hereditary osteodystrophy uncouples cell surface receptors from adenylyl cyclase. J Biol Chem 1994;269:25,387–25,391.

151. Sullivan KA, Miller RT, Masters SB, Beiderman B, Heideman W, Bourne HR. Identification of receptor contact site involved in receptor-G protein coupling. Nature 1987;330:758–760.

152. Rall T, Harris BA. Identification of the lesion in the stimulatory GTP-binding protein of the uncoupled S49 lymphoma. FEBS Lett 1987;224:365–371.

153. Nakamoto JM, Jones EA, Zimmerman D, Scott ML, Donlan MA, Van Dop C. A missense mutation in the Gs-α gene is associated with pseudohypoparathyroidism type I-A and gonadotropin-independent precocious puberty. Clin Res 1993; 41:40A (Abstract).

154. Iiri T, Herzmark P, Nakamoto JM, Van Dop C, Bourne HR. Rapid GDP release from Gs-α in patients with gain and loss of endocrine function. Nature 1994;371:164–167.

155. Farfel Z, Iiri T, Shapira H, Roitman A, Mouallem M, Bourne HR. Pseudohypoparathyroidism: a novel mutation in the βγ-contact region of G$_s$α impairs receptor stimulation. J Biol Chem 1996;271: 19,653–19,655.

156. Weinstein LS, Shenker A, Gejman PV, Merino MJ, Friedman E, Spiegel AM. Activating mutations of the stimulatory G protein in the McCune-Albright syndrome. N Engl J Med 1991;325: 1688–1695.

157. Weinstein LS. Other skeletal diseases resulting from G protein defects-fibrous dysplasia and McCune-Albright syndrome. In: Bilezikian JP, Raisz LG, Rodan GA, eds. Principles of Bone Biology. Academic, San Diego, 1996, pp. 877–888.

158. Tsang RC, Venkataraman P, Ho M, Steichen JJ, Whitsett J, Greer F. The development of pseudo-hypoparathyroidism. Involvement of progressively increasing serum parathyroid hormone concentrations, increased 1,25-dihydroxyvitamin D concentrations, and "migratory" subcutaneous calcifications. Am J Dis Child 1984;138:654–658.

159. Werder EA, Fischer JA, Illig R, et al. Pseudohypoparathyroidism and idiopathic hypoparathyroidism: relationship between serum calcium and parathyroid hormone levels and urinary cyclic adenosine-3',5'-monophosphate response to parathyroid extract. J Clin Endocrinol Metab 1978;46:872–879.

160. Barr DGD, Stirling HF, Darling JAB. Evolution of pseudohypoparathyroidism: An informative family study. Arch Dis Child 1994;70:337–338.

161. Balachandar V, Pahuja J, Maddaiah VT, Collipp PJ. Pseudohypoparathyroidism with normal serum calcium level. Am J Dis Child 1975;129:1092–1095.

162. Breslau NA, Notman DD, Canterbury JM, Moses AM. Studies on the attainment of normocalcemia in patients with pseudohypoparathyroidism. Am J Med 1980;68:856–860.

163. Breslau NA, Zerwekh JE. Relationship of estrogen and pregnancy to calcium homeostasis in pseudo-hypoparathyroidism. J Clin Endocrinol Metab 1986;62:45–51.

164. Zerwekh JE, Breslau NA. Human placental production of 1α,25-dihydroxyvitamin D3: biochemical characterization and production in normal subjects and patients with pseudohypoparathyroidism. J Clin Endocrinol Metab 1986;62:192–196.

165. Werder EA, Illig R, Bernasconi S, Kind H, Prader A. Excessive thyrotropin response to thyrotropin-releasing hormone in pseudohypoprathyroidism. Pediatr Res 1975;9:12–16.

166. Mallet E, Carayon P, Amr S, et al. Coupling defect of thyrotropin receptor and adenylate cyclase in a pseudohypoparathyroid patient. J Clin Endocrinol Metab 1982;54:1028–1032.

167. Levine MA, Jap TS, Hung W. Infantile hypothyroidism in two sibs: an unusual presentation of pseudohypoparathyroidism type Ia. J Pediatr 1985;107:919–922.

168. Weisman Y, Golander A, Spirer Z, Farfel Z. Pseudohypoparathyroidism type Ia presenting as congenital hypothyroidism. J Pediatr 1985;107:413–415.

169. Yokoro S, Matsuo M, Ohtsuka T, Ohzeki T. Hyperthyrotropinemia in a neonate with normal thyroid hormone levels: the earliest diagnostic clue for pseudo-hypoparathyroidism. Biol Neonate 1990;58:69–72.

170. Wolfsdorf JI, Rosenfield RL, Fang VS, Kobayashi R, Razdan AK, Kim MH. Partial gonadotrophin resistance in pseudohypoparathyroidism. Acta Endocrinol (Copenh) 1978;88:321–328.

171. Shapiro MS, Bernheim J, Gutman A, Arber I, Spitz IM. Multiple abnormalities of anterior pituitary hormone secretion in association with pseudohypoparathyroidism. J Clin Endocrinol Metab 1980;51: 483–487.

172. Shima M, Nose O, Shimizu K, Seino Y, Yabuuchi H, Saito T. Multiple associated endocrine abnormalities in a patient with pseudohypoparathyroidism type 1a. Eur J Pediatr 1988;147:536–538.

173. Carlson HE, Brickman AS, Bottazzo GF. Prolactin deficiency in pseudohypoparathyroidism. N Engl J Med 1977;296:140–144.

174. Brickman AS, Carlson HE, Deftos LJ. Prolactin and calcitonin responses to parathyroid hormone infusion in hypoparathyroid, pseudohypoparathyroid, and normal subjects. J Clin Endocrinol Metab 1981;53:661–664.

175. Kruse K, Gutekunst B, Kracht U, Schwerda K. Deficient prolactin response to parathyroid hormone in hypocalcemic and normocalcemic pseudohypoparathyroidism. J Clin Endocrinol Metab 1981;52:1099–1105.

176. Scott DC, Hung W. Pseudohypoparathyroidism type Ia and growth hormone deficiency in two siblings. J Pediatr Endocrinol Metab 1995;8:205–207.

177. Urdanivia E, Mataverde A, Cohen MP. Growth hormone secretion and sulfation factor activity in pseudohypoparathyroidism. J Lab Clin Med 1975;86:772–776.

178. Brickman AS, Carlson HE, Levin SR. Responses to glucagon infusion in pseudohypoparathyroidism. J Clin Endocrinol Metab 1986;63:1354–1360.

179. Carlson HE, Brickman AS. Blunted plasma cyclic adenosine monophosphate response to isoproterenol in pseudohypoparathyroidism. J Clin Endocrinol Metab 1983;56:1323–1326.

180. Carlson HE, Brickman AS, Burns TW, Langley PE. Normal free fatty acid response to isoproterenol in pseudohypoparathyroidism. J Clin Endocrinol Metab 1985;61:382–384.

181. Kaartinen JM, Käär M-L, Ohisalo JJ. Defective stimulation of adipocyte adenylate cyclase, blunted lipolysis, and obesity in pseudohypoparathyroidism 1a. Pediatr Res 1994;35:594–597.

182. Ridderskamp P, Schlaghecke R. Pseudohypoparathyroidism and adrenal insufficiency—a case of multiple endocrinopathy due to hormone resistance. Klin Wochenschr 1990;68:927–931.

183. Henkin RI. Impairment of olfaction and of the tastes of sour and bitter in pseudohypoparathyroidism. J Clin Endocrinol Metab 1968;28:624–628.

184. Weinstock RS, Wright HN, Spiegel AM, Levine MA, Moses AM. Olfactory dysfunction in humans with deficient guanine nucleotide-binding protein. Nature 1986;322:635–636.

185. Ikeda K, Sakurada T, Sasaki Y, Takasaka T, Furukawa Y. Clinical investigation of olfactory and auditory function in type I pseudohypoparathyroidism: participation of adenylate cyclase system. J Laryngol Otol 1988;102:1111–1114.

186. Doty RL, Fernandez AD, Levine MA, Moses A, McKeown DA. Olfactory dysfunction in type I pseudohypoparathyroidism: dissociation from $G_s\alpha$ deficiency. J Clin Endocrinol Metab 1997;82:247–250.

187. Jones DT, Reed RR. G_{olf}: an olfactory neuron specific-G protein involved in odorant signal transduction. Science 1989;244:790–795.

188. McLaughlin SK, McKinnon PJ, Margolskee RF. Gustducin is a taste-cell-specific G protein closely related to the transducins. Nature 1992;357:563–569.

189. Koch T, Lehnhardt E, Böttinger H, et al. Sensorineural hearing loss owing to deficient G proteins in patients with pseudohypoparathyroidism: results of a multicentre study. Eur J Clin Invest 1990;20:416–421.

190. Steinbach HL, Young DA. The roentgen appearance of pseudohypoparathyroidism (PH) and pseudo-pseudohypoparathyroidism (PPH). Differentiation from other syndromes associated with short metacarpals, metatarsals, and phalanges. Am J Roentgenol Radium Ther Nucl Med 1966;97:49–66.

191. Poznanski AK, Werder EA, Giedion A, Martin A, Shaw H. The pattern of shortening of the bones of the hand in pseudohypoparathyroidism and pseudopseudohypoparathyroidism—a comparison with brachydactyly E, Turner syndrome, and acrodysostosis. Radiology 1977;123:707–718.

192. Graudal N, Milman N, Nielsen LS, Niebuhr E, Bonde J. Coexistent pseudohypoparathyroidism and D brachydactyly in a family. Clin Genet 1986;30:449–455.

193. de Wijn EM, Steendijk R. Growth and maturation in pseudohypoparathyroidism: a longitudinal study in five patients. Acta Endocrinol (Copenh) 1982;101:223–226.

194. Alam SM, Kelly W. Spinal cord compression associated with pseudohypoparathyroidism. J R Soc Med 1990;83:50–51.

195. Goadsby PJ, Lollin Y, Kocen RS. Pseudopseudohypoparathyroidism and spinal cord compression. J Neurol Neurosurg Psychiatry 1991;54:929–931.

196. Okada K, Iida K, Sakusabe N, Saitoh H, Abe E, Sato K. Pseudohypoparathyroidism-associated spinal stenosis. Spine 1994;19:1186–1189.

197. Prendiville JS, Lucky AW, Mallory SB, Mughal Z, Mimouni F, Langman CB. Osteoma cutis as a presenting sign of pseudohypoparathyroidism. Pediatr Dermatol 1992;9:11–18.

198. Trueb RM, Panizzon RG, Burg G. Cutaneous ossification in Albright's hereditary osteodystrophy. Dermatology 1993;186:205–209.

199. Vortkamp A, Lee K, Lanske B, Segre GV, Kronenberg HM, Tabin CJ. Regulation of rate of cartilage differentiation by Indian hedgehog and PTH-related protein. Science 1996;273:613–622.

200. Karaplis AC, Luz A, Glowacki J, et al. Lethal skeletal dysplasia from targeted disruption of the parathyroid hormone-related peptide gene. Genes Dev 1994;8:277–289.

201. Lanske B, Karaplis AC, Lee K, et al. PTH/PTHrP receptor in early development and Indian hedgehog-regulated bone growth. Science 1996;273:663–666.

202. Candeliere GA, Glorieux FH, Prud'homme J, St.-Arnaud R. Increased expression of the c-*fos* proto-oncogene in bone from patients with fibrous dysplasia. N Engl J Med 1995;332:1546–1551.

203. Rüther U, Garber C, Komitowski D, Müller R, Wagner EF. Deregulated c-*fos* expression interferes with normal bone development in transgenic mice. Nature 1987;325:412–416.

204. Nanes MS, Boden S, Weinstein LS. Oligonucleotides antisense to Gsα promote osteoblast differenti-
     ation. Endocrine Society 77th Annual Meeting Program and Abstracts. 1995;62–60 (Abstract).
205. Wang H, Watkins DC, Malbon CC. Antisense oligodeoxynucleotides to $G_s\alpha$-subunit sequence accel-
     erate differentiation of fibroblasts to adipocytes. Nature 1992;358:334–337.
206. Hamann A, Flier JS, Lowell BB. Decreased brown fat markedly enhances susceptibility to diet-
     induced obesity, diabetes and hyperlipidemia. Endocrinology 1996;137:21–29.
207. Wilson LC, Leverton K, Oude Luttikhuis MEM, et al. Brachydactyly and mental retardation: an Albright
     hereditary osteodystrophy-like syndrome localized to 2q37. Am J Hum Genet 1995;56:400–407.
208. Phelan MC, Rogers RC, Clarkson KB, et al. Albright hereditary osteodystrophy and del(2)(q37.3) in
     four unrelated individuals. Am J Med Genet 1995;58:1–7.
209. Farfel Z, Bourne HR. Pseudohypoparathyroidism: mutation affecting adenylate cyclase. Miner
     Electrolyte Metab 1982;8:227–236.
210. Schipani E, Weinstein LS, Bergwitz C, et al. Pseudohypoparathyroidism type Ib is not caused by
     mutations in the coding exons of the human parathyroid hormone (PTH)/PTH-related peptide recep-
     tor gene. J Clin Endocrinol Metab 1995;80:1611–1621.
211. Fukumoto S, Suzawa M, Takeuchi Y, et al. Absence of mutations in parathyroid hormone (PTH)/PTH-
     related protein receptor complementary deoxyribonucleic acid in patients with pseudohypopara-
     thyroidism type Ib. J Clin Endocrinol Metab 1996;81:2554–2558.
212. Silve C, Suarez F, El Hessni A, Loiseau A, Graulet AM, Gueris J. The resistance to parathyroid
     hormone of fibroblasts from some patients with type Ib pseudohypoparathyroidism is reversible with
     dexamethasone. J Clin Endocrinol Metab 1990;71:631–638.
213. Suarez F, Lebrun JJ, Lecossier D, Escoubet B, Coureau C, Silve C. Expression and modulation of the
     parathyroid hormone (PTH)/PTH-related peptide receptor messenger ribonucleic acid in skin fibroblasts
     from patients with type Ib pseudohypoparathyroidism. J Clin Endocrinol Metab 1995;80: 965–970.
214. Winter JS, Hughes IA. Familial pseudohypoparathyroidism without somatic anomalies. Can Med
     Assoc J 1980;123:26–31.
215. Izraeli S, Metzker A, Horev G, Karmi D, Merlob P, Farfel Z. Albright hereditary osteodystrophy with
     hypothyroidism, normocalcemia, and normal Gs protein activity: a family presenting with congenital
     osteoma cutis. Am J Med 1992;43:764–767.
216. Hedeland H, Berntorp K, Arheden K, Kristoffersson U. Pseudohypoparathyroidism type I and
     Albright's hereditary osteodystrophy with a proximal 15q chromosomal deletion in mother and
     daughter. Clin Genet 1992;42:129–134.
217. Rao DS, Parfitt AM, Kleerekoper M, Pumo BS, Frame B. Dissociation between the effects of endo-
     genous parathyroid hormone on adenosine 3′,5′-monophosphate generation and phosphate reabsorption
     in hypocalcemia due to vitamin D depletion: an acquired disorder resembling pseudohypopara-
     thyroidism type II. J Clin Endocrinol Metab 1985;61:285–290.
218. Matsuda I, Takekoshi Y, Tanaka M, Matsuura N, Nagai B, Seino Y. Pseudohypoparathyroidism type
     II and anticonvulsant rickets. Eur J Pediatr 1979;132:303–308.
219. Rodriguez HJ, Villarreal H,Jr., Klahr S, Slatopolsky E. Pseudohypoparathyroidism type II: restoration
     of normal renal responsiveness to parathyroid hormone by calcium administration. J Clin Endocrinol
     Metab 1974;39:693–701.
220. Yamada K, Tamura Y, Tomioka H, Kumagai A, Yoshida S. Possible existence of anti-renal tubular
     plasma membrane autoantibody which blocked parathyroid hormone-induced phosphaturia in a
     patient with pseudohypoparathyroidism type II and Sjögren's syndrome. J Clin Endocrinol Metab
     1984;58:339–343.
221. Davies SJ, Hughes HE. Familial acrodysostosis: can it be distinguished from Albright's hereditary
     osteodystrophy. Clin Dysmorphol 1992;1:207–215.
222. Mallette LE, Kirkland JL, Gagel RF, Law WM Jr, Heath H III. Synthetic human parathyroid hormone
     (1-34) for the study of pseudohypoparathyroidism. J Clin Endocrinol Metab 1988;67:964–972.
223. Stirling HF, Darling JAB, Barr DGD. Plasma cyclic AMP response to intravenous parathyroid hor-
     mone in pseudohypoparathyroidism. Acta Paediatr Scand 1991;80:333–338.
224. Singhellakis P, Pappas P, Nicolou CH, Ikkos D. Separation of pseudohypoparathyroidism into types I
     and II using only basal nephrogenous cAMP determinations. Endocrinologie 1991;29:67–71.
225. Gejman PV, Weinstein LS. Detection of mutations and polymorphisms of the $G_s\alpha$ gene by denaturing
     gradient gel electrophoresis. In: Iyengar R, ed. Methods in Enzymology, 237th ed. Academic,
     Orlando, 1994, 308–321.
226. Slater S. An evaluation of the metacarpal sign (short fourth metacarpal). Pediatrics 1970;46:468–471.

227. Kruse K, Kracht U, Wohlfart K, Kruse U. Biochemical markers of bone turnover, intact serum parathyroid hormone and renal calcium excretion in patients with pseudohypoparathyroidism and hypoparathyroidism before and during vitamin D treatment. Eur J Pediatr 1989;148:535–539.

228. Yamamoto M, Takuwa Y, Ogata E. Effects of endogenous and exogenous parathyroid hormone on tubular reabsorption of calcium in pseudohypoparathyroidism. J Clin Endocrinol Metab 1988;66:618.

229. Mizunashi K, Furukawa Y, Sohn HE, Miura R, Yumita S, Yoshinaga K. Heterogeneity of pseudo-hypoparathyroidism type I from the aspect of urinary excretion of calcium and serum levels of parathyroid hormone. Calcif Tissue Int 1990;46:227–232.

230. Davies SJ, Hughes HE. Imprinting in Albright's hereditary osteodystrophy. J Med Genet 1993;30: 101–103.

231. Campbell R, Gosden CM, Bonthron DT. Parental origin of transcription from the human GNAS1 gene. J Med Genet 1994;31:607–614.

232. Schuster V, Kress W, Kruse K. Paternal and maternal transmission of pseudohypoparathyroidism type Ia in a family with Albright hereditary osteodystrophy: no evidence of genomic imprinting. J Med Genet 1994;31:84.

3

$G\alpha_s$-Activating Mutations

A Cause of Acromegaly, Thyroid Adenomas, Fibrous Dysplasia, and the McCune-Albright Syndrome

Allen M. Spiegel, MD

CONTENTS

INTRODUCTION
IDENTIFICATION OF ACTIVATING MUTATIONS IN $G\alpha_s$
CONCLUSIONS
ACKNOWLDGMENTS
REFERENCES

INTRODUCTION

G_s was the first G protein to be purified and characterized biochemically in detail. It is expressed in all mammalian cells, and is highly conserved not only in all vertebrates, but also in invertebrates, such as *Drosophila* and *Caenorhabditis elegans*. G_s couples receptors for numerous peptide hormones and monoamines to stimulation of adenylyl cyclase. Although it is now clear that G-protein $\beta\gamma$-subunits can independently modulate adenylyl cyclase (positively or negatively depending on the adenylyl cyclase subtype), it is the $G\alpha_s$-subunit that is the principal stimulator of adenylyl cyclase activity *(1,2)*. Resultant cyclic adenosine monophosphate (cAMP) formation activates cAMP-dependent protein kinase A (PKA), causing phosphorylation of key intracellular proteins. Brief elevation in cAMP causes acute changes in cellular function; a more sustained increase in cAMP can lead to longer term alterations in cellular function, at least in part by modulating gene expression through cAMP-responsive transcription factors, such as cAMP response element binding protein (CREB). Not all of the actions of $G\alpha_s$ are necessarily mediated by cAMP activation of PKA. cAMP may act directly in certain cell types by regulating cyclic nucleotide-gated ion channels *(3)*. There have also been suggestions that some actions of $G\alpha_s$ are independent of cAMP *(4,5)*.

Given its central role in signal transduction in many different cell types, it is not surprising that alterations in $G\alpha_s$ function have emerged as an important pathophysiologic mechanism in a number of different disorders. Heterozygous germline loss-of-function mutations in the $G\alpha_s$ gene cause Albright hereditary osteodystrophy and the associated

From: *Contemporary Endocrinology: G Proteins, Receptors, and Disease*
Edited by: A. M. Spiegel Humana Press Inc., Totowa, NJ

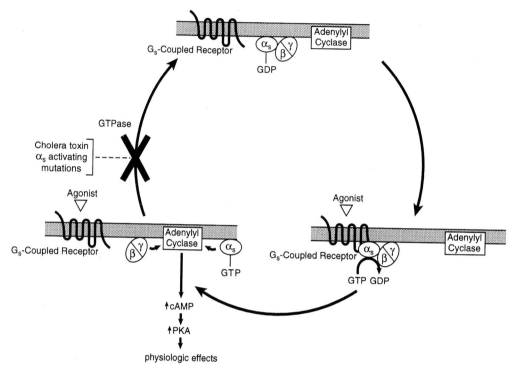

Fig. 1. The G_s protein GTPase cycle. In the basal, inactive state, the $G\alpha_s$-subunit contains tightly bound GDP, and is associated as a heterotrimer with the $\beta\gamma$-dimer. Interaction with the intracellular portion of an agonist-bound, activated, receptor leads to release of bound GDP and binding of ambient GTP. Binding of GTP leads to dissociation of G protein from receptor, and of $G\alpha_s$-subunit from $\beta\gamma$. GTP-bound $G\alpha_s$ activates adenylyl cyclase. The $\beta\gamma$-dimer independently regulates adenylyl cyclase activity. Intrinsic GTPase activity of $G\alpha_s$ leads to hydrolysis of bound GTP to GDP with liberation of inorganic phosphate. This causes dissociation of $G\alpha_s$ from adenylyl cyclase and reassociation with $\beta\gamma$. Cholera toxin covalently modifies its substrate $G\alpha_s$, causing constitutive activation and agonist-independent cAMP formation. Mutations identified in $G\alpha_s$ *(see text)* can also lead to constitutive activation by inhibiting GTPase activity.

hormone resistance syndrome, pseudohypoparathyroidism (*see* Chapter 2). The lethal secretory diarrhea characteristic of cholera infection is caused by covalent modification of $G\alpha_s$ in intestinal lining cells catalyzed by an exotoxin elaborated by the pathogen. The toxin hydrolyzes nicotinomide adanime dinucleotide (NAD) transferring the adenosine diphosphate (ADP)-ribose moiety to the guanidine side chain of arginine 201 of $G\alpha_s$ (four splice variants of $G\alpha_s$ have been identified, which do not differ significantly in function; residue numbers vary for each splice variant; by convention, the numbering used refers to the 394 amino acid form of the protein). Cholera toxin-catalyzed ADP ribosylation of $G\alpha_s$ inhibits the protein's intrinsic guanosine triphosphatase (GTPase) activity. This in turn leads to constitutive activation with resultant persistent stimulation of cAMP formation (Fig. 1). In the small intestine, the only organ affected by the noninvasive cholera bacteria, elevated cAMP, alters mucosal chloride and water secretion leading to diarrhea.

GTPase inhibition caused by cholera toxin-catalyzed covalent modification of arginine 201 of $G\alpha_s$ provided the clue that mutations of this residue could have similar effects. Site-directed mutagenesis of arginine 201 or of glutamine 227 (Fig. 2) to almost any

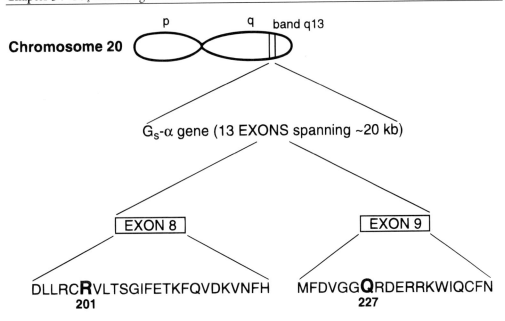

Fig. 2. Location of Gα_s-activating mutations. (Top) The human Gα_s gene has been mapped to the distal long arm of chromosome 20 (20q13). Middle: The gene contains 13 exons and spans ~20 kb. (Bottom) Exons 8 and 9 encode sequences highly conserved in all G-protein α-subunits, including arginine 201 and glutamine 227 of Gα_s.

other amino acid reduces GTPase activity *(6)*. Glutamine 227 is the equivalent of glutamine 61 in the *ras* proto-oncogene. Mutations in this position in ras have been identified in a wide variety of human tumors, and are known to activate ras constitutively by inhibiting GTPase activity. A glutamine equivalent to residue 227 in Gα_s is found in nearly all members of the GTPase superfamily, and based on X-ray crystallography-determined 3-D structure, is involved in binding the γ-phosphate of GTP. Perturbation of this binding by mutation interferes with the normal GTPase mechanism. An arginine equivalent to residue 201 of Gα_s is not present in ras or other low-mol-wt GTP binding proteins, but is conserved in all heterotrimeric G-protein α-subunits. 3-D structural studies of a GDP-bound Gα_{i1}-subunit activated by ALF_4^- (which mimics the γ-phosphate of GTP) show that the arginine equivalent to arginine 201 of Gα_s is directly involved in the mechanism of GTP hydrolysis *(7)*. Appreciation of the critical importance of the rate of GTPase activity in modulating G-protein function, and a detailed understanding of the biochemistry of the GTPase reaction provided the basis for identification of disease-causing mutations in Gα_s.

IDENTIFICATION OF ACTIVATING MUTATIONS IN Gα_S

Pituitary Somatotroph Tumors Causing Acromegaly

Studies by Spada et al. *(8)* showed that a subset of GH-secreting pituitary adenomas are characterized by high levels of in vitro GH release. Membranes from these tumors showed increased adenylyl cyclase activity not further activated by a variety of stimulators, including GHRH, which under physiologic conditions activates adenylyl cyclase through its G_s-coupled receptor *(8)*. Landis et al. *(6)* subsequently identified heterozygous missense mutations in $G\alpha_s$ (arginine 201 to either histidine or cysteine and glutamine 227 to either arginine or leucine) in tumor DNA *(6,8)*. Since genomic DNA from peripheral blood of such patients showed only the normal sequence, the mutations are of somatic origin. As discussed, such mutations reduce intrinsic GTPase activity, leading to constitutive activation of $G\alpha_s$ and then of adenylyl cyclase. Such mutations act in a dominant fashion and led to designation of the mutated $G\alpha_s$ as the *gsp* oncogene *(8)*.

cAMP is mitogenic in certain cell types, particularly endocrine cells, such as somatotrophs, thyroid, and adrenal cortical cells *(9)*. While stimulating cell proliferation, cAMP maintains differentiated functions, such as hormone synthesis and secretion. The phenotype expected from a somatic mutation causing excessive cAMP production in a somatotroph is a benign proliferation characterized by excessive growth hormone (GH) secretion. This is exactly what is observed in the subset of acromegalic subjects with tumors harboring activating $G\alpha_s$ mutations. Interestingly, transgenic mice expressing active cholera toxin in somatotrophs (driven by a rat GH promoter) show pituitary hyperplasia, excessive GH secretion, and gigantism *(10)*. In this model, toxin-catalyzed modification of arginine 201 of $G\alpha_s$ rather than a mutation causes a similar phenotype.

Subsequent studies have shown that ~40% of somatotroph tumors from patients with acromegaly harbor activating $G\alpha_s$ mutations at either arginine 201 or glutamine 227 *(11)*. Essentially all tumors studied biochemically and shown to have constitutively activated cAMP formation are found to harbor activating $G\alpha_s$ mutations *(8)*. In theory, activating mutations of the growth hormone releasing hormone (GHRH) receptor could result in the same phenotype. Although such mutations of the thyroid-stimulating hormone (TSH) receptor have indeed been identified in thyroid adenomas (*see* Thyroid and Other Tumors and Chapter 7), they have not been found in the GHRH receptor.

Few clinical differences between somatotroph tumors with and without $G\alpha_s$ mutations have been observed. Mutation-positive tumors tend to be smaller, but basal GH levels were higher in one study *(12)* and lower in another *(13)* by comparison with a mutation-negative group. In vitro studies suggest that $G\alpha_s$ mutation-positive tumors preserve responsiveness to inhibition of GH secretion by somatostatin *(14)*. These in vitro results agree with in vivo results, suggesting preserved response to inhibitory agonists, such as somatostatin and dopamine *(12)*. Evidently, despite constitutive $G\alpha_s$ activation, adenylyl cyclase is still susceptible to inhibition through G_i-coupled receptors in such tumor cells. $G\alpha_s$ mutation-positive somatotroph tumors have also been shown to secrete increased amounts of glycoprotein hormone α-subunit *(15)*.

Other Types of Pituitary Tumor

In addition to somatotrophs in which GH secretion is stimulated by GHRH-activated cAMP production, adrenocorticotropic hormone (ACTH) secretion in corticotrophs is stimulated by the G_s-coupled corticotropin-releasing hormone (CRH) receptor. In thyrotrophs, lactotrophs, and gonadotrophs, in contrast, the receptors for their respective hypothalamic stimulators are not G_s-coupled. In theory, one might expect to find a similar proportion of $G\alpha_s$ mutations in ACTH-producing corticotroph tumors as in somatotroph tumors, but this has not been observed. In the first large study identifying $G\alpha_s$ mutations in 18 of 42 somatotroph tumors, no such mutations were found in 24 other pituitary tumors (12 prolactinomas, 2 TSH-secreting, 7 ACTH-secreting, and 3 non-secreting) studied *(11)*.

Subsequent studies have identified Gα$_s$ mutations in a small number of pituitary tumors other than somatotrophs. Two of 21 nonfunctioning pituitary tumors showed such mutations in one study *(16)*. Gα$_s$ mutations were identified in 2 of 32 corticotroph tumors in another study *(17)*. In a study of nine thyrotroph tumors, no Gα$_s$ mutations were identified nor were any mutations identified in components of the physiologically important TRH stimulatory pathway, including the TRH receptor, and either Gα$_q$ or Gα$_{11}$ *(18)*.

Thyroid and Other Tumors

Expression of mutationally activated (glutamine 227 to leucine) Gα$_s$ in FRTL5 cells, a rat thyroid cell line, stimulates growth while maintaining differentiated function (19). On this basis, one would predict that autonomously functioning thyroid adenomas ("hot nodules") would be likely to harbor somatic Gα$_s$ mutations. Subsequent studies have confirmed this, but the correlation between the presence of Gα$_s$ mutation and thyroid tumor type has not been perfect. In addition to pituitary tumors, Lyons et al. *(11)* searched for Gα$_s$ mutations in a variety of benign and malignant endocrine and nonendocrine neoplasms. A single thyroid tumor of 25 studied was the only nonpituitary tumor to show a Gα$_s$ mutation. In one study, 5 of 13 autonomously functioning adenomas showed Gα$_s$ mutations, but none were identified in 16 nonfunctioning adenomas, 6 papillary, and 3 follicular carcinomas *(20)*. In another study of differentiated thyroid carcinomas in which adenylyl cyclase activity was measured, three of the tumors (two microfollicular and one papillary) with high basal cyclase activity were positive for Gα$_s$ mutations *(21)*. Overall, the incidence of Gα$_s$ mutations in thyroid tumors appears to be quite low, 1/100 in one of the largest studies performed *(22)*. Many of these tumors, however, may harbor activating TSH receptor mutations, which have the same biochemical effect (*see* Chapter 7). TSH receptor-activating mutations occur both as somatic and germline events. In the former, a single thyroid neoplasm, such as a follicular adenoma, occurs identical to the situation for an activating Gα$_s$ mutation. Germline-activating TSH receptor mutations cause diffuse thyroid enlargement and hyperfunction. Germline-activating Gα$_s$ mutations have not been identified. Unlike the localized expression of the TSH receptor gene, ubiquitous expression of an activated Gα$_s$ gene might well be lethal (*see* McCune-Albright Syndrome and Fibrous Dysplasia).

Somatic Gα$_s$ mutations have also rarely been identified in other endocrine tumors. An arginine 201 cysteine mutation was found in 1 of 19 adrenocortical adenomas tested in one study *(23)*, but in another study of 18 adrenocortical tumors of varying type, no mutations were found *(24)*, nor were any found in parathyroid or endocrine pancreatic tumors *(23,25)*.

McCune-Albright Syndrome (MAS) and Fibrous Dysplasia

McCune and Albright independently described several cases of a sporadic disease of unknown etiology with prominent features, including cafe-au-lait skin hyperpigmentation, bone lesions (polyostotic fibrous dysplasia), precocious puberty, and other endocrinopathies (*see* ref 26 and references therein for review). The pattern of cutaneous hyperpigmentation led to the suggestion that MAS, as it came to be known, is caused by a somatic mutation occurring early in development and leading to a mosaic distribution of mutation-bearing cells *(27)*. It was further suggested that this mutation would be lethal if inherited in the germline.

Adrenal Adenoma

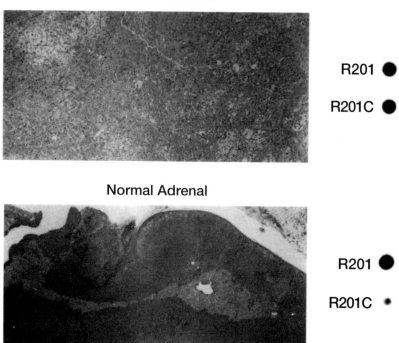

R201 ●

R201C ●

Normal Adrenal

R201 ●

R201C ·

Fig. 3 Identification of arginine 201 mutation in adrenal adenoma from subject with McCune-Albright syndrome. (Top) Adrenal adenoma. Bottom: Apparently normal contralateral adrenal. Allele-specific oligonucleotide hybridization was used to test for arginine 201 mutation of $G\alpha_s$. Exon 8 of $G\alpha_s$ was amplified from genomic DNA of each adrenal cortex using the polymerase chain reaction. Oligonucleotides used for hybridization correspond to normal sequence or to arginine 201 cysteine (R201C) mutation. The DNA from adrenal adenoma shows heterozygous wild-type and mutant sequence, whereas the mutant sequence is present at much lower level in DNA from apparently normal adrenal. Since normal DNA used as control shows no hybridization to the mutant oligonucleotide under the conditions used (see Fig. 4C), the slight hybridization to the mutant oligonucleotide seen with DNA from normal adrenal likely reflects a small number of mutant-bearing cells.

Endocrine studies in subjects with MAS showed a wide spectrum of hyperfunctional endocrinopathies, including gigantism/acromegaly, hyperthyroidism, hyperadrenocorticism, and precocious puberty (the latter predominantly in females, but also documented in males). In any given patient, one or more of these endocrine disturbances might be present in association with the characteristic skin and bone lesions. With the advent of radioimmunoassay, the pathophysiology of the endocrinopathies was defined. Each represented autonomous hyperfunction as reflected in suppressed levels of the corresponding trophic hormone, e.g., suppressed gonadotropins with precocious puberty. The ability of cAMP to stimulate endocrine cell growth and function prompted Weinstein et al. *(26)* to hypothesize that the MAS could be caused by an activating somatic mutation of $G\alpha_s$ occurring early in development. In each case they studied (four in the initial report *[26]*, but more than 30 subsequently), they identified arginine 201 mutations (either to histidine or cysteine). These were present as predicted in a mosaic distribution with heterozygous mutant present in DNA from overtly pathologic tissue and low to undetectable levels of

A

Fig. 4. (A) A girl with McCune-Albright syndrome. This young girl shows the classic triad of cafe-au-lait skin pigmentation (note the patchy skin spots), polyostotic fibrous dysplasia (note the "shepherd's crook" deformity of the left femur), and precocious puberty. **(B)** Photomicrograph (hematoxylin and eosin stained) showing a bone biopsy from a fibrous dysplasia lesion. The interface between normal bone (left) with normal marrow elements and the dysplastic area (right) with fibrous tissue in the marrow space and abnormal bone spicules ("Chinese writing" appearance) is shown. **(C)** Identification of arginine 201 mutations of $G\alpha_s$ in DNA from dysplastic bone. Methods used are as in legend to Fig. 3. The dysplastic bone samples show heterozygous normal (wild-type) arginine 201 and either arginine 201 histidine (R201H) or arginine 201 cysteine (R201C) mutations. The mutation is not detectable in DNA from peripheral blood cells from the same subjects. A normal bone DNA sample is shown as a control.

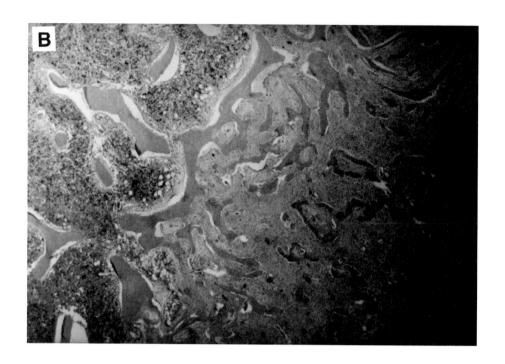

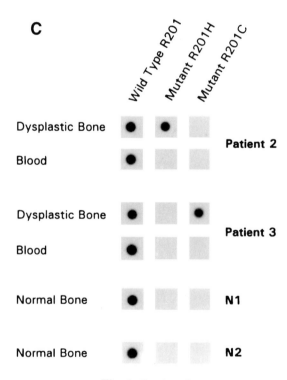

Fig. 4. *Continued*

mutant in DNA from other tissues (Figs. 3 and 4). Interestingly, although both arginine 201 and glutamine 227 somatic mutations in the Gα$_s$ gene have been identified in subjects with focal somatotroph or thyroid tumors, only arginine 201 mutations have been identified to date in MAS. The glutamine 227 mutation more powerfully inhibits GTPase activity than the arginine 201 mutation; perhaps only focal expression of this more powerfully activating mutation is compatible with normal development.

Arginine 201 mutations have subsequently been identified in a variety of affected tissues from subjects with MAS, including hyperpigmented skin *(28)* and dysplastic bone *(29,30)*. The mutation has been found in a pituitary tumor from a 6-yr-old boy with gigantism as a feature of MAS *(31)*, and in nodular hyperplastic adrenalcortical tissue from an infant with Cushing's syndrome and fibrous dysplasia *(32)*. Shenker et al. *(33)* identified the arginine 201 mutation in a much wider distribution (e.g., heart and liver in addition to numerous endocrine organs) in a subset of MAS subjects with severe endocrine and nonendocrine manifestations, including early death. They speculate that such cases are caused by occurrence of the somatic mutation particularly early in development, resulting in a much wider distribution.

At the other extreme are cases of monostotic fibrous dysplasia in which bone lesions typical of those seen in MAS occur in isolated form without the associated skin and endocrine manifestations. Identification of the arginine 201 Gα$_s$ mutation in dysplastic cells from monostotic lesions *(34)* places monostotic fibrous dysplasia in the same category as isolated somatotroph tumors in subjects with acromegaly.

There may be other examples of isolated occurrence of components of MAS. Girls with gonadotropin-independent precocious puberty analogous to that occurring in MAS have been described, but their ovaries could not be analyzed to determine the molecular basis for autonomous gonadal hyperfunction *(35)*. A unique cause of gonadotropin-independent precocious puberty was identified in two males in association with classic features of Albright herditary osteodystrophy, including hormone resistance. This puzzling combination of hormone resistance and testicular Leydig cell hyperfunction was caused by a Gα$_s$ mutation, alanine 366 to serine *(36)*. The mutant protein is unstable at normal body temperature leading to loss-of-function and hormone resistance (*see* Chapter 2), but at the lower temperature prevalent in the testes, the protein is stable and activated as a result of agonist-independent release of GDP (*see* Fig. 1).

Autonomous endocrine hyperfunction and even skin hyperpigmentation can all be explained by constitutive Gα$_s$ activation with resultant increased cAMP production. Each of the cell types involved is ordinarily stimulated by agonists binding to G$_s$-coupled receptors, so that mutational activation mimics the effect of agonist. In skin melanocytes, for example, the melanocortin type 1 receptor when activated by MSH increases cAMP and causes increased pigmentation (*see* Chapter). The mechanism whereby Gα$_s$ mutation causes the fibrous dysplasia bone lesion is much less clear. One hypothesis is that the mutation occurs in an osteoblast precursor cell and stimulates proliferation while blocking full differentiation. According to this hypothesis, the fibroblast-like cells that fill the marrow space of dysplastic bone lesions are in fact undifferentiated "preosteoblasts." Excessive expression of the *fos* gene, normally expressed only early in osteoblast development, has been found in fibrous dysplasia bone lesions from subjects with MAS harboring arginine 201 mutations *(37)*. Since cAMP is known to stimulate *fos* gene expression, this provides one mechanism whereby Gα$_s$-activating mutations could block osteoclast differentiation. Fibrous dysplasia bone cells with Gα$_s$-activating mutations have also been shown to secrete increased amounts of IL-6, a potent osteoclast activator whose production is increased by parathyroid hormone (PTH) and parathyroid-hormone-related protein (PTHrP)-stimulated cAMP *(38)*. This mechanism may explain the osteo-clastic resorption observed in fibrous dysplasia lesions. Rare cases of osteogenic sarcoma occurring in subjects with fibrous dysplasia have been reported. Whether this represents malignant transformation of a benign lesion and the role if any of the $G\alpha_s$ activating mutation are unclear.

Myxomas, often occurring in muscle overlying a fibrous dysplasia bone lesion, have been reported in subjects with MAS. Interestingly, an activating $G\alpha_s$ mutation has been shown to disrupt normal differentiation of cultured myogenic cells *(4)*. Since $G\alpha_s$-activating mutations have been identified in myxomas from subjects with MAS (Shenker A., personal communication), the pathogenesis may be similar to that postulated for the fibrous dysplasia lesions, i.e., the mutation in a myogenic precursor cell stimulates proliferation and blocks differentiation.

A report of typical features of MAS in a subject with a strong family history of multi-ple endocrine neoplasia type 1 (MEN 1) has suggested a possible overlap between the two diseases *(39)*. The subject herself did not have features of MEN 1, so this could simply be a coincidence, but another report found an arginine 201 to cysteine $G\alpha_s$ mutation in the pituitary adenoma, but not parathyroid and pancreatic tumors, of a subject with typical MEN 1 *(40)*. Another study found the same mutation in a variety of endocrine tumors from several patients with multiple endocrine tumors, but not necessarily classic MEN 1 *(41)*. The significance of this observation is unclear, particularly since another study of 13 sub-jects with MEN 1 found no evidence of $G\alpha_s$ mutation in any of 18 tumors studied *(42)*. Identification of the MEN 1 tumor suppressor gene on 11q13 and study of its biologic function should help define any possible pathogenetic connection to $G\alpha_s$ mutation.

CONCLUSIONS

Identification of $G\alpha_s$-activating mutations in subjects with acromegaly, thyroid tumors, fibrous dysplasia, and MAS has defined a novel pathogenetic mechanism involving unregulated cAMP production in affected tissues with resultant hyperprolifer-ation and hyperfunction. This discovery has led directly to recognition that activating mutations of an "upstream" component in the signal transduction pathway, the G_s-coupled receptor for thyrotropin in thyroid tumors (Chapter 7), and for LH in familial male preco-cious puberty (Chapter 8) can cause disease in a similar way.

Although mutation identification has provided a much better understanding of patho-genesis of previously poorly understood diseases, such as MAS, it has not yet had a major impact on clinical evaluation and treatment. Since there are no major differences in clini-cal characteristics of acromegalics with or without $G\alpha_s$-activating mutations in their soma-totroph tumors, the diagnostic importance of mutation identification is unclear. In subjects with atypical features of MAS, mutation identification could be helpful in making the diagnosis, but since it is not clear that treatment would be affected, tissue biopsy may not be warranted simply for the purpose of mutation analysis.

Elucidation of the pathogenetic importance of $G\alpha_s$-activating mutations in these disorders should lead to newer, more effective forms of treatment directed at reducing excess cAMP production or blocking its distal effects. Any pharmacologic approach to reducing cAMP production will of course have to consider the critical role of this ubiquitous second messenger in so many different cells. As more novel approaches, including gene transfer, become practical, one can envision targeting individual lesions with vectors carrying genes for dominant negative forms of cAMP-dependent protein kinase to block the effects of excessive cAMP. Such an approach to the crippling bone lesions of fibrous dysplasia for which there is no currently satisfactory treatment is particularly appealing. In Chapter 5, Malbon and colleagues describe experimental studies using antisense approaches to reduce synthesis of specific G-protein α-subunits, and suggest that such methods could be applied to treatment of MAS. Undoubtedly other methods, including development of ribozymes specific for mutated Gα$_s$ genes, will be developed in the future. Only with successful development of such novel therapeutics will the full impact of the discovery of Gα$_s$-activating mutations be realized.

ACKNOWLEDGMENTS

I am grateful to Andrew Shenker and Lee Weinstein who collaborated in studies on the McCune-Albright syndrome. I also thank Andrew Shenker for preparation of material in Figs. 3 and 4.

REFERENCES

1. Neer EJ. Heterotrimeric G proteins: organizers of transmembrane signals. Cell 1995;80:249–257.
2. Dessauer CW, Posner BA, Gilman AG. Visualizing signal transduction: receptors, G-proteins, and adenylate cyclases. Clin Sci 1996;91:527–537.
3. Biel M, Zong X, Distler M, Bosse E, Klugbauer N, Murakami M, Flockerzi V, Hofmann F. 1994 Another member of the cyclic nucleotide-gated channel family, expressed in testis, kidney, and heart. Proc Natl Acad Sci USA 1994;91:3505–3509.
4. Tsai CC, Saffitz JE, Billadello JJ. Expression of the Gs protein alpha-subunit disrupts the normal program of differentiation in cultured murine myogenic cells. J Clin Invest 1997;99:67–76.
5. Wolfgang WJ, Roberts IJ, Quan F, O'Kane C, Forte M. Activation of protein kinase A-independent pathways by G$_s$ alpha in Drosophila. Proc Natl Acad Sci USA 1996;93:14,542–14,547.
6. Landis CA, Masters SB, Spada A, Pace AM, Bourne HR, Vallar L. GTPase inhibiting mutations activate the alpha chain of Gs and stimulate adenylyl cyclase in human pituitary tumours. Nature 1989;340:692–696.
7. Coleman DE, Berghuis AM, Lee E, Linder ME, Gilman AG, Sprang SR. Structures of active conformations of G$_{ia1}$ and the mechanism of GTP hydrolysis. Science 1994;265:1405–1412.
8. Spada A, Vallar L, Faglia G. G protein oncogenes in pituitary tumors. Trends Endocrinol Metab 1992;3:355–360.
9. Dumont JE, Jauniaux J-C, Roger PP. The cyclic AMP-mediated stimulation of cell proliferation. Trends Biochem Sci 1989;14:67–71.
10. Burton FH, Hasel KW, Bloom FE, Sutcliffe JG. Pituitary hyperplasia and gigantism in mice caused by a cholera toxin transgene. Nature 1991;350:74–77.
11. Lyons J, Landis CA, Harsh G, Vallar L, Grünewald K, Feichtinger H, Duh Q-Y, Clark OH, Kawasaki E, Bourne HR, McCormick F. Two G protein oncogenes in human endocrine tumors. Science 1990;249:655–659.
12. Spada A, Arosio M, Bochicchio D, Bazzoni N, Vallar L, Bassetti M, Faglia G. Clinical, biochemical, and morphological correlates in patients bearing growth hormone-secreting pituitary tumors with or without constitutively active adenylyl cyclase. J Clin Endocrinol Metab 1990;71:1421–1426.
13. Landis CA, Harsh G, Lyons J, Davis RL, McCormick F, Bourne HR. Clinical characteristics of acromegalic patients whose pituitary tumors contain mutant Gs protein. J Clin Endocrinol Metab 1990;71:1416–1420.
14. Adams EF, Lei T, Buchfelder M, Petersen B, Fahlbusch R. Biochemical characteristics of human pituitary somatotropinomas with and without gsp mutations: in vitro cell culture studies. J Clin Endocrinol Metab 1995;80:2077–2081.

15. Harris PE, Alexander JM, Bikkal HA, Hsu DW, Hedley-Whyte ET, Klibanski A, Jameson JL. Glycoprotein hormone alpha-subunit production in somatotroph adenomas with and without Gs alpha mutations. J Clin Endocrinol Metab 1992;75:918–923.

16. Tordjman K, Stern N, Ouaknine G, Yossiphov Y, Razon N, Nordenskjold M, Friedman E. Activating mutations of the Gs alpha-gene in nonfunctioning pituitary tumors. J Clin Endocrinol Metab 1993;77:765–769.

17. Williamson EA, Ince PG, Harrison D, Kendall-Taylor P, Harris PE. G-protein mutations in human pituitary adrenocorticotrophic hormone-secreting adenomas. Eur J Clin Invest 1995;25:128–131.

18. Dong Q, Brucker-Davis F, Weintraub BD, Smallridge RC, Carr FE, Battey J, Spiegel AM, Shenker A. Screening of candidate oncogenes in human thyrotroph tumors: absence of activating mutations of the Gα-q, Gα-11, Gα-s, or thyrotropin-releasing hormone receptor genes. J Clin Endocrinol Metab 1996;81:1134–1140.

19. Muca C, Vallar L. Expression of mutationally activated G alpha s stimulates growth and differentiation of thyroid FRTL5 cells. Oncogene 1994;9:3647–3653.

20. O'Sullivan C, Barton CM, Staddon SL, Brown CL, Lemoine NR. Activating point mutations of the gsp oncogene in human thyroid adenomas. Mol Carcinog 1991;4:345–349.

21. Suarez HG, du Villard JA, Caillou B, Schlumberger M, Parmentier C, Monier R. gsp mutations in human thyroid tumours. Oncogene 1991;6:677–679.

22. Esapa C, Foster S, Johnson S, Jameson JL, Kendall-Taylor P, Harris PE. G protein and thyrotropin receptor mutations in thyroid neoplasia. J Clin Endocrinol Metab 1997;82:493–496.

23. Yoshimoto K, Iwahana H, Fukuda A, Sano T, Itakura M. Rare mutations of the Gs alpha subunit gene in human endocrine tumors. Mutation detection by polymerase chain reaction-primer-introduced restriction analysis. Cancer 1993;72:1386–1393.

24. Reincke M, Karl M, Travis W, Chrousos GP. No evidence for oncogenic mutations in guanine nucleotide-binding proteins of human adrenocortical neoplasms. J Clin Endocrinol Metab 1993;77:1419–1422.

25. Vessey SJ, Jones PM, Wallis SC, Schofield J, Bloom SR. Absence of mutations in the Gs alpha and Gi2 alpha genes in sporadic parathyroid adenomas and insulinomas. Clin Sci 1994;87:493–497.

26. Weinstein LS, Shenker A, Gejman PV, Merino MJ, Friedman E, Spiegel AM. Activating mutations of the stimulatory G protein in the McCune-Albright syndrome. N Engl J Med 1991;325:1688–1695.

27. Happle R. The McCune-Albright syndrome: a lethal gene surviving by mosaicism. Clin Genet 1986;29:321–324.

28. Schwindinger WF, Francomano CA, Levine MA. Identification of a mutation in the gene encoding the alpha subunit of the stimulatory G protein of adenylyl cyclase in McCune-Albright syndrome. Proc Natl Acad Sci USA 1992;89:5152–5156.

29. Shenker A, Weinstein LS, Sweet DE, Spiegel AM. An activating Gsa mutation is present in fibrous dysplasia of bone in the McCune-Albright syndrome. J Clin Endocrinol Metab 1994;79:750–755.

30. Malchoff CD, Reardon G, MacGillivray DC, Yamase H, Rogol AD, Malchoff DM. An unusual presentation of McCune-Albright syndrome confirmed by an activating mutation of the Gs alpha-subunit from a bone lesion. J Clin Endocrinol Metab 1994;78:803–806.

31. Dotsch J, Kiess W, Hanze J, Repp R, Ludecke D, Blum WF, Rascher W. Gs alpha mutation at codon 201 in pituitary adenoma causing gigantism in a 6-year-old boy with McCune-Albright syndrome. J Clin Endocrinol Metab 1996;81:3839–3842.

32. Boston BA, Mandel S, LaFranchi S, Bliziotes M. Activating mutation in the stimulatory guanine nucleotide-binding protein in an infant with Cushing's syndrome and nodular adrenal hyperplasia. J Clin Endocrinol Metab 1994;79:890–893.

33. Shenker A, Weinstein LS, Moran A, Pescovitz OH, Charest NJ, Van Wyk JJ, Merino MJ, Feuillan PP, Spiegel AM. Severe endocrine and non-endocrine manifestations of the McCune-Albright syndrome associated with activating mutations of the stimulatory G protein, Gs. J Pediatr 1993;123:509–518.

34. Shenker A, Chanson P, Weinstein LS, Chi P, Spiegel AM, Lomri A, Marie PJ. Osteoblastic cells derived from isolated lesions of fibrous dysplasia contain activating somatic mutations of the Gs alpha gene. Hum Mol Genet 1995;4:1675, 1676.

35. Feuillan PP, Jones J, Oerter KE, Manasco PK, Cutler GB, Jr. Luteinizing hormone-releasing hormone (LHRH)-independent precocious puberty unresponsive to LHRH agonist therapy in two girls lacking features of the McCune-Albright syndrome. J Clin Endocrinol Metab 1991;73:1370–1373.

36. Iiri T, Herzmark P, Nakamoto JM, Van Dop C, Bourne HR. Rapid GDP release from G_{sa} in patients with gain and loss of endocrine function. Nature 1994;371:164–168.

37. Candeliere GA, Glorieux FH, Prud'homme J, St-Arnaud R. Increased expression of the c-fos proto-oncogene in bone from patients with fibrous dysplasia. N Engl J Med 1995;332:1546–1551.

38. Yamamoto T, Ozono K, Kasayama S, Yoh K, Hiroshima K, Takagi M, Matsumoto S, Michigami T, Yamaoka K, Kishimoto T, Okada S. Increased IL-6 production by cells isolated from the fibrous bone dysplasia tissues in patients with McCune-Albright syndrome. J Clin Invest 1996;98:30–35.

39. O'Halloran DJ, Shalet SM. A family pedigree exhibiting features of both multiple endocrine neoplasia type 1 and McCune-Albright syndromes. J Clin Endocrinol Metab 1994;78:523–525.

40. Hosoi E, Yokogoshi Y, Hosoi E, Yokoi K, Sano T, Saito S. A pituitary specific point mutation of codon 201 of the Gs alpha gene in a pituitary adenoma of a patient with multiple endocrine neoplasia (MEN) type 1. Endocrinol Jpn 1992;39:319–324.

41. Williamson EA, Johnson SJ, Foster S, Kendall-Taylor P, Harris PE. G protein gene mutations in patients with multiple endocrinopathies. J Clin Endocrinol Metab 1995;80:1702–1705.

42. Sakurai A, Katai M, Furihata K, Hashizume K. Gs alpha mutation may be uncommon in patients with multiple endocrine neoplasia type 1. J Clin Endocrinol Metab 1996;81:2394–2396.

4

Ulcerative Colitis in Mice Lacking $G\alpha_{i2}$

Uwe Rudolph, MD *and Lutz Birnbaumer,* PHD

CONTENTS

INTRODUCTION
RESULTS
DISCUSSION
REFERENCES

INTRODUCTION

Functions Ascribed to $G\alpha_{i2}$ and Other PTX Substrates

"G_i" has first been identified as a negative regulator of adenylyl cyclase, one of the best-studied G-protein-coupled systems, and thus been named the "inhibitory" G protein. The α-subunit of G_i is adenosine diphosphate (ADP)-ribosylated by pertussis toxin and thus functionally uncoupled from the corresponding receptors. Three closely related cDNAs coding for $G\alpha_{i1}$, $G\alpha_{i2}$, and $G\alpha_{i3}$ have been cloned, and the corresponding proteins been identified by suptype-specific antibodies and purified. Recently, a putatively pertussis toxin-insensitive carboxy-terminal splice variant of $G\alpha_{i2}$ was discovered in the Golgi apparatus *(1)*.

The first biological function that could be ascribed to purified native G_i-proteins was the stimulation of inwardly rectifying K^+ channels of heart and endocrine cells *(2,3)*. As tested with recombinant proteins, all three G_is were able to mediate this effect. G_is also stimulate adenosine triphosphate (ATP)-sensitive K^+ channels in pancreatic cells and heart *(4)*. Surprisingly, it was difficult to demonstrate that G_is are indeed coupled to adenylyl cyclase in an inhibitory fashion *(5)*. $G\alpha_{i2}$ has further been demonstrated to be involved in the differentiation of F9 teratocarcinoma cells into primitive endoderm *(6)*, the regulation of fibroblast proliferation *(7)*, in the stimulation of the mitogen-activated protein (MAP) kinase pathway *(8)*, and has been demonstrated to be a proto-oncogene in Rat-1 cells. Rat-1 cells transfected with mutationally activated $G\alpha_{i2}$ form tumors in nude mice *(9)*. Furthermore, mutationally activated $G\alpha_{i2}$ has been found in human adrenal and ovarian tumors *(10)*. It has also been demonstrated that murine melanoma

From: *Contemporary Endocrinology: G Proteins, Receptors, and Disease*
Edited by: A. M. Spiegel, Humana Press Inc., Totowa, NJ

K-1735 cells are gowth-inhibited in vitro and in vivo by a dominant negative mutant $G\alpha_{i2}$ *(11)*. Although an involvement of $G\alpha_{i2}$ in the regulation of proliferative pathways has clearly been demonstrated, it is not known whether $G\alpha_{i1}$ and $G\alpha_{i3}$ may also serve similar functions.

A variety of functions have been ascribed to G_is on the basis of the pertussis toxin sensitivity of the respective pathways without identification of the specific subtype involved. These include stimulation of phohspholipase A_2 by the α_1-adrenergic receptor in FRTL-5 thyroid cells *(12)*, increase in phospholipase C activity in rat liver by EGF *(13)*, stimulation of a phosphotyrosine phosphatase in pancreatic (MIA PaCa-2) cells *(14)*, mediation of action of CSF-1 in promacrophages *(15)*, mediation of tumor necrosis factor (TNF) action in promacrophages *(16)*, zona pellucida-induced acrosome reaction of capacitated sperm cells *(17)*, negative regulation of vesicle budding from Golgi membranes *(18)*, mitogen-induced intracellular alkalinization in lung (CCL39) fibro-blasts *(19)*, stimulation of DNA synthesis by lysophosphatidic acid *(20)*, endosomal acidification *(21)*, maintenance of the differentiated state of cultered primary hepatocytes *(22)*, chemotactic peptide-induced signaling in leukocytes *(23)*, thymocyte maturation *(24)*, T-cell homing *(25)*, and regulation of cell proliferation *(26)*.

Experimentation has recently been expanded to study the functions of G proteins in vivo. Moxham et al. *(27)* developed transgenic mice expressing RNA antisense specific for $G\alpha_{i2}$ under the control of the phosphoenolpyruvate carboxykinase (PEPCK) promoter in selected tissues (fat, liver, kidney) after birth. The amount of fat and liver tissues was significantly reduced in these mice, which also displayed a failure to thrive and had an approx. 30% reduction in body weight at 6 and 12 wk of age, indicating systemic consequences of the absence of $G\alpha_{i2}$ in selected organs.

RESULTS

Generation of Mice Lacking $G\alpha_{i2}$

To learn more about the in vivo roles of $G\alpha_{i2}$, we decided to generate mice that are completely $G\alpha_{i2}$-deficient via homologous recombination in embryonic stem cells. Targeting vectors were constructed that have been described elsewhere *(28)*. Briefly, a mouse genomic $G\alpha_{i2}$ clone was isolated from a λ phage library, suitable sequences subcloned into plasmid vectors, and a neomycin resistance marker inserted into the *Nco*I site in exon 3. This targeting vector was then electroporated into AB1 embryonic stem stells *(29)*, and clones that had integrated the targeting vector in the predicted fashion at the $G\alpha_{i2}$ locus were injected into mouse blastocysts, which were then implanted into pseudopregnant foster mothers. The resulting male chimeras were bred to C57 BL6/J and 129SvEv wild-type females, and the transmission of the mutant allele monitored by Southern blotting *(30)*. Heterozygous mice were then intercrossed, and mice homo-zygous for the mutant allele obtained on both a crossbred and an inbred background. In order to ascertain that the mutated allele is a true null allele, the absence of $G\alpha_{i2}$ was demonstrated by both pertussis toxin-catalyzed [^{32}P]-ADP-ribosylation and by immunoblotting *(31,32)*.

Phenotype of Mice Lacking $G\alpha_{i2}$

DEVELOPMENT IN PERI- AND POSTNATAL PERIOD

Embryos resulting from intercrosses of crossbred (129SvEv × C57BL/6J) hetero-zygotes were genotyped on day 14. 11 +/+, 26 +/−, and 9 −/− crossbred embryos consistent with a Mendelian $1:2:1$ distribution were found. However, 4 wk after birth, the ratio was $86:142:34$ for crossbred and $61:116:24$ for inbred (129SvEv) embyros, indicating that a significant number of homozygous mutant embryos is lost between these two observation points. Since there were practically no losses after the perinatal period, homozygous mutant animals are lost either in late embryonic development or in the perinatal period. The processes underlying this potentially very interesting observation are currently not known.

Homozygous mutant animals apparently develop normally in the early postnatal period. At 4 wk of age, there is no detectable weight difference compared to wild-type animals. However, starting at 6 wk of age, the homozygous mutants fall below the weight of wild-type animals. Substantial mortality was observed: the mean age at spontaneous death was 21.2 ± 2.1 wk for 19 crossbred homozygous mutant mice and 14.7 ± 1.8 wk for 7 inbred homozygous mutant mice. Heterozyous mutant animals were indistinguishable from wild-type animals (which also holds true for the pathology; *see below*), indicating that the insertion of the neomycin resistance expression cassette does not produce a dominant phenotype.

ULCERATIVE COLITIS

Macroscopic examination of the abdominal situs of homozygous mutants revealed colons with irregular dilatations and focally thickened inflamed walls of the descending or of the entire colon (megacolon). In one mouse, a perforation and localized peritonitis was found. In a single case, there was also a marked dilatation and congestion of the duodenum. Otherwise, the small intestines were unremarkable, as were the other organs. Some mice in advanced stages also developed a rectal prolapse.

Microscopic examination of an inital series of 26 crossbred and inbred homozygous mutant mice revealed colitis of increasing frequency and severity in 21 mice *(31)*. Every mouse that was 13 wk or older had chronic active inflammation of the colon, and every colon was most heavily inflamed distally. In the early stages, an increased number of lymphocytes and plasma cells was present in the lamina propia slightly separating the crypts, as well as some collections of neutrophils in the lumen (crypt abscesses), whereas crypt architecture was normal and the epithelial lining intact; there was a minimal reduction in the quantity of mucus in the goblet cells. In later stages, the neutrophils permeated and destroyed individual crypts, and goblet cells were depleted of mucus (Fig. 1). Acute ulcerations were also found. The intensity and extent of colitis generally progressed with age. Two mice also displayed a small intestinal inflammation.

All inbred 129SvEv $G\alpha_{i2}$-deficient mice consistently develop colitis. On 129SvEv × Balb/c and 129Sv × C3H/HeN backgrounds, the frequency and severity of disease remained high. However, when breeding the mutated allele on a 129SvEv × C57BL/6 background for several generations, the incidence of disease, which was also less severe, was low, indicating that, in addition to the $G\alpha_{i2}$ gene, other disease susceptibility genes play a role in development of colitis in these mice (Gregory R. Harriman, personal communication).

ADENOCARCINOMA OF THE COLON

Homozygous mutant mice with colonic ulcerations displayed foci of regenerative proliferation throughout the full thickness of the mucosa, in some cases penetrating into the submucosa. In eight mice (i.e., 31% of $G\alpha_{i2}$-deficient mice in this series), there were highly

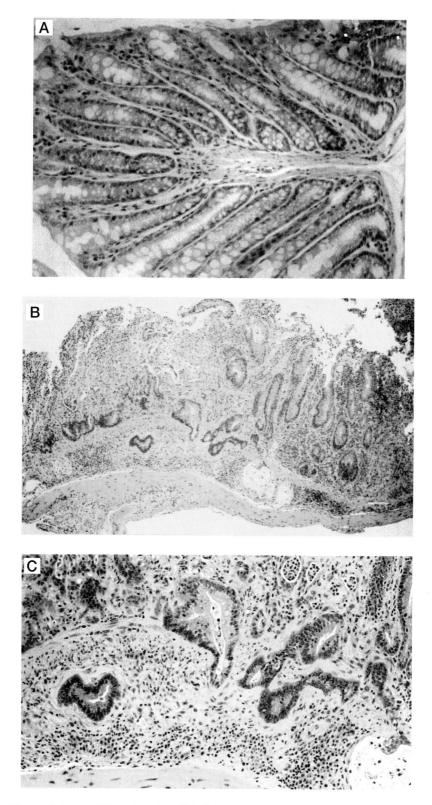

Fig. 1. Histopathology of $G\alpha_{i2}$–/– mice. **(A)** Colon of a 9-wk-old wild-type mouse. The glands (crypts), which are lined with goblet cells containing mucus, are straight and regular with little intervening stroma (lamina propria). The border of the epithelial surface is intact. **(B,C)** Sigmoid of a 23-wk-old α_{i2}–/– mouse. The surface epithelium has been replaced by an inflammatory exudate. Large pools of mucus can be seen in the submucosa. Complex and distorted glands have broken through the muscularis mucosae, suggesting an invasive adenocarcinoma.

atypical glands showing back-to-back growth without intervening stroma, loss of nuclear polarity, and severe crowding, indicating cancer of the colon *(31)*. These cancers were in all regions of the colon; in three mice, two separate cancerous foci were found. In one mouse, the cecum was nodular grossly, and this was owing to an invasive mucin-producing carcinoma with flattened neoplastic cells surrounding the large pools of mucus in the deep submucosa and muscularis. No metastatic dissemination was observed in any animal.

Inbred homozygous mutant mice raised in an SPF barrier facility also developed ulcerative colitis and adenocarcinoma of the colon, thus largely excluding common mouse pathogens as the cause of the observed phenotype.

T- AND B-CELL MATURATION AND FUNCTION

Flow cytometric analysis revealed a two- to fourfold increase in the proportion of α_{i2}–/–thymocytes with $CD4^+8^-$ or $CD4^-8^+$ single positive phenotype and a threefold increase in cells expressing high-intensity CD3-staining characteristic of mature thymocytes. Spleen and lymph node α_{i2}–/– T-cells were indistinguishable from normal controls. α_{i2}–/– Thymocytes exhibited hightened proliferation in response to stimulation by immobilized anti-CD3ε (with or without addition of the phorbol ester PMA), staphylococcal enterotoxin A, and Balb/c ($H-2^d$) T-depleted splenocytes in mixed lymphocyte reactions, consistent with the increased frequency of mature thymocytes. Immobilized anti-CD3ε (with or without PMA) or PMA/ionomycin stimulated α_{i2}–/– thymocytes to produce several-fold increased IL-2, IFN-γ and TNF, but not IL-4 levels, even after normalization of cytokine levels to 100% $CD3^{hi}$ cells of control and mutant populations. α_{i2}–/– peripheral T-cells produced IL-2, IFN-γ and TNF levels that were elevated up to 80-fold over those of wild-type T-cells, depending on cytokine and stimulus; IL-4 was more modestly enhanced. Thus, peripheral α_{i2}–/– T-cells migrate properly to spleen and lymph nodes, but retain a hyperresponsive cytokine production profile *(31)*. It is currently not clear whether the alterations in the immune system play a role in the pathogenesis of the ulcerative colitits observed in the $G\alpha_{i2}$-deficient mice.

Analysis of the B-cell phenotype in bone marrow and spleen of $G\alpha_{i2}$-deficient mice did not reveal any substantial defects in B-cell development (except for an increase in granulocytes in spleen as well as in peripheral blood in 8-wk-old animals). Plasma IgM levels were unaffected, whereas plasma IgG and IgA levels were elevated approximately twofold.

Analysis of immunoglobulins in large and small intestinal secretions showed that IgA predominates in both α_{i2}+/+ and α_{i2}–/– mice, but was elevated in α_{i2}–/– mice. IgG was markedly (ca. 60-fold) elevated in the large intestine of α_{i2}–/– mice and more modestly (approximately fivefold) in the small intestine, whereas IgM was elevated only in the large intestine *(33)*. This pattern corresponds to the pathological process primarily affecting the large intestine.

The mucosal immune system of the $G\alpha_{i2}$-deficient mice was examined in detail by Hörnquist et al. *(33)*. Large intestinal lamina propria lymphocytes displayed a large increase in memory $CD4^+$ T-cells ($CD44^{hi}$, $CD45RB^{lo}$, $CD62L^{lo}$). In addition, the mucosal homing receptor integrin β7 was increased on mucosal, but not on systemic $CD4^+$ T-cells. There were increases in production of proinflammatory Th1-type cytokines (IFN-γ, IL-1β, IL-6,TNF) and also of IL-12 mRNA, the key cytokine that directs the immune response toward a Th1-dominated response. Th-2-type cytokines were not increased.

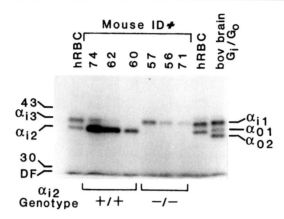

Fig. 2. PTX-catalyzed [^{32}P]-ADP-ribosylation of normal and Gα_{i2}-deficient RBC membranes. Red blood cell membrane aliquots from three $\alpha_{i2}+/+$ mice (74,60,62) and three $\alpha_{i2}-/-$ mice (57,56,71) were [^{32}P]-ADP-ribosylated with pertussis toxin and subjected to 4–8M urea gradient/9% polyacrylamide SDS-PAGE and subsequent autoradiography essentially as described previously *(32)*. Human red blood cell membranes (containing α_{i2} and α_{i3}) and a bovine G$_i$/G$_o$ preparation have been included as controls.

ALTERED G-PROTEIN SUBUNIT EXPRESSION AND ADP-RIBOSYLATION PATTERNS

The α-subunits of G$_i$ and G$_o$ proteins are substrates for pertussis toxin catalyzed ^{32}P-ADP-ribosylation. Folllowing SDS-PAGE on a double urea and polyacrylamide gradient, Gα_{i2} has a higher mobility than Gα_{i1} and Gα_{i3} (which have an about equal mobility). Gα_{o1} comigrates with Gα_{i2} or displays an intermediate mobility running between Gα_{i2} and Gα_{i1}/Gα_{i3}. Gα_{o2} migrates faster than Gα_{i2} *(34)*. Red blood cell membranes from $\alpha_{i2}+/+$ mice contain Gα_{i2} and Gα_{i3}, whereas red blood cell membranes from $\alpha_{i2}-/-$ mice contain Gα_{i3}, but not Gα_{i2} (Fig. 2). Membranes from $\alpha_{i2}+/+$ adipocytes display two bands corresponding to Gα_{i2} and Gα_{i1}/Gα_{i3}. In membranes from $\alpha_{i2}-/-$ adipocytes, however, only one band corresponding to Gα_{i1}/Gα_{i3} was visible. The absence of a band corresponding to Gα_{i2} also indicates the absence of detectable amounts of Gα_{o1} or Gα_{o2} *(32)*. Likewise, labeling of skeletal muscle membranes showed two bands in $\alpha_{i2}+/+$ membranes and only one (the upper) in $\alpha_{i2}-/-$ membranes, indicating the absence of detectable amounts of Gα_{o1} or Gα_{o2} (Fig. 3B). Similar results were obtained with skeletal muscle homogenates (Fig. 3A). The presence of Gα_o species in these tissues has been controversial *(35–37)*. In both thymus and fibroblast homogenates, it was noticed that the labeling intensity of the Gα_{i2} band appeared to be reduced with respect to that of the Gα_{i3} band in $\alpha_{i2}+/-$ as compared to $\alpha_{i2}+/+$ samples *(32)*.

Primary embryonic fibroblasts derived from matings of inbred heterozygotes were immortalized by transfection with Simian Virus 40 (SV40) T-antigen. Western analysis with α_{common}, β_{common}, Gα_{i2}, and Gα_{i3} polyclonal antibodies revealed:

1. That Gα_{i2} is not expressed in $\alpha_{i2}-/-$ fibroblasts;
2. A parallel reduction in the abundance of Gα- and Gβ-subunits to about 50%; and
3. A ca. 30–50% increase of Gα_{i3} in $\alpha_{i2}-/-$ cell homogenates compared to $\alpha_{i2}+/+$ cell homogenates *(32)*.

These results indicate that the inactivation of the Gα_{i2} gene may lead to compensatory changes in cell homeostasis.

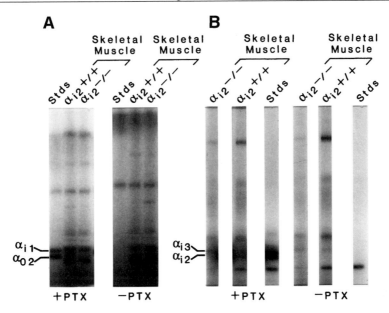

Fig. 3. Pertussis toxin substrates in skeletal muscle homogenates (**A**) and membranes (**B**). Skeletal muscle was excised from the back and homogenized in 10 vol of homogenization medium *(32)*. For preparations of membranes, the homogenate was centrifuged at 365*g* for 10′ at 4°C. The loose sediment was discarded, the supernatant centrifuged at 27,300*g* for 10′ at 4°C, and the pellet resuspended in homogenization medium. Pertussis toxin-catalyzed [^{32}P]-ADP-ribosylation was performed as described in the legend to Fig. 2. Reactions without pertussis toxin served as controls to identify nonspecific labeling. Standards were bovine G_i/G_o (A) and human red bood cell membranes (B).

INHIBITORY REGULATION OF ADENYLYL CYCLASE

In heart homogenates from crossbred α_{i2}+/+ mice, isoproterenol-stimulated adenylyl cyclase activity is inhibited by ca. 32% in the presence of 100 μ*M* carbachol. In contrast, in heart homogenates from crossbred α_{i2}–/– mice, the inhibition is reduced to ca. 12% *(32)*. Thus, hormonal inhibition of adenylyl cyclase can still be achieved in α_{i2}–/– heart homogenates, but only to a significantly reduced degree, indicating that native $G\alpha_{i1}$ and/or $G\alpha_{i3}$ is able to mediate this effect, but cannot fully substitute for the loss of $G\alpha_{i2}$. Inhibition of isoproterenol-stimulated adenylyl cyclase was also examined in adipocyte membranes prepared from individual animals. In α_{i2}+/+ membranes, the adenylyl cyclase could be inhibited with prostaglandin E2, phenylisopropyladenosine, and nicotinic acid. Inactivation of $G\alpha_{i2}$ resulted in two distinct phenotypes: in 5 of 10 animals, there was a blunting of the inhibitory responses, which were reduced by roughly 50%. In the other five animals, the inhibitory responses were indistinguishable from wild-type *(32)*. It is noteworthy, however, that animals showing no effect on inhibition of adenylyl cyclase in fat cells displayed a blunted carbachol-induced inhibition of adenylyl cyclase in heart homogenates. It is possible that the incomplete penetrance of the phenotype in the adipocytes is owing to the fact that the experiments were performed with 129SvEv × C57BL/6J crossbred mice and that the genetic background is at least partially responsible for the variability. In order to test whether the residual adenylyl cyclase inhibition is mediated by pertussis toxin-sensitive or pertussis toxin-insensitive G proteins, we inhibited isoproterenol-stimulated adenylyl cyclase activity in SV40-transformed fibroblasts

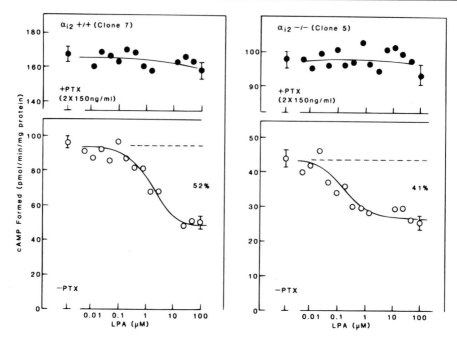

Fig. 4. Inhibition of adenylyl cyclase in SV40-transformed $\alpha_{i2}+/+$ and $\alpha_{i2}-/-$ fibroblast homogenates. The hormone-stimulated enzyme (10 μM GTP, 10 μM isoproterenol) was inhibited with the indicated concentrations of LPA. cAMP formation is plotted against the LPA concentration. The open circles represent data points obtained without pretreatment, and the closed circles represent data points obtained with pretreatment of the cells with 2×150 ng/mL pertussis toxin overnight.

with increasing concentrations of lysophosphatitid acid (LPA). In both $\alpha_{i2}+/+$ and $\alpha_{i2}-/-$ fibroblasts, a significant inhibition (ca. 40–50%) of cAMP formation was found, which could be almost completely inhibited by pretreatment of the cells with pertussis toxin (Fig. 4). These results further support the notion that $G\alpha_{i1}$ and/or $G\alpha_{i3}$ mediates hormonal inhibition of adenylyl cyclase. It is of particular interest that we functionally demonstrated the coupling of four receptors to $G\alpha_{i2}$ as well as to other $G\alpha_i$ proteins. Furthermore, Raymond et al. *(38)* reported that cAMP accumulation can still be inhibited in ES cells devoid of $G\alpha_{i2}$ via a transfected α_{2A}-adrenergic receptor, whereas Simonds et al. *(39)* were able to block α_2-adrenergic inhibition of adenylyl cyclase in platelet membranes by preincubation with a C-terminal $G\alpha_{i2}$ antibody. These findings may indicate that receptor–G-protein interactions are selective rather than specific and that the specificity observed by Kleuss et al. *(40–42)* is not necessarily the rule. It is possible that a receptor–G-protein–effector interaction may be dependent on the subcellular distribution of the components involved, leading to specificity at the subcellular level.

DISCUSSION

Moxham et al. *(27)* expressed in transgenic mice an antisense RNA to $G\alpha_{i2}$ in a hybrid RNA construct involving rat phosphoenolpyruvate carboxykinase sequences whose expression was specific for liver, fat, and kidney, and was induced at birth. A major characteristic of these mice was a failure to thrive. Tissue weights of fat and liver were significantly decreased, as was the body weight (approx 30% at 6 and 12 wk and approx 20% at 18 wk) (*See* Chapter 5). The body weight of $G\alpha_{i2}$-deficient knockout mice is, however, indistinguishable from wild-type controls at 4 wk of age. It is surprising that a >90% suppression of $G\alpha_{i2}$ in selected organs of $G\alpha_{i2}$ antisense mice may have a more drastic effect in early postnatal development than a standard gene knockout. This may be owing, for example, to differences in the genetic background or with adaptation processes. With tissues derived from the $G\alpha_{i2}$ antisense mice, it was also demonstrated that inhibition of cAMP accumulation in adipocytes by phenylisopropyladenosine is attenuated *(43)*. Other experiments suggest that phospholipase C signaling is enhanced in adipocytes from the $G\alpha_{i2}$ antisense mice and in cell lines transfected with the $G\alpha_{i2}$ antisense construct *(44)*; the molecular basis and the potential physiological relevance of these observations are not clear. Most interestingly, it has been reported that the $G\alpha_{i2}$ antisense mice have elevated fasting serum insulin levels, an abnormal glucose tolerance, and insulin resistance, and thus, constitute an animal model for noninsulin-dependent diabetes mellitus (NIDDM) *(45)*. It could be demonstrated that suppression of $G\alpha_{i2}$ increases the protein tyrosine phosphatase activity and attenuates insulin-stimulated tyrosine phosphorylation of insulin receptor substrate 1 (IRS-1) in vivo, thus providing a potential molecular explanation for the phenotypic alterations *(45)*. It is currently not known whether $G\alpha_{i2}$ knockout mice display a similar phenotype.

Using pertussis toxin as a tool to block G_i function, apparently conflicting results have been obtained in in vitro studies with regard to activation and inhibition of T-cells. This might be owing to effects of the B-oligomer of pertussis toxin, which may produce mitogenesis in T-cells independent of the ADP-ribosyltransferase activity of the S1-subunit. Therefore, Perlmutter and collaborators *(25)* expressed the S1-subunit in transgenic mice in the T-cell lineage from the lymphocyte-specific *lck* promoter to define the role of G_i-proteins in T-cell signal transduction. They demonstrated that the pertussis toxin substrates (G_{i2} and G_{i3}) are profoundly depleted in transgenic thymocytes. Treatment of the transgenic thymocytes with mitogenic stimuli leads to increases in intracellular free Ca^{2+} concentrations and IL-2 secretion indistinguishable from wild-type controls, indicating that G_i-proteins are not required for T-cell activation. However, mature T-cells accumulated in the thymus and failed to migrate to peripheral lymphoid organs, suggesting that G_i proteins are involved in thymocyte emigration *(24,25)*. The S1-transgenic mice displayed an increase in CD4$^+$CD8$^-$ and CD4$^-$CD8$^+$ single positive thymoctes with high-intensity CD3 staining, as was also observed for the $G\alpha_{i2}$-deficient mice. This similarity also includes increased expression of the lymph node homing receptor, Mel-14, and greater proportions of J11d$^-$ and CD44^{lo} cells. Despite these striking similarities indicating an increased proportion of mature T-cells in the thymus similar to those that are normally found in peripheral lymphoid organs, S1-transgenic T-cells display a profound deficiency in the population of the spleen (rarely more than 15% of wild-type controls up to 10 wk of age), whereas in $G\alpha_{i2}$-deficient mice, the population of the spleen by T-cells was normal. This discrepancy in the phenotype may point to a crucial role for $G\alpha_{i3}$ (or a combined action of $G\alpha_{i2}$ and $G\alpha_{i3}$) in lymphocyte homing to peripheral organs. Inactivation of $G\alpha_{i3}$ by gene targeting should prove or disprove this hypothesis. It might also be possible that the S1-subunit exerts toxic effects in thymocytes. Since S1-transgenic thymocytes display no increase of the intracellular cAMP concentration, it appears unlikely that the inhibition of adenylyl cyclase activity by G_i

proteins plays an essential role for emigration. In S1-transgenic thymocytes, IL-2 secretion after stimulation by T-cell-activating signals was indistinguishable from normal controls. However, in $G\alpha_{i2}$-deficient thymoctes, it was significantly increased. The reasons for this difference in the phenotypes are unclear. One potential explanation is that the inactivation of G_i proteins in S1-transgenic thymocytes may not be complete, and thus, potential essential functions of G_i proteins in T-cell activation may be "rescued" by residual G_i. It was not reported directly whether the S1-transgenic mice also developed a colonic inflammation. However, there are indications that they did not (46). Thus, it is unlikely that the accumulation of single positive mature T-cells in the thymus is solely responsible for the development of the gut inflammation in $G\alpha_{i2}$-deficient mice. It is noteworthy, however, that the S1 transgenic mice were backcrosses to C57BL/6, a background that may suppress the development of colitis in the $G\alpha_{i2}$-deficient mice. The partially overlapping and partially distinct phenotpye of S1-transgenic mice and $G\alpha_{i2}$-deficient mice may be of help in the delineation of the functions of G_i-proteins in the immune system.

Mice with targeted disruptions of IL-2, IL-10, $\alpha\beta$ T-cell receptor, and MHC class II develop a chronic inflammation of the bowel (47–49). In contrast, RAG-1 mice, which are lacking both functional B-cells and T-cells, do not develop a colonic inflammation (49). However, there are important differences between these mouse strains. By 9 wk of age, 50% of the IL-2-deficient mice had died of an early disease consisting of splenomegaly, lymphadenopathy, and severe anemia. The remaining animals developed an ulcerative colitis limited to the colon and rectum and widespread amyloidosis (liver, spleen, kidneys). IL-10-deficient mice developed a chronic enterocolitis predominantly affecting duodenum, adjoining jejunum, and colon; in addition to weight loss, they have severe anemia. In the mice lacking functional $\alpha\beta$ T-cells, the inflam-mation was limited to colon and rectum, but there was no mucosal ulceration present. Of 224 $\alpha\beta$ T-cell-deficient mice, three developed tumors (a benign adenomatous polyp in the colon of a 6-mo-old mouse, a rectal adenocarcinoma in an 11-mo-old mouse and a thymic lymphoma in a 7-mo-old mouse). Of all models cited, only in the $G\alpha_{i2}$-deficient mice is adenocarcinoma of the colon a typical feature of the bowel disease. SCID mice reconstituted with CD45RB[hi] CD4[+] cells also developed a chronic inflammation of the bowel, which could be prevented by cotransfer of the reciprocal CD45RB[lo] CD4[+] T cells (50,51). Taken together, these findings indicate that intact mucosal immune function is necessary for homeostasis in the intestinal mucosa.

Hermiston and Gordon (52) expressed a dominant negative N-Cadherin lacking an extracellular domain (NCADΔ) from the fatty acid binding protein gene (Fabp) that is active in the small intestine in undifferentiated crypt epithelial cells and the enterocytes, mucin-producing goblet cells, enteroendocrine cells, and Paneth cells in chimeric mice derived from ES cells. Expression of NCADΔ along the entire crypt-villus axis led to characteristic histopathological changes, such as transmural inflammation, numerous lymphoid aggregates, lymphangiectasia, cryptitis, crypt abscesses, goblet cell depletion, Paneth cell hyperplasia, perturbed crypt-villus architecture, and aphtoid as well as larger linear mucosal ulcers, reminiscent of Crohn's disease. In addition, the chimeras also developed adenomas (in inflamed and noninflamed patches), which did not progress to carcinomas. Cadherins are transmembrane glycoproteins mediating adhesive interaction between cells. It has been determined previously that NCADΔ expressed in postmitotic enterocytes causes loss of endogenous N-cadherin from the cell surface, disruption of cell–cell and cell–matrix contacts, increased rates of cell migration, and precocious entry of enterocytes into a death program *(53)*. The mechanisms responsible for the association of inflammatory bowel disease and intestinal neoplams are not known. The NCADΔ chimeras demonstrate that a distinct molecular defect, namely the perturbation of endogenous cadherins in the crypt epithelium, may lead to both inflammation and neoplasia. Thus, mice deficient for immunoregulatory molecules develop inflammation, but apparently no neoplasia, whereas the NCADΔ mice develop both. It will be interesting to see whether the inflammatory bowel disease in the Gα_{i2}-deficient mice is owing to perturbation of the immune system and/or to a local effect on the gut epithelium. In addition, it may be possible to determine why the Gα_{i2}-deficient mice develop neoplasia, whereas others do not.

ACKNOWLEDGMENTS

The authors thank their collaborators Susan S. Rich (T-cell analysis), Gregory R. Harriman (B-cell analyis), and Milton J. Finegold (Histopathology) for their contributions to the analysis of the phenotype of the Gα_{i2}-deficient mice.

REFERENCES

1. Montmayeur JP, Borrelli E. Targeting of Gαi2 to the Golgi by alternative spliced carboxyl-terminal region. Science 1994;263:95–98.
2. Yatani A, Codina J, Sekura RD, Birnbaumer L, Brown AM. Reconstitution of somatostatin and muscarinic receptor mediated stimulation of K$^+$ channels by isolated G$_k$ protein in clonal rat anterior pituitary cell membranes, Mol Endocrinol 1987;1:283–289.
3. Yatani A, Mattera R, Codina J, Graf R, Okabe K, Padrell E, Iyengar R, Brown AM, Birnbaumer L. The G protein-gated atrial K$^+$ channel is stimulated by three distinct G$_{i\alpha}$ subunits. Nature 1988;336: 680–682.
4. Kirsch G, Codina J, Birnbaumer L, Brown AM. Coupling of ATP-sensitive K$^+$ channels to purinergic receptors by G proteins in rat venticular myocytes. Am J Physiol 1990;259:H820–H826.
5. Taussig R, Iñiguez-Lluhi JA, Gilman AG. Inhibition of adenylyl cyclase by G$_{i\alpha}$. Science 1993;261: 218–221.
6. Watkins DC, Johnson GL, Malbon CC. Regulation of the differentiation of teratocarcinoma cells into primitive endoderm by Gα_{i2}. Science 1992;258:1373–1375.
7. Hermouet S, Merendino JJ, Gutkind JS, Spiegel AM. Activating and inactivating mutations of the α subunit of G$_{i2}$ protein have opposite effects on proliferation of NIH 3T3 cells. Proc Natl Acad Sci USA 1991;88:10,455–10,459.
8. Gupta SK, Gallego C, Johnoson G, Heasley LE. MAP kinase is constitutively activated in gip2 and src transformed Rat-1a fibroblasts. J Biol Chem 1992;267:7987–7990.
9. Pace AM, Wong YH, Bourne HR. A mutant α subunit of G$_{i2}$ induced neoplastic transformation of Rat-1 cells. Proc Natl Acad Sci USA 1991;88:7031–7035.
10. Lyons J, Landis CA, Harsh G, Vallar L, Grünewald K, Feichtinger H, Duh QY, Clark OH, Kawasaki E, Bourne HR, McCormick F. Two G protein oncogenes in human endocrine tumors. Science 1990;249:655–659.
11. Hermouet S, Aznavoorian S, Spiegel AM. *In vitro* and *in vivo* growth inhibition of murine melanoma K-1735 cells by a dominant negative mutant α subunit of the Gi2α protein. Cell Signal 1996;8:159–166.
12. Burch RM, Luini A, Axelrod J. Phospholipase A$_2$ and phospholipase C are activated by distinct GTP-binding proteins in response to alpha$_1$-adrenergic stimulation in FRTL-5 cells. Proc Natl Acad Sci USA 1986;83:7201–7205.
13. Yang L, Baffy G, Rhee SG, Manning D, Hansen CA, Williamson JR. Pertussis toxin-sensitive G$_i$ protein involvement in epidermal growth factor-induced activation of phospholipase C-γ in rat hepatocytes. J Biol Chem 1991;266:22,451–22,458.
14. Pan MG, Florio T, Stork PJS. G protein activation of a hormone-stimulated phosphatase in human tumor cells. Science 1992;256:1215–1217.
15. Imamura K, Kufe D. CSF-1 Induced Na$^+$ influx Into human monocytes involves activation of a pertussis toxin sensitive GTP-binding protein. J Biol Chem 1988;263:14,093–14,098.

16. Imamura K, Sherman ML, Spriggs D, Kufe D. Effect of tumor necrosis factor on GTP binding and GTPase activity in HL-60 and L929 Cells. J Biol Chem 1988;263:1–7.

17. Endo Y, Lee MA, Kopf G. Evidence for the role of a guanine nucleotide binding regulatory protein in the zona pellucida-induced mouse sperm acrosome reaction. Dev Biol 1987;119:210–216.

18. Leyte A, Barr FA, Kehlenbach RH, Huttner, WB. Mutliple trimeric G-proteins on the trans-Golgi network exert stimulatory and inhibitory effects on secretory vesicle formaton. EMBO J 1992;11:4795–4804.

19. Paris S, Pouysségur J. Pertussis toxin inhibits thrombin-induced activation of phosphoinositide hydrolysis and Na^+/H^+ exchange in hamster fibroblasts. EMBO J 1986;5:55–60.

20. van Corven EJ, Groenink A, Jalink K, Eichholtz T, Molenaar WH. Lysophosphatidate-induced cell proliferation: identification and dissection of signaling pathways mediated by G proteins. Cell 1989;50:45–54.

21. Gurich RW, Codina J, DuBose TD Jr. A potential role for guanine nucleotide-binding protein (G protein) in the regulation of endosomal proton transport. J Clin Invest 1991;87:1547–1552.

22. Itoh H, Okajima F, Ui M. Conversion of adrenergic mechanisms from an α- to a β-type during primary culture of rat hepatocytes. Accompanying decreases in the function of the inhibitory guanine nucleotide regulatory component of adenylate cyclase identified as the substrate of islet-activating protein. J Biol Chem 1984;259:15,464–15,473.

23. Wu D, LaRosa GJ, Simon MI. G protein-coupled signal transduction pathways for interleukin-8. Science 1993;261:101–103.

24. Chaffin KE, Perlmutter RM. A pertussis toxin-sensitive process controls thymocyte emigration. Eur J Immunol 1991;21:2565–2573.

25. Chaffin KE, Beals CR, Wilkie TM, Forbush KA, Simon MI, Perlmutter RM. Dissection of thymocyte signaling pathways by in vivo expression of pertussis toxin ADP-ribosyltransferase. EMBO J 1990;9: 3821–3829.

26. Hildebrandt JD, Stolzenberg E, Graves J. Pertussis toxin alters growth characteristics of Swiss 3T3 cells. FEBS Lett 1986;203:87–90.

27. Moxham CM, Hod Y, Malbon CC. Induction of $G\alpha_{i2}$-specific antisense RNA in vivo inhibits neonatal growth. Science 1993;260:991–995.

28. Rudolph U, Bradley A, Birnbaumer L. Targeted inactivation of the $G_{i2}\alpha$ gene with replacements and insertion vectors: analysis in a 96-well plate format. Methods Enzymol 1994;237, 366–386.

29. McMahon AP, Bradley A. The Wnt-1 (int-1) proto-oncogene is required for development of a large region of the mouse brain. Cell 1990;62:1073–1085.

30. Rudolph U, Brabet P, Hasty P, Bradley A, Birnbaumer L. Disruption of the $G_{i2}\alpha$ locus in embryonic stem cells and mice: a modified hit and run strategy with detection by a PCR dependent on gap repair. Transgenic Res 1993;2:345–355.

31. Rudolph U, Finegold MJ, Rich SS, Harriman GR, Srinivasan Y, Brabet P, Boulay G, Bradley A, Birnbaumer L. Ulcerative colitis and adenocarcinoma of the colon in $G\alpha_{i2}$-deficient mice. Nature Genet 1995;10:143–150.

32. Rudolph U, Spicher K, Birnbaumer L. Adenylyl cyclase inhibition and altered G protein subunit expression and ADP-ribosylation patterns in tissues and cells from $G\alpha_{i2}$–/– mice. Proc Natl Acad Sci USA 1996;93:3209–3214.

33. Hörnquist CE, Lu X, Rogers-Fani PM, Rudolph U, Shappell S, Birnbaumer L, Harriman GR. $G\alpha_{i2}$-deficient mice with colitis exhibit a local increase in memory $CD4^+$ T cells and pro-inflammatory Th1-type cytokines. J Immunol 1997;158:1068–1077.

34. Codina J, Grenet D, Chang KJ, Birnbaumer L. Urea gradient/SDS-PAGE: a useful tool in the investigation of signal transducing G proteins. Journal of Receptor Research 1991;11:587–601.

35. Homburger V, Brabet P, Audigier Y, Pantaloni C, Bockaert J, Rouot B. Immunological localization of the GTP binding protein G_o in different tissues of vertebrates and invertebrates. Mol Pharmacol 1987;31:313–319.

36. Toutant M, Gabrion J, Vandaele S, Peraldi-Roux S, Barhanin J, Bockaert J, Rouot B. Cellular distribution and biochemical characterization of G proteins in skeletal muscle: comparative location with voltage-dependent calcium channels. EMBO J 1990;9:363–369.

37. Hinsch KD, Rosenthal W, Spicher K, Binder T, Gausepohl H, Frank R, Schultz G, Joost, HG. Adipocyte plasma membranes contain two G_i subtypes but are devoid of G_o. FEBS Lett 1988;238:191–196.

38. Raymond JR, Arthur JM, Casanas SJ, Olsen CL, Gettys TW, Mortensen RM. α_{2A} Adrenergic receptors inhibit cAMP accumulation in embryonic stem cells which lack $G_{i\alpha2}$. J Biol Chem 1994;269: 13073–13075.

39. Simonds WF, Goldsmith PK, Codina J, Unson CG, Spiegel AM. G_{i2} mediates α_2-adrenergic inhibition of adenylyl cyclase in platelet membranes: in situ identification with G_α C-terminal antibodies. Proc Natl Acad Sci USA 1989;86:7809–7813.

40. Kleuss C, Hescheler J, Ewel C, Rosenthal W, Schultz G, Wittig B. Assignment of G protein subtypes to specific receptors inducing inhibition of calcium currents. Nature 1991;353:43–48.

41. Kleuss C, Scherübl H, Hescheler J, Schultz G, Wittig B. Different β-subunits determine G protein interaction with transmembrane receptors. Nature 1992;358:424–426.

42. Kleuss C, Scherübl H, Hescheler J, Schultz G, Wittig B. Selectivity in signal transduction determined by γ subunits of heterotrimeric G proteins. Science 1993;259:832–834.

43. Moxham CM, Hod Y, Malbon CC. $G_{i\alpha2}$ mediates the inhibitory regulation of adenylylcyclase in vivo: analysis intransgenic mice with $G_{i\alpha2}$ suppressed by inducible antisense RNA. Dev Genet 1993; 14:266–273.

44. Watkins DC, Moxham CM, Morris J, Malbon CC. Suppression of $G_{i\alpha2}$ enhances phospholipase C signalling. Biochem J 1994;299:593–596.

45. Moxham CM, Malbon CC. Insulin action impaired by deficiency of the G-protein subunit $G_{i\alpha2}$. Nature 1996;379:840–844.

46. Spiegel A. G protein knockout hits the gut. Nature Med 1993;1:522–524.

47. Sadlack B, Merz H, Schorle H, Schimpl A, Feller AC, Horak I. Ulcerative colitis-like disease in mice with a disrupted interleukin-2 gene. Cell 1993;75:253–261.

48. Kühn R, Löhler J, Rennick D, Rajewsky K, Müller W. Interleukin-10-deficient mice develop chronic enterocolitis. Cell 1993;75:263–274.

49. Mombaerts P, Mizoguchi E, Grusby MJ, Glimcher LH, Bhan AK, Tonegawa S. Spontaneous development of inflammatory bowel disease in T cell receptor mutant mice. Cell 1993;75:275–282.

50. Morrissey PJ, Charrier K, Braddy S, Liggitt D, Watson JD. CD4[+] T cells that express high levels of CD45RB induce wasting disease when transferred into congenic severe combined immunodeficient mice. Disease development is prevented by cotransfer of purified CD4[+] T cells. J Exp Med 1993; 178:237–244.

51. Powrie F, Leach MW, Mauze S, Caddle LB, Coffman RL. Phenotypically distinct subsets of CD4[+] T cells induce or protect from chronic intestinal inflammation in C.B-17 scid mice. Int Immunol 1993;5:1461–1471.

52. Hermiston ML, Gordon JI. Inflammatory bowel disease and adenomas in mice expressing a dominant negative N-cadherin. Science 1995;270:1203–1207.

53. Hermiston ML, Gordon JI. In vivo analysis of cadherin function in the mouse intestinal epithelium: essential roles in adhesion, maintenance of differentiation, and regulation of programmed cell death. J Cell Biol 1995;129:489–506.

5

G Proteins Regulating Insulin Action and Obesity

Analysis by Conditional, Targeted Expression of Antisense RNA in vivo

Craig C. Malbon, PhD, Patricia Galvin-Parton, MD, Hsien-yu Wang, PhD, Jun Hua Guo, MD, and Christopher M. Moxham, PhD

CONTENTS

INTRODUCTION

This chapter introduces a novel approach to the study of G-protein function in vivo in which transgenic mice are created that harbor a conditional, tissue-specific expression vector that can produce RNA antisense to target mRNA(s). The central role of G proteins in transmembrane signaling from the superfamily of G-protein-linked receptors (GPLRs) to a less populous class of effector molecules that includes adenyl cyclase, phospholipase C (PLC), and various ion channels needs little explanation (see earlier review articles 1–10). Much less obvious is the pivotal role G proteins play in more complex biological processes, such as growth and development. Infectious diseases such as cholera and whooping cough, for example, express elements of their pathology via covalent modification (mono-adenosine diphosphate [ADP]-ribosylation) of G-protein targets. In

From: *Contemporary Endocrinology: G Proteins, Receptors, and Disease*
Edited by: A. M. Spiegel Humana Press Inc., Totowa, NJ

endocrine tissues, mutations of specific G-protein subunits have been shown to induce tumor growth *(11)*. Finally, genetic mutations of G proteins have been linked to pseudo-hypoparathyroidism, McCune-Albright syndrome (MAS), and Albright's hereditary osteodystrophy in humans *(12)*.

Recent work from several laboratories has provided insights into G-protein function in vivo by using transgenic mice *(13–15)*. The roles of G proteins in cellular differentiation have been illuminated in a variety of systems, including stem cell progression to primitive endoderm *(16–19)*, neurite outgrowth *(20,21)*, and adipogenesis *(22–25)*, and are not described here. The bulk of the chapter is devoted to describing novel approaches to the study of G-protein function in vivo, using transgenic mice and describing recent examples in which G proteins have been shown to control early neo-natal growth, development, and aspects of insulin action relevant to diabetes in humans. The prospects for developing new therapies for human disease based on the use of tissue-specific inducible expression vectors are explored.

INDUCIBLE, TISSUE-SPECIFIC ABLATION OF G-PROTEIN SUBUNITS

In view of the fundamental role of G proteins in cell signaling, the study of G-protein biology in vivo by gene inactivation through homologous recombination ("knockout") should yield lethality. In addition, the widespread expression of several G-protein sub-units in tissues, including the hypothalamus, in which transmembrane signaling controls the secretion of a diverse group of powerful hormones has highlighted the possibility that a constellation of effects that are difficult to interpret as being directly related to the absence of a G-protein subunit may occur in a "knock-out" mouse. For these reasons, we developed a different approach that combines tissue-specific elements of a promoter, conditional induction, and expression of RNA antisense to G-protein subunits to explore G-protein function in vivo *(13,14)*.

Since our primary goal was to obtain viable transgenic mouse pups for analysis, we sought a conditional promoter that was silent *in utero* but robustly expressed at birth. The construct must provide tissue-specific expression to avoid the pleotrophic changes that are derivative of changes that might occur if a G protein were inactivated in endocrine tissue, such as the hypothalamus. G-protein signaling in liver and adipose tissue offers a rich diverse field for study, and these tissues were specifically targeted in our original design. The ability to regulate the expression of the transgene in vivo is another entry on our "wish list" of considerations for this approach. Repression and/or induction of the transgene would provide an additional set of opportunities to examine the effects of conditional expression of a G-protein subunit in vivo. Analysis of the promoters and tissue-specific elements for application to our set of criteria yielded few alternatives, but the gene for phosphoenolpyruvate carboxykinase (PEPCK) seemed the most promising. The PEPCK gene offers the advantages outlined in Table 1, including conditional expression, tissue-specific expression, and the potential for repression and/or induction in vivo.

The next phase of expression vector development involved combining the advantages offered by the PEPCK gene for conditional, targeted expression with antisense RNA technology *(26–29)*. The antisense RNA/DNA approach is not new but remains in its infancy *(26)*. The use of complementary, or "antisense," RNA and DNA sequences to block the expression of a gene product succeeds through base-pairing of DNA–RNA or the formation of RNA duplexes that are degraded rapidly *(29)*. The selection of the proper sequence

Table 1
Criteria for Conditional, Tissue-Specific Antisense RNA
Expression in Vivo and Features of PEPCK Gene Expression

Consideration	PEPCK gene expression
Developmental restriction	Undetectable expression *in utero*
	Initial appearance after birth
Tissue-specific expression	Predominant expression in liver, kidney, and adipose tissue.
Regulated expression	
Inducers	Glucagon, catecholamines (via cAMP)
	Glucocorticoids (liver and kidney)
	Thyroid hormones (synergistic with cAMP)
	Retinoic acid (liver)
	Metabolic acidosis (kidney)
	High-protein diet (via glucagon)
Repressors	Insulin
	Glucocorticoids (adipose)
	Metabolic alkalosis (kidney)
	High-carbohydrate diet (via insulin)

and size of the antisense is crucial, driven by the need to achieve specificity. Optimally, probes of 20 to 30 bases offer a level of specificity that declines as the length increases, owing to inadvertent and unintentional pairing with other target mRNA species. For G proteins, studies with oligodeoxynucleotides in cell culture have validated this operating premise, whether the oligos are added to the medium *(20,22)* or microinjected directly into the nucleus *(30,31)*. Although many researchers select a sequence that includes the initiator codon ATG within its boundaries, it has been shown in several studies that this is not a prerequisite *(30)*. The selection of sequences 5′ vs 3′ of the initiator codon is dictated largely by the need for specificity. For G-protein subunits, sequences just 3′ to the ATG often are shared among members of closely related families, such as $G_{\alpha i2}$, so that 5′ sequences with greater diversity are required *(7)*. This point implies an important additional advantage of the antisense RNA approach over gene inactivation by homologous recombination: Antisense RNA can be designed to target specifically more than one member of a family of gene products by selecting a conserved region that is common to all family members *(14)*. This approach requires great caution and some knowledge of the basis for conservation, since one can easily mistake a sequence shared by $G_{\alpha i}$ family members for a structural domain that may be common to any guanosine triphosphate (GTP)-binding protein. Thus, there exist boundaries of specificity that restrict the targeting of some sequences to a few alternatives. As experience with antisense RNA expression accumulates, further understanding of these boundaries will emerge.

For G proteins, not only oligodeoxynucleotides *(20–22,30,31)* but also antisense RNA driven by retroviral expression vectors *(16–18)* have been employed successfully to ablate specific subunits. With this information, it was possible to select with great confidence a sequence capable of targeting $G_{\alpha i2}$. The next challenge in merging antisense technology with conditional, tissue-specific elements of the PEPCK gene was positioning the insert. The marked stability of PEPCK mRNA *(13)* and the well-known

pPCK-AS-X

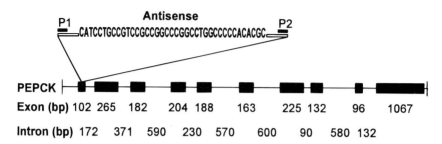

Fig. 1. pPCK-AS-X vector for conditional, tissue-specific expression of antisense RNA in vivo. The elements conferring tissue-specific, conditional antisense RNA expression are present in the 5′-promoter region. Stability of the antisense mRNA is enhanced by the presence of mRNA stabilizing sequences in the 3′-untranslated region.

lesser stability of short sequences of RNA *(28,29)* led to a strategy in which one inserts the antisense sequence into the gene to take advantage of the inducibility, tissue-specific expression, and mRNA stability while eliminating expression of the normal gene product and ensuring that the expressed "hybrid" mRNA has the antisense region available for hybridization with the targeted mRNA *(14)*. These conditions were met by inserting the antisense sequence into exon 1 of the PEPCK gene (Fig. 1), creating an inducible, tissue-specific expression vector that was silent *in utero* and active at birth. At birth, the activation of PEPCK is so robust that its mRNA can account for 2–3% of the mRNA.

After we achieved on paper the goals outlined for this strategy, one other element required attention before the creation of transgenic mice harboring this pPCK-ASG$_{\alpha i2}$ construct: field testing. The initial design identified the need for a cell culture system capable of indicating whether the approach that appeared highly feasible could be demonstrated operationally before introduction into preimplantation embryos. The rat hepatoma FTO-2B cell line displays the capacity to support the induction of PEPCK gene expression in response to cyclic adenosine monophosphate (cAMP) *(14)*. Thus, constructs employing this strategy could be screened after stable transfection of FTO-2B cells with pPCK-AS constructs and induction with cAMP for 6–12 d. Stable transfection of FTO-2B cells with pPCK-ASG$_{\alpha i2}$ followed by induction with cAMP analogs stably suppressed the expression of G$_{\alpha i2}$ and nearly abolished the inhibitory adenyl cyclase pathway that is regulated by G$_{\alpha i2}$ *(13,14)*. Subsequent studies with a variety of constructs have demonstrated repeatedly the ability of this system to act as a sensitive screen with which to check the feasibility of constructs based on the PEPCK gene promoter. In addition, the potential ability to target a specific G-protein subunit in a tissue-specific and conditional manner may offer a new strategy for the treatment of patients suffering from the effects derivative of the expression of aberrant G proteins, such as MAS *(12)* and various endocrine tumors *(11)*.

G$_{\alpha i2}$-DEFICIENCY

G$_{\alpha i2}$ *and Growth*

Microinjection of the conditional, tissue-specific pPCK-ASG$_{\alpha i2}$ expression vector into preimplantation mouse embryos yielded mice that harbored the transgene *(13,14)*.

As planned, all the pups were virtually identical at birth, including those harboring the pPCK-ASG$_{\alpha i2}$ transgene, which is silent *in utero*. The transgenic mice can be identified readily by polymerase chain reaction (PCR) amplification and Southern analysis of samples of tail DNA. Five pPCK-ASG$_{\alpha i2}$ founders were identified after two rounds of injection. Sampling various tissues for the expression of the pPCK-ASG$_{\alpha i2}$ transgene revealed tissue-specific expression in liver and adipose tissue but not in brain, lung, heart, and other nontargeted tissues. Immunoblotting revealed marked suppression of G$_{\alpha i2}$ in the liver and adipose tissue. This loss of G$_{\alpha i2}$ was maintained throughout the lifetime of the mice, which was normal. The transgenic mice were viable and procreated. Within the first month of life, however, the pPCK-ASG$_{\alpha i2}$ transgenic mice displayed a marked reduction in growth. This runted phenotype was prominent in all the founder lines and the mice derivative of the founders that carry the transgene. Most displayed a body mass more than 35% smaller than that of their nontransgenic littermates *(13)*. Radiological analysis of the mice revealed skeletal dimensions of long bones that were not significantly different from those of the normal littermates *(14)*. These were the first data to suggest that neonatal growth can be influenced in a dramatic fashion by G$_{i\alpha2}$-deficiency in key metabolic tissues, such as adipose tissue and liver.

$G_{\alpha i2}$ and Insulin Action

The phenotype of the pPCK-ASG$_{i\alpha2}$ transgenic mice deficient in G$_{i\alpha2}$ was so runted that investigation of the metabolic consequences of the G$_{i\alpha2}$ deficiency became a primary goal *(32)*. The fasting serum insulin levels were found to be elevated in transgenic (0.46 ± 0.03 ng/ml, $n = 6$) mice compared with control mice (0.28 ± 0.01 ng/mL, $n = 6$), while fasting blood glucose levels were found to be equivalent in control and transgenic mice (55 ± 5 and 58 ± 4 mg/dl, $n = 6$, respectively). Transgenic mice displayed impaired glucose tolerance in response to the administration of a bolus of glucose (Fig. 2). Serum glucose levels declined to <80 mg/dL within 30 min of glucose loading for control mice (littermates), whereas for the transgenic mice the return to these levels required 60–120 min after loading.

The inability of the G$_{i\alpha2}$-deficient mice to tolerate glucose led to an assessment of the insulin tolerance of these mice compared with their normal littermates. A rapid and sustained hypoglycemia was observed in fasted control mice challenged with insulin but not in the pPCK-ASG$_{i\alpha2}$ transgenic mice (Fig. 2). In combination, the poor glucose tolerance, the blunted insulin response, and the runted phenotype reflected many of the features of type II diabetes mellitus in humans, which is noninsulin-dependent (NIDDM). If correct, the hypothesis linking G$_{i\alpha2}$ deficiency to a form of NIDDM will illuminate a new dimension of G-protein function in which G proteins are intimately involved in the actions of growth factors *(32)*, including insulin, insulin-like growth factor (IGF)-I, and perhaps others. The fact that G$_{i\alpha2}$ deficiency was associated with blunted insulin action was an unexpected and insightful derived from the study of G-protein action in vivo.

Insight into the nature of the insulin resistance observed in the pPCK-ASG$_{i\alpha2}$ transgenic mice was gained through the study of three cardinal insulin-sensitive responses: inhibition of lipolysis, increased glucose transport, and activation of glycogen synthase. In regard to lipolysis, the ability of increasing concentrations of insulin to counter the lipolytic effects of isoproterenol was markedly blunted in adipocytes isolated from the pPCK-ASG$_{i\alpha2}$ transgenic mice (Fig. 3). Since the adipocytes of the pPCK-ASG$_{i\alpha2}$ transgenic mice lack G$_{i\alpha2}$ and display a blunted inhibitory adenyl cyclase, the counter-regulatory influence of insulin on lipolysis was measured in adipocytes from control mice

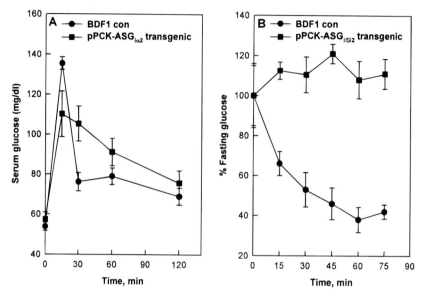

Fig. 2. pPCK-ASG$_{i\alpha2}$ transgenic mice are hyperinsulinemic and have impaired tolerance to glucose loading (**A**) and insulin (**B**) in vivo. Control and transgenic mice were fasted overnight and administered glucose (2.5 mg/g wbw, *ip* injection) or insulin (0.75 IU/kg wbw, *ip* injection) for determinations of glucose and insulin tolerance, respectively. At the times indicated after glucose or insulin injection, glucose levels were measured in blood samples from mouse tails using a One Touch Glucometer (LifeScan, Milpitas, CA).

in the presence of a submaximal concentration of isoproterenol, providing levels of intracellular cAMP that were equivalent to those of the unstimulated adipocytes from the transgenic mice. At equivalent levels of intracellular cAMP, the ability of insulin to counterregulate lipolysis remains dramatically blunted in the G$_{i\alpha2}$-deficient cells (Fig. 3).

Increased glucose uptake is a cardinal response stimulated by insulin. The uptake of 3-*O*-methyl-glucose by adipocytes provided a measure of the hexose transport capacity of the cells in the absence and presence of insulin (Fig. 4). Insulin stimulated an increase of approx 30-fold in hexose transport in adipocytes from control mice, whereas in G$_{i\alpha2}$-deficient adipocytes insulin provoked a very poor response. Basal glucose transport rates (fmol/cell/min, $n = 6$), in contrast, were 0.12 ± 0.03 for control and 0.08 ± 0.02 for transgenic mouse adipocytes. Clamping the cAMP levels of the adipocytes from control mice to those of the unstimulated adipocytes from the pPCK-ASG$_{i\alpha2}$ transgenic mice lacking G$_{i\alpha2}$ did not change the basic observation that G$_{i\alpha2}$ deficiency of adipocytes provokes insulin resistance with regard to hexose transport as well as lipolysis. Complementary studies performed in vivo with mice that were given insulin intravenously and the translocation of the insulin-sensitive GLUT4 transporter from the microsomal membranes to the plasma membrane confirmed the observations derived from the measurement of hexose transport. GLUT4 transporters of G$_{i\alpha2}$-deficient adipocytes were not recruited to the plasma membrane in response to insulin.

Glycogen deposition in liver and skeletal muscle is achieved by converting glycogen synthase from a glucose-6-phosphate (G6P)-dependent (D-form) to an independent enzyme (I-form) that displays enhanced activity at physiological concentrations of G6P. Insulin is the primary agent responsible for the activation of glycogen synthase and was

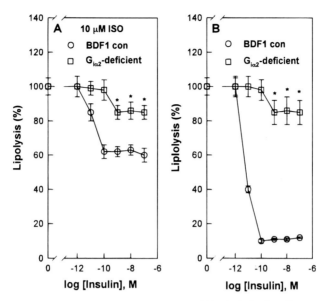

Fig. 3. $G_{i\alpha2}$ deficiency (□) abolishes counterregulation of lipolysis by insulin compared with control mice (○) after challenge with a maximal lipolytic dose of isoproterenol (**A**). The antilipolytic action of insulin is abolished even when the intracellular levels of cAMP in fat cells from control mice (○) are normalized to those of the transgenic mice (□) with 25 nM isoproterenol (**B**), demonstrating that increased cAMP cannot account for the insulin resistance induced by $G_{i\alpha2}$ deficiency (**B**).

studied in vivo in mice after the iv administration of insulin. Insulin stimulates a rapid increase in the amount of I-form synthase in the liver (Fig. 5) and skeletal muscle of control mice. Insulin produces a maximal stimulation of glycogen synthase within 3 min of administration. For pPCK-ASG$_{i\alpha2}$ transgenic mice, glycogen synthase activity in liver (Fig. 5) or skeletal muscle was refractory to stimulation by insulin, although the total amount of synthase activity was not affected.

The precise molecular basis of this insulin resistance is unknown, but several observations implicate $G_{i\alpha2}$ with phosphotyrosine protein phosphatases *(32)*. Insulin action involves signaling via a cascade that includes tyrosine kinase activation, recruitment of adapter molecules such as IRS-1 and Grb2, regulation of *ras*, and downstream activation of members of the Mitogen-Activated Protein (MAP) kinase regulatory network *(33)*. The ability of $G_{i\alpha2}$ deficiency to influence such a wide array of downstream responses suggests that it exerts this influence through steps proximal to the insulin receptor that are common to hexose transport, glucose metabolism, and glycogen synthase activation. Clearly, $G_{i\alpha2}$ deficiency can result in a constellation of metabolic changes closely associated with those of NIDDM in humans *(34)*. Recent work has shown a substantial increase in PTP-1B phosphotyrosine phosphatase activity in adipocytes lacking $G_{i\alpha2}$ *(32)*. Interestingly, the activity of a second PTP, *Syp*, is not influenced *(32)*. Further studies will be required to investigate the basis of the linkage between $G_{i\alpha2}$ and insulin action.

$G_{\alpha i2}$, Ulcerative Colitis, and Adenocarcinoma of the Colon

Although it seems that homozygous knockouts of G-protein subunits should be lethal, at least for $G_{\alpha i2}$, this is not the case. Rudolph and colleagues *(15)* reported the successful creation of mice deficient in $G_{\alpha i2}$ by homologous recombination in embryonic stem cells.

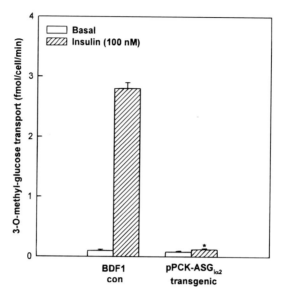

Fig. 4. $G_{i\alpha2}$ deficiency abolishes insulin-stimulated glucose transport in isolated adipocytes as well as the insulin-stimulated recruitment of GLUT 4 (not shown). Adipocytes were isolated by collagenase digestion and incubated in the absence or presence of insulin (100 nM), and the initial rates of 3-O-methyl glucose transport were measured.

As in the earlier work in which $G_{\alpha i2}$ deficiency was targeted to liver, adipose tissue, and skeletal muscle *(13,14)*, the true knockout mice displayed a runted phenotype *(15)*. Unlike the mice harboring the pPCKASG$_{\alpha i2}$ transgene for the production of RNA anti-sense to $G_{\alpha i2}$ in target tissues that displayed normal longevity, the homozygous knockout mice deficient in $G_{\alpha i2}$ developed a diffuse colitis that was lethal. In addition to develop-ing colitis, some animals went on to display the clinical and histopathologic features of human ulcerative colitis, including adenocarcinoma of the colon (see Chapter 1). These important studies may provide new insights into the pathogenesis of ulcerative colitis. The way in which $G_{\alpha i2}$ deficiency provokes colitis and adenocarcinoma is not known.

INDUCIBLE, TISSUE-SPECIFIC EXPRESSION OF G-PROTEIN SUBUNITS

Recent studies reviewed elsewhere in this volume (Chapter 3) have provided com-pelling evidence that the occurrence of mutations in G-protein α-subunits in which constitutive activation results can be linked to a variety of human diseases with complex pathologies, perhaps best exemplified by McCune-Albright syndrome. Because of the limitations of clinical analysis of these human diseases, the development of animal models in which activating mutations of G proteins can be investigated in vivo is criti-caly important to the eventual understanding of these disease states and novel therapies for such diseases. To address this interesting possibility we describe ongoing efforts in our laboratory specifically aimed at solving this problem.

On the basis of our experience with the PEPCK gene construct, we have developed the expression vector shown in Fig. 6. This vector offers the same advantages outlined with

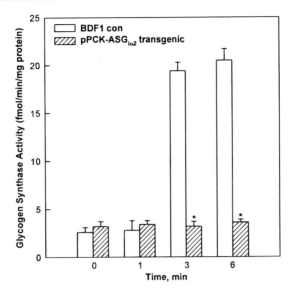

Fig. 5. Hepatic glycogen synthase activation by insulin (5 IU iv injection) in vivo is markedly impaired by $G_{i\alpha2}$ deficiency. At the times indicated after insulin administration in vivo, hepatic glycogen synthase activity was determined by measurement of the incorporation of [^{14}C]-UDP-glucose into glycogen in the absence (I-form) and presence (total) of G6P (10 mM). The results are presented as the glycogen synthase activity measured in the absence of G6P (I-form). Total glycogen synthase activity was not unchanged by $G_{i\alpha2}$ deficiency (not shown).

respect to the expression of antisense RNA for tissue-specific, inducible expression of constitutively activated mutants of G-protein α-subunits *(13,14)*. The mutations in G-protein α-subunits that provide a constitutively activated state do this by virtue of the ability of the mutation to attenuate the guanosine triphosphatase (GTPase) activity intrinsic to the molecule. For $G_{\alpha i2}$, the Q205L mutation provides for a robust, activated state of the sub-unit *(16,17,23)*. Therefore, we selected the Q205L $G_{\alpha i2}$ mutant as the initial target for expression in vivo.

The construct pPCK-Q205LG$_{\alpha i2}$ was screened for its ability to be induced via the PEPCK promoter, using the FTO-2B rat hepatoma cells described *(14)*. The initial results in stably transfected FTO-2B cells demonstrate the successful expression of the Q205L $G_{\alpha i2}$ mutant in response to induction by cAMP. The level of expression of the Q205L $G_{\alpha i2}$ mutant ranged from one to twofold over the level of expression of endogenous $G_{\alpha i2}$ in these cells *(35)*. Thus, the construct can provide expression of a G-protein α-subunit in an inducible fashion via the PEPCK promoter.

The successful expression of Q205L $G_{\alpha i2}$ in the cell line employed for screening prompted us to introduce the construct into transgenic mice. The construct was microinjected into the preimplantation embryos, and the blastula stage derived was carried by pseudopregnant recipient mice to full development *in utero*. The micro-injections succeeded in introducing the transgene in approx 20% of the offspring. The mice harboring the Q205L $G_{\alpha i2}$-expressing transgene were identified by PCR of tail DNA. The mice have been bred for several generations and display normal viability and growth. Characterization of the mice expressing Q205 L $G_{\alpha i2}$ in target tissues is under way.

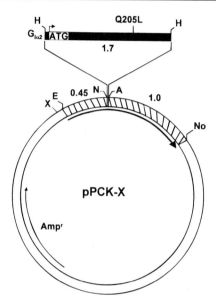

Fig. 6. The pPCK-X vector designed for conditional, tissue-specific overexpression of Q205LG$_{i\alpha2}$ constitutively active mutant in vivo. The vector utilizes both the 5′-promoter sequences providing the tissue specificity and conditional gene expression in tandem with the mRNA stabilizing sequences present in the 3′-untranslated region (UTR).

G$_{\alpha q}$-DEFICIENCY

We adopted the same strategy of inducible, antisense RNA used to suppress G$_{\alpha i2}$ in vivo *(14,15)* to ablate G$_{\alpha q}$ in a tissue-specific manner, creating loss-of-function mutants in adipose tissue and liver, which are major sites of G$_{\alpha q}$ expression *(36)*. FTO-2B hepatoma cells that were stably transfected with pPCK-AS G$_{q\alpha}$ were screened after induction of the promoter with the chlorophenylthio analog of cAMP (CPT-cAMP, 25 μM). Levels of G$_{\alpha i2}$, G$_{\alpha s}$, and G$_{\beta 2}$ were unaffected by induction of pPCK-AS G$_{\alpha q}$, whereas staining with an antibody to G$_{\alpha q}$ revealed total ablation of G$_{q\alpha}$ by d 12 after induction *(36)*. Induction of a pPCK-ASG$_\alpha$ vector that harbored the sense as compared to the antisense sequence for G$_{\alpha q}$ in this case resulted in a null phenotype, i.e., G$_{\alpha q}$ expression was unaffected. G$_{\alpha q}$ activates PLCβ; in the liver. Suppression of Gαq in FTO-2B hepatoma cells resulted in a decline of basal PLC activity from 2.7 ± 0.6 to 1.0 ± 0.3 ($n = 6$, pmol IP3/μg cellular protein) and abolished PLC stimulation in response to either angiotensin II or epinephrine *(36)*.

The pPCK-ASG$_{\alpha q}$ construct can be excised as a 7.0-kb *Eco* RI-*Bam* HI fragment microinjected into single-cell, preimplantation embryos, and the microinjected embryos can be transferred into pseudopregnant recipients. BDF1 mice harboring the transgene have been identified by PCR of tail DNA. Five independent founder lines have been identified from two rounds of microinjection and implantation. Immunoblotting of crude membranes from fat, liver, brain, and lung subjected to sodium dodecyl sulfate-polymerase chain reaction and stained with a G$_{\alpha q}$-specific antiserum reveals the absence of G$_{\alpha q}$ in targeted tissues, including fat and liver. Immunoblotting of brain and lung, tissues in which the PEPCK vector is not activated, in contrast, reveals normal levels of G$_{\alpha q}$. The expression of G$_{\alpha i2}$, G$_{\beta 2}$, and G$_{\alpha 11}$ is not significantly altered in the transgenic mice.

$G_{\alpha q}$ Deficiency and Growth

Necropsy and histology of the transgenic mice were performed. The frank obesity observed in the mice harboring the pPCK-ASG$_{\alpha q}$ transgene was prominent. At 5 wk of age, the transgenic mice were noticeably heavier than their control littermates (36). By 2 mo, the transgenic mice displayed about twice the ratio of fat-whole body mass. Equally notable was the dramatic increase in adiposity, i.e., fat cell number, that occurred in the transgenic mice lacking G$_{\alpha q}$ in liver and adipose tissue. These observations demonstrate a linkage between G$_{\alpha q}$ and growth and show for the first time the ability of the loss of a specific G-protein α-subunit to alter a fundamental aspect of early development, in this case adipogenesis.

$G_{\alpha q}$ Deficiency and Lipolysis

Signaling by loss-of-function G$_{\alpha q}$-deficient adipocytes has been examined and compared to that of adipocytes of control BDF1 littermates. G$_{\alpha q}$ deficiency abolishes IP3 and diacylglycerol (DAG) accumulation in response to a variety of hormones that activate PLC (36). Only G$_{\alpha q}$, not G$_{\alpha 11}$, is suppressed in these target tissues, suggesting that these G-protein subunits found together in liver and other tissues cannot be redundant with respect to PLC activation in vivo. Unexpectedly, study of the pharmacology of the lipolytic response of G$_{\alpha q}$-deficient adipocytes added a new dimension to our understanding of the hormonal regulation of lipolysis. Stimulation by mixed α/β-adrenergic catecholamines such as noradrenaline was noticeably absent from the lipolytic response of the G$_{\alpha q}$-deficient adipocytes. Exhaustive studies with both agonists and antagonists of α- and β-adrenergic pharmacology demonstrated the presence of an α-adrenergic stimulation of lipolysis that was totally absent in the G$_{\alpha q}$-deficient cells (36). Furthermore, the ability of adrenaline or isoproterenol to stimulate cAMP accumulation was found to be blunted in G$_{\alpha q}$-deficient adipocytes. These observations suggest that alpha-adrenergic agents that operate by means of PLC activation can increase IP3 and DAG levels, stimulating increased cAMP accumulation and lipolysis through a pathway atypical of the stimulatory adenyl cyclase pathway. Further studies will be required to establish the basis for this novel element of lipolysis, but clearly, PLC activation and protein kinase C activation play prominent roles.

Adipocytes develop in early neonatal life, and studies have suggested that obesity in adult humans correlates with neonatal weight and adiposity. In obese adults and children, adiposity cannot be reduced by dieting, suggesting that multiplication of fat cells in early life may predispose individuals to lifelong obesity. The absence of G$_{q\alpha}$ resulted in neonatal fat accumulation and a hyperadiposity that was sustained throughout adult life. Recently, G proteins have been shown to play prominent roles in differentiation and neonatal growth. The absence of G$_{\alpha q}$ abolished an important stimulatory control of lipolysis, apparently predisposing the mice to marked obesity. G$_{\alpha q}$ may play a critical role in controlling obesity, suggesting that mutations at this level contribute to obesity in humans.

NEW THERAPIES FOR McCUNE-ALBRIGHT SYNDROME (MAS)

The successful development of an expression vector with the qualities of conditional expression and tissue specificity merged with antisense RNA technology provides a new method for the parallel development of new therapeutic approaches to disease states in which a mutant gene product is responsible for the pathology (Fig. 7). The

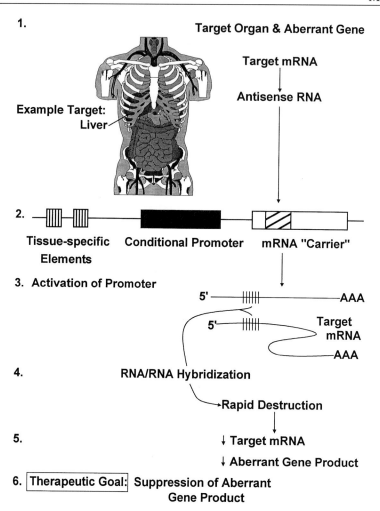

Fig. 7. Novel strategies for the use of conditional, tissue-specific expression of antisense RNA to treat human disease states characterized by the expression of aberrant gene products. Application of this approach requires identification and cloning of the aberrant gene product to facilitate the design of the antisense RNA target sequence. The desired target tissue affected by the aberrant gene product (e.g., liver) is selected. After construction of the expression vector and delivery to the target tissue, the transcribed antisense RNA binds to its target mRNA encoding the aberrant gene product and forms an RNA/RNA duplex molecule. Formation of the RNA/RNA dimer promotes degradation, leading to decreased mRNA levels and thus decreased translation of the aberrant gene product.

MAS is a sporadic disease characterized by precocius puberty, *cafe au lait* pigmentation, monoostotic (or polyostotic) fibrous dysplasia, and a variety of endocrinopathies, including hyperparathyroidism, acromegaly, hepatomegaly, Cushing's syndrome, and hyperthyroidism. The hyperactivity of specific endocrine tissues appears to result from the constitutive activation of $G_{\alpha s}$ *(37,38)* adenyl cyclase, and increased accumulation of cAMP *(39)*. An MAS patient is a mosaic with respect to the pattern of expression of the mutant G protein, a property consistent with a somatic activating mutation of $G_{\alpha s}$ occurring at an early stage of development. More recent studies suggest that MAS may be the cause, though it was not identified as such, of early death in childhood *(40)*. Thus, MAS is probably only one example of the occurrence of an activating mutation of a G protein that results in endocrinopathies and aberrations in early childhood development.

In combination, antisense RNA technology and conditional, tissue-specific expression vectors offer a new approach to treating severe endocrine and nonendocrine manifestations of diseases such as MAS. Theoretically, the mosaic character of MAS provides an opportunity to address tissue-specific manifestations that may be life-threatening, such as hepatobiliary disease and cardiac disease. Tissue-specific elements can be assembled to provide expression limited to target sites, as we have shown for tissue-specific expression in liver, adipose tissue, and skeletal muscle with the pPCK-AS vector. Further engineering and/or discovery of tissue-specific expression elements that complement the therapeutic targets will be a primary task. Tissue-specific expression of transgenes has been reported for a number of tissues, and so one can anticipate that designing an expression vector to accommodate the tissues in which antisense RNA must be expressed to ablate the products of mutant genes will not pose no insurmountable problems.

Conditional expression offers an additional safeguard in gene therapy. Because it was useful in avoiding the lethality of knockouts targeting gene products necessary for development *in utero*, the PEPCK promoter demonstrated the feasibility of this approach. One can envision a variety of other opportunities for conditional expression based on the two-hybrid system in yeast used to probe protein-protein interactions *(41)*. The DNA-binding and activation domains of a promoter could be constructed to hybridize on the binding of a small organic molecule that already has been approved for use in humans by the FDA. Thus, expression of RNA antisense to the mRNA of the mutant G protein could be conditional, based on the administration of a small molecule drug, providing an additional safeguard to that provided by the use of tissue-specific elements for expression. The selection of the proper vector for gene therapy is beyond the scope of this chapter, but it should be noted that Moloney murine leukemia virus-based vectors have been employed successfully to express transgenes with PEPCK gene elements in mice *(42)*. Though speculative, the use of conditional, tissue-specific vectors to express RNA antisense to mRNA of mutant proteins appears to add a novel dimension to gene therapy that is readily adaptable to a host of human disease states, including MAS.

FUTURE PROSPECTS

Recent advances in the application of molecular biology probes to the diagnosis of G-protein involvement in human disease states portend an expansion of our understanding of the extent to which spontaneous or inherited mutations of G proteins are responsible for human pathophysiologies. From the work briefly reviewed in this chapter, it should be clear that mutations in the genes encoding G-protein α-subunits can and do result in reduced expression or the expression of mutant forms that are constitutively "turned on." Much as molecular biology provides the tools for diagnosis, it also provides avenues by which the underlying pathology can be treated. Although further information and understanding of tissue-specific elements, inducible promoters, and reliable vectors will be required to exploit the potential for the use of antisense RNA as a therapeutic tool with which to treat human disease, ample evidence exists for its feasibility *in vivo*. In many ways we should admire the ability of bacteria such as

Vibrio cholera and *Bordetella pertussis* to exploit by trial and error the repertoire of signaling pathways, arriving at the specific G-protein subunit target through which entire complex biological pathways can be regulated to facilitate the spread of infection. In this manner we can learn from our understanding of underlying pathologies to develop new approaches with which to rectify these mutations in the expression and/or function of G proteins.

REFERENCES

1. Gilman AG. G proteins: transducers of receptor-generated signals. Annu Rev Biochem 1987; 56:615–649.
2. Johnson G, Dhanasekaran N. The G-protein family and their interaction with receptors. Endocr Rev 1989;10:317–331.
3. Bourne HR, Sanders DA, McCormick F. The GTPase superfamily: a conserved switch for diverse cell functions. Nature 1990;348:125–132.
4. Birnbaumer L, Abramowitz J, Brown AM. Receptor-effector coupling by G proteins. Biochim Biophysics Acta 1990;1031:163–224.
5. Kaziro Y, Itoh H, Kozasa T, Nakafuku M, Satoh, T. Structure and function of signal-transducing GTP-binding proteins. Annu Rev Biochem 1991;60:349–400.
6. Bourne HR, Sanders DA, McCormick F. The GTPase superfamily: conserved structure and molecular mechanism. Nature 1991;349:117–127.
7. Simon MI, Strathmann MP, Gautam N. Diversity of G proteins in signal transduction. Science 1991;252:802–808.
8. Hadcock JR, Malbon CC. Regulation of receptor expression by agonist: transcriptional and post-transcriptional controls. Trends Neurosci 1991;14:242–247.
9. Hepler JR, Gilman AG. G proteins. Trends Biochem. Sci. 1992;17:383–387.
10. Clapham DE, Neer EJ. New roles for G protein β/γ dimers in transmembrane signalling. Nature 1993;365:403–406.
11. Lyons J, Landis CA, Harsh G, Vallar L, Grunewald K, Feichtinger H, Duh QY, Clark OH, Kawasaki E, Bourne HR, and McCormick F. Two G protein oncogenes in human endocrine tumors. Science 1990;249:655–659.
12. Milligan G, Wakelam M. (eds). G-proteins, Signal Transduction and Disease. Academic, New York, 1992.
13. Moxham CM, Hod Y, Malbon CC. Induction of $G_{i\alpha 2}$-specific antisense RNA *in vivo* inhibits neonatal growth. Science 1993;260:991–995.
14. Moxham CM, Hod Y, and Malbon CC. $G_{i\alpha 2}$ mediates the inhibitory regulation of adenylylcyclase in vivo: analysis in transgenic mice with $G_{i\alpha 2}$ suppressed by inducible antisense RNA. Dev Genet 1993;14:266–273.
15. Rudolph U, Finegold MJ, Rich SS, Harriman GR, Srinivasan Y, Brabet G, Bradley A, and Birnbaumer, L. Ulcerative colitis and adenocarcinoma of the colon in $G_{i\alpha 2}$-deficient mice. Nat Genet 1995;10: 143–150.
16. Watkins DC, Johnson GL, and Malbon CC. $G_{i\alpha 2}$ regulates differentiation of stem cells to primitive endoderm in F9 teratocarcinoma cells. Science 1992;258:1373–1375.
17. Gao P, Watkins DC, and Malbon CC. Expression of constitutively-active mutant $G_{s\alpha}$ (G225T) or of a null-mutant of $G_{i\alpha 2}$ (G203T) induce differentiation of teratocarcinoma stem cells to primitive endoderm. Am J Physiol 1995;268:C1460-C1466.
18. Gao P, Malbon CC. $G_{i\alpha 2}$ regulates stem cell differentiation via phospholipase C and MAP kinase pathways. J Biol Chem, 196;271:9002–9009.
19. Gao P, Malbon CC. Differentiation of F9 teratocarcinoma stem cells to primitive endoderm is regulated by the $G_{i\alpha 2}/G_{s\alpha}$ axis via phospholipase C and not adenylylcyclase. J Biol Chem 1996;271: 30,692–30,698.
20. Strittmater SM, Valenzuela D, Kennedy TE, Neer EJ, and Fishman MC. $G_{o\alpha}$ is a major growth cone protein subject to regulation by GAP-43. Nature 1990;344:836–841.
21. Igarashi M, Strittmater SM, Vartanen H, and Fishman MC. Mediation by G-proteins of signals that cause collapse of growth cones. Science 1993;259:77–79.
22. Wang H-Y, Watkins DC, Malbon CC. Antisense oligodeoxynucleotides to G_s protein α-subunit sequence accelerate differentiation of fibroblasts to adipocytes. Nature 1992;358:334–337.

23. Su H-L, Malbon CC, and Wang H-Y. Increased expression of $G_{i\alpha2}$ in mouse embryo fibroblast 3T3-L1 cells promotes terminal differentiation to adipocytes. Am J Physiol 1993;34:C1729–C1735.

24. Wang H-Y, and Malbon CC. The $G_{s\alpha}/G_{i\alpha2}$ axis controls adipogeneisis independently of adenylyl-cyclase. Int J Obes 1995;19:197–203.

25. Wang H-Y, Johnson GL, and Malbon CC. $G_{s\alpha}$ and adipogenesis: analysis of regulation using $G_{s\alpha}/G_{i\alpha2}$ chimeric α-subunit expression. J Biol Chem 1996;271:22,022–22,029.

26. Haseloff J, and Gerlach WL. Dominant-negative control of gene expression. Nature 1988; 334:585–591.

27. Miller PS. Effects of a trinucleotide ethyl phosphotriester, $G^m p(Et)G^m$ p(Et)U, on mammalian cells in culture. Biochemistry 1989;16:1988–1996.

28. Crooke ST, Bennett CF. Progress in antisense therapeutics. Ann Rev Pharmacol Toxicol 1996; 36:107–129

29. Agrawal S, (ed.). Antisense therapeutics. Humana, Totowa, NJ, 1996.

30. Kleuss C, Scherubl H, Hescheler J, Schultz G, and Wittig B. Different β-subunits determine G-protein interaction with transmembrane receptors. Nature 1992;358:424–426.

31. Kleuss C, Scherubl H, Hescheler J, Schultz G, and Wittig B. Selectivity in signal transduction determined by γ-subunits of heterotrimeric G proteins. Science 1993;259:832–843.

32. Moxham CM, and Malbon CC. Insulin action impaired by deficiency of the G-protein $G_{i\alpha2}$. Nature 1996;379:840–845.

33. White MF, Kahn CR. The insulin signaling system. J Biol Chem 1994;269:1–4.

34. Reaven GM. Pathophysiology of insulin resistance in human disease. Physiol Rev 1995;75:473–486.

35. Chen JF, Guo JH, Moxham CM, Wang, H-Y, and Malbon CC. Conditional, tissue-specific expression of Q205L $G_{i\alpha2}$ in vivo mimics insulin action. J Mol Med 1997;75:283–289.

36. Galvin-Parton PA, Chen X, Moxham CM, and Malbon CC. Induction of Gαq-specific antisense RNA in vivo causes increased body mass and hyperadiposity. J Biol Chem 1997;272:4335–4341.

37. Weinstein LS, Shenker A, Gejman PV, Merino MJ, Friedman E, and Spiegel AM. Activating mutations of the stimulatory G protein in the McCune Albright syndrome. N Engl J Med 1991;325:1688–1695.

38. Schwindinger WF, Francomano CA, and Levine MA. Identification of a mutation in the gene encoding the alpha subunit of the stimulatory G protein of adenylyl cyclase in McCune-Albright syndrome. Proc Natl Acad Sci USA 1992;89:5152–5156.

39. Schnabel P, and Bohm M. Mutations of signal-transducing G proteins in human disease. J Mol Med 1995;73:221–228.

40. Shenker A, Weinstein LS, Moran A, Pescovitz OH, Charest NJ, Boney CM, Van Wyk JJ, Merino MJ, Feuillan PP, and Spiegel AM. Severe endocrine and non-endocrine manifestations of the McCune-Albright syndrome associated with activating mutations of stimulatory G protein Gs. J Pediatr 1993;123:509–518.

41. Fields S, and Sternglanz R. The two-hybrid system: an assay for protein–protein interactions. Trends Genet 1994;10:286–292.

42. Hatzoglou M, Lamers W, Bosch F, Wynshaw-Boris A, Clapp DW, Hanson RW. Hepatic gene transfer in animals using retroviruses containing the promoter from the gene for phsophoenolpyruvate carboxykinase. J Biol Chem 1990;265:17,285–17,293.

6

Gα₁₂- and Gα₁₃-Subunits of Heterotrimeric G-Proteins

A Novel Family of Oncogenes

J. Silvio Gutkind, PhD, Omar A. Coso, PhD, and Ningzhi Xu, MD

CONTENTS

PROLIFERATIVE SIGNALING THROUGH G-PROTEIN-COUPLED RECEPTORS

Certain polypeptide growth factor receptors possess an intrinsic protein tyrosine kinase activity *(1)*, and a large body of information implicates these receptors in normal and aberrant cell growth. As such, a number of oncogenes have been found to code for altered forms of these receptors *(2–4)*, their ligands *(5)*, or for molecules thought to participate in their growth-promoting pathways *(6)*. Another family of structurally related cell-surface receptors is linked to heterotrimeric G-proteins, and this class of receptors has been traditionally linked to tissue-specific, fully differentiated cell functions, such as photoreception, chemoreception, and neurotransmission *(7)*. However, G-protein-coupled receptors (GPCRs) are also expressed in most proliferating cells, and they have been implicated in embryogenesis and growth stimulation *(8)*. Furthermore, the vast majority of GPCRs identified so far exhibit a common structural

From: *Contemporary Endocrinology: G Proteins, Receptors, and Disease*
Edited by: A. M. Spiegel, Humana Press Inc., Totowa, NJ

motif consisting of the presence of seven transmembrane-spanning domains *(7)*, a property that was also predicted for the protein product of the *mas* oncogene on the basis of its nucleotide sequence *(9)*. This finding provided the first link between cellular transformation and GPCRs.

The mechanisms by which GPCRs control cell proliferation are still poorly understood. Inhibition of adenylyl cyclase has been observed in cells responding to certain growth-promoting agents acting on GPCRs, such as serotonin, thrombin, or lysophosphatidic acid. However, these mitogens can also trigger a variety of other biochemical responses *(10–13)*, and there is no formal proof that induction of DNA synthesis results from decreasing intracellular levels of cAMP. In contrast, several lines of investigation have implicated phosphatidylinositol bis-phosphate (PIP_2) hydrolysis as a critical component of mitogenesis. Mitogens acting through a structurally diverse set of cell-surface receptors, such as those for thrombin, serotonin, bombesin, endothelin, bradykinin, or platelet-derived growth factor (PDGF), all induce PIP_2 hydrolysis on addition to quiescent cells expressing their respective receptors *(8)*. However, this signaling pathway might not be sufficient to explain their growth-promoting effect, since certain mutated PDGF receptors impaired for mitogenesis are still capable of potently eliciting PIP_2 hydrolysis *(14)*. Furthermore, a number of agonists acting on GPCRs coupled to the PIP_2 turnover pathway do not stimulate growth when added alone to quiescent cells *(15)*.

In our laboratory, we have used the expression of human muscarinic receptors for acetylcholine (mAChRs) in NIH 3T3 cells as a model for studying proliferative signaling through GPCRs. The mAChR family consists of five distinct, but highly related subtypes (m1–m5), which are encoded by five separate genes *(16–18)*. mAChRs subtypes can be divided into two functionally distinct groups: m1, m3, and m5 mAChRs, which couple through G proteins of the G_q class to phospholipase C-β and PIP_2 metabolism, and m2 and m4 mAChRs, which couple through pertussis toxin-sensitive G proteins of the G_i subfamily to the inhibition of adenylyl cyclases *(18,19)*. In this biological system, mAChRs subtypes coupled to G_q (m1, m3, m5) can effectively transduce mitogenic signals *(20)* and, when persistently activated, can induce malignant transformation *(21)*. Similarly, G_q-coupled receptors for serotonin or noradrenaline can behave as ligand-dependent oncogenes when expressed in murine or rat fibroblasts *(22,23)*. In contrast, those mAChRs coupled to the inhibition of adenylyl cyclase (m2 and m4) fail to induce the transformed phenotype *(21)*.

WHEREAS AN ACTIVATED MUTANT OF $G\alpha_{i2}$ ALTERS THE GROWTH PROPERTIES OF NIH 3T3 CELLS, AN ACTIVATED MUTANT OF $G\alpha_Q$ IS FULLY ONCOGENIC IN THESE CELLS

In view of the remarkably different biological properties of G-protein-coupled receptors and their distinct coupling specificity, we and others explored whether constitutively activated mutants of $G\alpha_q$ and $G\alpha_{i2}$ could mimic the effect of activating the m1 and the m2 class of GPCRs, respectively. These experiments were based on the observation that all G-protein α-subunits exhibit a number of highly conserved regions *(24)*. One of them, the G-3 region, is involved in binding and hydrolysis of GTP, and has the Gα consensus sequence DVGGQ. Replacing the glutamine residue for leucine (QL mutant) constitutively activates the α-subunit of G_s *(25)*. Furthermore, mutation of the corresponding sequence in the *ras* gene (codon 61) increases steady-state levels of GTP-bound p21[ras] and unmasks its oncogenic potential *(26)*. Accordingly, α_{i2} and α_q were mutated at codons corresponding to the G-3 region. For α_q, cDNAs that encoded leucine instead of glutamine at position 209 (α_q-Q209L), and for α_{i2}, cDNAs that encoded leucine instead of glutamine at position 205 (α_{i2}-Q205L) were generated. As discussed above, mutation of glutamine 209 or 205 for leucine in Gα_q or Gα_{i2}, respectively, would be expected to produce a constitutively activated G protein.

In our experiments, on transfection into NIH 3T3 cells, only α_q-Q209L or the human *ras* oncogene induced focus formation *(27,28)*. However, *ras* displayed a higher focus-forming activity, and these foci were larger and more diffuse than α_q-Q209L-induced foci, which exhibited a compact and punctuate appearance (Fig. 1). Although control cells grew in monolayer and showed the characteristic fusiform morphology, α_q-Q209L-transfected NIH 3T3 cells were rounded, displayed refractile cell bodies, and grew in a crisscross pattern. This morphology was not observed in cells transfected with wild type (wt) or other mutated forms of α_q or α_{i2}. Particularly, cells transfected with α_{i2}-Q205L grew more densely, but in no case did foci of transformation arise even when cells were cultured for up to 3 wk post-confluence.

The acquisition of anchorage-independent growth of fibroblasts correlates well with their malignant potential. Thus, transfected NIH 3T3 cells were assayed for their ability to form colonies in semisolid media. As shown in Fig. 2, only α_q-Q209L and *ras*-transfected cells formed large colonies in soft agar. *ras*-Transfected cells plated with greater efficiency, and colonies were larger (Table 1). NIH 3T3 cells expressing α_{i2}-Q205L formed very few colonies in soft agar, they were smaller in size, and they exhibited a compact morphology (Fig. 2, Table 1), although selected clones expressing very high levels of α_{i2}-Q205L protein grew more efficiently in soft agar *(27)*.

The same cell lines were studied for their ability to form tumors in nude mice. Mice injected with *ras*-transfected cells or α_q-Q209L formed large tumors. Tumors were evident as early as 1 wk postinjection for *ras*- or after 2 wk for α_q-Q209L-transfected cells (Table 1). Some animals injected with NIH 3T3 cells expressing the α_{i2}-Q205L protein also developed tumors, although they were evident much later (4 wk postinjection) and were smaller in size. Thus, by several criteria, including focus induction, focus formation on a lawn of contact-inhibited fibroblasts, morphology, anchorage-independent growth, and tumorigenicity, cells transfected with the α_q-Q209L cDNA are fully malignant.

As discussed, the activation of G_i-coupled receptors fails to induce reinitiation of DNA synthesis or transformation when expressed in NIH 3T3 cells. In line with that observation, we and others have demonstrated that constitutively activated Gα_{i2} induces alterations in cell growth, but fails to induce a fully transformed phenotype when expressed in mouse fibroblasts *(27,29)*. Nevertheless, somatic mutations in α_s and α_{i2} genes have been recently found in human tumors *(25,30,31)*. Interestingly, such tumors were restricted to those tissues where mutated α_s and α_{i2} could mimic mitogenic effects of trophic hormones that normally stimulate or inhibit adenylyl cyclase (*see below*). On the other hand, the activated mutant of Gα_q induces cellular transformation. It has been shown that this family of G-protein α-subunits can at least mediate receptor-activated PIP$_2$-PLC *(32,33)*. Thus, continuous activation of the PIP$_2$-PLC pathway might result in cellular transformation. However, the focus-forming activity of m1 receptors, which couple to PIP$_2$-PLC, is several orders of magnitude higher than that of activated G$_q$. This discrepancy could be explained by the dual transforming and toxic effect of activated G$_q$ *(28)*, or alternatively, other biochemical pathways might be

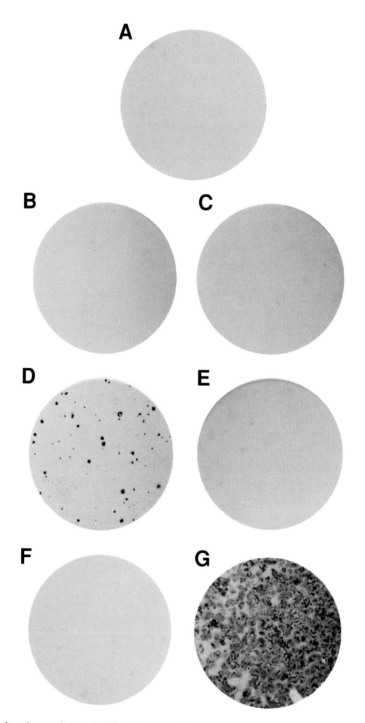

Fig. 1. Focus-forming activity of WT and mutated Gα cDNAs. NIH 3T3 cells were transfected with 2 μg of pZN (**A**), pZNα$_q$-wt (**B**), pZNα$_q$-G207T (**C**), pZNα$_q$-Q209L (**D**), pZNα$_{i2}$-wt (**E**), pZNα$_{i2}$-Q205L (**F**), or 0.2 μg of pT24 plasmid DNA (**G**). Cultures were maintained in DMEM plus 10% calf serum, and plates were stained 3 wk after transfection. Data are from ref *28*.

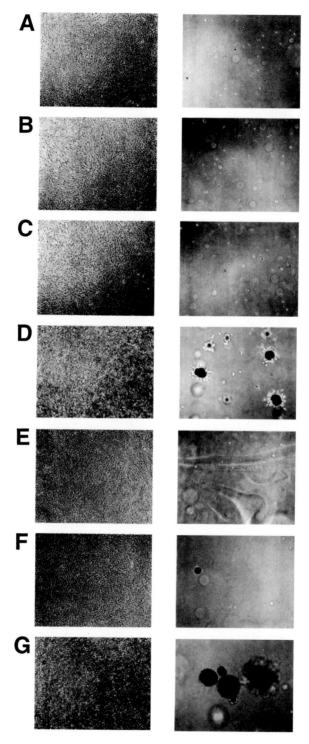

Fig. 2. Morphology and soft agar growth of G418-resistant NIH 3T3 cell transfectants. Cultures transfected with pZN (**A**), pZNα$_q$-wt (**B**), pZNα$_q$-G207T (**C**), pZNα$_q$-Q209L (**D**), pZNα$_{i2}$-wt (**E**), pZNα$_{i2}$-Q205L (**F**), or pT24 (**G**) plasmids were G418-selected and photographed when nearly confluent (left panel) (×10). Human *ras* transfectants were not treated with G418. Cells were trypsinized and aliquots containing $1–5 \times 10^3$ transfected cells were plated in 0.3% agar containing DMEM plus 10% calf serum. Photographs were taken after 15 d of growth (right panel) (×10). Data are from ref. *28*.

Table 1
Focus-Forming Activity of WT and Mutated α-Subunits of G_i and G_q Proteins[a]

DNA construct	Focus-forming activity/μg DNA	Colony-forming activity/μg DNA
pZN	<1	>500
pZNα$_q$-wt	<1	236 ± 18
pZNα$_q$-G207T	<1	235 ± 28
pZNα$_q$-Q209L	27 ± 8	4 ± 1
pZNα$_{i2}$-wt	<1	346 ± 24
pZNα$_{i2}$-Q205L	<1	320 ± 44
pT24	2160 ± 172	ND[b]

[a] Wt or mutated Gα$_q$ or Gα$_{i2}$ cDNAs were inserted into an expression vector, pZipNeoSV(X) (pZN), and 0.05–2 μg of plasmid DNA were transfected into NIH 3T3 murine fibroblasts, using the human *ras* oncogene (pT24) as control. Cultures were scored for both colony-forming activity, in the presence of G418 (Gibco, Gaithersburg, MD), or for focus formation 2–3 wk after transfection. Data shown represent mean values ± SE of triplicate plates from three independent experiments. Data are from ref. *28*.
[b] ND, not determined.

activated by transforming m1 receptors, which, in addition to PIP$_2$-hydrolysis, would result in higher transforming efficiency. If that were the case, then G proteins in addition to those inducing PIP$_2$ hydrolysis might also harbor oncogenic potential as well as participate in the m1-transforming pathway.

POTENT TRANSFORMING ACTIVITY OF THE Gα$_{12}$- AND Gα$_{13}$-SUBUNITS DEFINES A NOVEL FAMILY OF ONCOGENES

During the course of these studies, a new family of G proteins was discovered on amplification of sequences from a mouse brain cDNA library by the polymerase chain reaction (PCR) technique, using degenerated oligonucleotides corresponding to regions highly conserved among all G proteins *(34)*. This new family was termed G$_{12}$, and includes G$_{12}$ and its highly homologous G protein, G$_{13}$. These G proteins appear to be ubiquitously expressed, and they exhibit 67% of amino acid identity with each other, but only 35–44% of amino acid identity to α-subunits of other classes, such as G$_i$ and G$_q$ *(34)*. Interestingly, the finding that *concertina* (*cta*), a *Drosophila* gene involved in embryogenesis, is closely related to α$_{12}$ provided an early indication that this G protein class might be involved in growth regulation *(35)*. *cta* was first identified by an embryonic lethal, loss-of-function mutation that disrupts ventral furrow formation in *Drosophila* embryos. This information, and the limited transforming capacity of activated G$_q$ and G$_i$ prompted us to ask whether this novel class of G proteins harbors oncogenic potential.

We mutated mouse α$_{12}$ and α$_{13}$ at codons corresponding to the G3 region, as described for G$_{i2}$ and G$_q$, generating cDNAs that encoded leucine instead of glutamine at position 229 for α$_{12}$ (α$_{12}$-QL) or in position 226 for α$_{13}$ (α$_{13}$-QL) *(36,37)*. We also generated an "inactive" Gα$_{12}$ by replacing alanine instead of glycine at position 228 (α$_{12}$-GA). As shown in Table 2, α$_{12}$-wt, α$_{12}$-QL, α$_{13}$-wt, and α$_{13}$-QL induced focus formation (*see* Fig. 3). Whereas α$_{12}$-wt and α$_{13}$-wt foci were observed only when >1 μg of

Table 2
Tumorigenicity of NIH 3T3 Transfected with WT and Mutated α-Subunits of the G₁₂ or G₁₃ Protein

Gene	Focus-forming[a] activity/μg DNA	Tumors[b]/ injection	Latency d	>1 cm by 40 d
neo	<1	0/10	>40	0/10
α_{12}-wt	5 ± 1	7/10	14–21	3/10
α_{12}-GA	<1	0/10	>40	0/10
α_{12}-QL	813 ± 50	10/10	7–14	9/10
α_{13}-wt	5 ± 2	2/10	21–28	0/10
α_{13}-QL	325 ± 20	10/10	14–21	9/10
v-raf	2030 ± 15	10/10	7–14	10/10
T24	680 ± 42	10/10	7–14	10/10

[a] Plasmid DNA (0.05–2 μg) was transfected into NIH 3T3 cells, and cultures were scored for focus formation 2–3 wk after transfection. Data shown represent mean values ± SE of triplicate plates from three independent experiments. Data are from ref. 37.

[b] Tumors were scored as positive when >5 mm in diameter. Latency is defined as the time interval required for palpable tumor to arise.

DNA was transfected/plate, α_{12}-QL and α_{13}-QL were remarkably potent transforming genes, nearly as potent as v-raf or the human ras oncogene (Table 2). In contrast, a putative inactive α_{12}, α_{12}-GA, lacked transforming activity.

All transfected cells overexpressed proteins encoded by their respective expression plasmids (36,37). These cells did not exhibit alterations in the metabolism of PIP₂, nor endogenous levels of cAMP affected (36). In addition, cells expressing wt or activated mutants of Gα₁₂ or Gα₁₃ were highly tumorigenic in vivo (Table 2). Similar results were obtained by a number of laboratories (38,39) on transfection into mouse or rat fibroblasts.

We have compared the relative transforming efficiency in NIH 3T3 cells of activated mutants representing all four known G protein families (40). As shown in Table 3, activated mutants of both members of the Gα₁₂ class are the highest transforming G proteins in these murine fibroblasts. Furthermore, overexpression of wt α_{12} or α_{13} is itself transforming, a feature unique among the G proteins tested to date. Thus, taken together, these findings strongly suggest that genes for α_{12} and α_{13} can be considered oncogenes. Whether the G₁₂ family of proto-oncogenes is the target for genetic alterations leading to naturally occurring neoplasia, as well as whether the G₁₂ family of G proteins mediates transformation by G-protein coupled receptors is currently being investigated (see below).

THE G₁₂ CLASS OF G PROTEINS: BIOCHEMICAL PATHWAYS

The potent biological activity of the novel G₁₂ class of G proteins, and its limited primary sequence similarity to other classes of G proteins controlling PIP₂ hydrolysis or adenylyl cyclases prompted many laboratories to investigate which receptors can couple to G₁₂, as well as to search for biologically relevant downstream effector molecules. To date, this is still a very active area of research, and we will attempt to summarize the most important findings in this area.

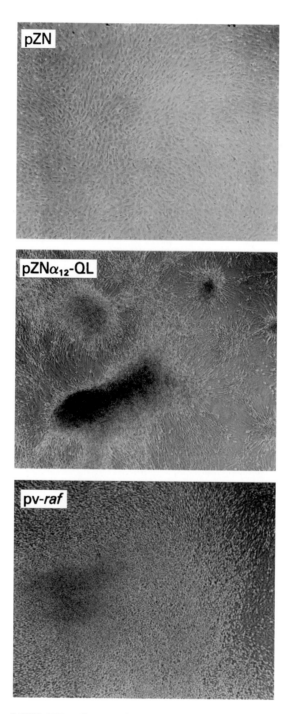

Fig. 3. Morphology of NIH 3T3 cells transfected with the activated mutant of $G\alpha_{12}$. Cultures transfected with pZN, pZNα_{12}-QL or pv-*raf* plasmids were photographed 3 wk after transfection (×10). Data are from ref. *36*.

Table 3
Focus-Forming Activity of Activated Mutants of G-Protein α-Subunits
When Expressed in NIH 3T3 Cells

α-Subunit Family	Members	Tested for focus-forming activity	Transforming activity in NIH 3T3 cells[a]	Gene designation
α_s	α_s, α_{olf}	α_s	–	gsp[b,c]
α_i	α_{i1}, α_{i2}, α_{i3}, α_o, α_t, α_{gus}	α_{12}	–/+	gip[b,d]
		α_{i1}	–/+	
		α_{i3}	–	
		α_o	+	
α_q	α_q, α_{11}, α_{14}, α_{15}, α_{16}	α_q	+	gqp
α_{12}	α_{12}, α_{13}	α_{12}	+++	gep
		α_{13}	+++	

[a] –, <1 Focus/μg DNA; –/+, <1 focus/μg DNA, but increased serum independent growth.
+, 1–50 foci/μg DNA; ++, 50–250 foci/μg DNA; +++, 250–1000 foci/μg DNA.
[b] Activated mutants have been idenified in human tumors (*see text*).
[c] Decreases serum dependency for growth when expressed in Swiss 3T3 cells *(64)*.
[d] Induces focus formation in Rat-2 cells *(29)*.

Receptors Coupled to G$_{12}$

The lack of a defined biochemical response specific for G$_{12}$ and G$_{13}$ has hampered the ability to identify receptors that utilize these G proteins for transducing extracellular signals. However, a number of novel approaches have been recently used to address this issue. For example, Offermans and coworkers *(40)* took advantage of the observation that receptor activation catalyzes the exchange of guanine nucleotides in the interacting Gα-subunits. Using membranes from human platelets and a radioactive photo affinity-labeling analog of GTP, [^{32}P]-azidoanilido GTP, they showed that agonists acting on thrombin and thromboxane A$_2$ receptors rapidly induce the exchange of GDP for GTP in G$_{12}$ *(40)*. Thus, these receptors might utilize G$_{12}$ and/or G$_{13}$ to couple to yet-to-be-identified pathways. Similar studies, using receptors and G$_{12}$ proteins expressed in insect cells on infection with baculoviral vectors, have revealed that the m1 class of receptors can also induce nucleotide exchange on G$_{12}$ (D. Manning, personal communication).

Additional evidence that G$_{12}$ participates in the biological responses elicited by thrombin was obtained in the human 1321N1 astrocytoma cell line *(41)*. In these cells, thrombin elevates the expression of AP-1-dependent genes, including the c-*jun* proto-oncogene, and the reinitiation of DNA synthesis *(41)*. Thrombin receptors are known to be coupled to G$_i$, but these effects were shown to be insensitive to pertussis toxin treatment, suggesting that a G protein distinct from G$_i$ participated in those responses. In line with those observations, activated G$_q$ and G$_{12}$, but not G$_i$, enhanced the expression of a reporter plasmid containing AP-1 regulatory elements *(41)*. Furthermore, microinjection of anti-G$_{12}$ antibodies blocked thrombin-induced DNA synthesis *(41)*.

Electrophysiological studies revealed that G$_{13}$ also participates in the coupling of bradykinin receptors to a voltage-dependent Ca^{2+} channel *(42)*. In the neuroblastoma-glioma hybrid cell line NG108-15, bradykinin activates a transient K$^+$ current through G$_q$-proteins, and, concomitantly, inhibits a voltage-dependent Ca^{2+} current through a distinct pertussis-toxin-insensitive G protein. Only the latter response was abolished by pretreatment of isolated membranes with anti-G_{13}-specific antibodies. These findings suggest that bradykinin receptors can couple to G_{13}, and since bradykinin is a potent mitogen in certain cell lines (8), it is conceivable that G_{13} and/or G_{12} also participates in the growth-stimulatory effects of this polypeptidic ligand. Taken together, we can conclude that G_{12} participates in mitogenic signaling through thrombin, and perhaps, additional G-protein-coupled receptors.

Downstream Effectors

The identities of effector molecules that interact directly with G_{12} or G_{13} are still unknown. As discussed above, procedures involving blocking antibodies suggest that G_{13} regulates the inhibition of voltage-dependent Ca^{2+} channels in response to bradykinin (42). Whether this G protein directly interacts with the channel is still unclear and warrants further investigation. As discussed below, other studies utilizing activated mutants of α_{12} and α_{13} have provided evidence supporting a role for these novel G proteins regulating a number of signaling pathways, including phospholipase A_2, Na^+/H^+ exchanger, c-Jun N-terminal kinase (JNK), and cytoskeletal components.

PHOSPHOLIPASE A_2

First, experimental observations led to the conclusion that these G proteins do not regulate adenylyl cyclases or PIP_2-specific phospholipase C. In our laboratory, we have observed a dramatic increase in serum-induced phospholipase A_2 activity, as judged by the accumulation of free arachidonic acid in response to serum (36). However, co-expression of $cPLA_2$ and activated forms of G_{12} and G_{13} did not enhance arachidonic acid release (N. X. and J. S. G., unpublished observation). Furthermore, we observed that NIH 3T3 cells transformed by activated mutants of G_{12} express approximately threefold more $cPLA_2$ protein than vector transfected cells, and that G_{12} enhances expression of a reporter plasmid containing the $cPLA_2$ promoter (N. X. and J. S. G., unpublished results). Thus, although G_{12} might control the expression of $cPLA_2$, this second messenger-generating enzyme appears not to be a direct target for G_{12} function.

Na^+/H^+ EXCHANGERS

In human embryonic kidney 293 cells, it was known that β-adrenergic stimulation activates the Na^+/H^+ exchanger (NHE). However, this effect was not mimicked by expression of activated $G\alpha_s$, nor blocked by pertussis toxin pretreatment (43). While searching for pertussis-toxin-insensitive G proteins, it was found that activated mutants of α_q and α_{13} stimulate the activity of NHE-1 (43). When similar studies were performed in Cos-1 cells, it was observed that activated forms of α_q, α_{12}, and α_{13} elevated the activity of an amiloride-sensitive exchanger activity (44). Since PKC stimulation might be sufficient to activate active NHE fully, further experimentation in this system showed that α_q and α_{12}, but not α_{13}, utilize a PKC-dependent pathway to stimulate the NHE activity in Cos-1 cells (44). However, α_q, but not α_{12} activates PIP_2-specific phospholipase C and, consequently, elevates $[Ca^{2+}]$ and diacylglycerol, both potent stimulators of PKC. These findings suggest that G_{12} might stimulate PKC through another lipid-mediator-generating system, such as phospholipase A_2 (*see above*), phosphatidylcholine-specific phospholipase C, or phospholipase D. Furthermore, in recent studies utilizing stable transfected renal epithelial MDCK cells, it has been shown that α_{13} wt overexpression or expression of its activated QL form led to enhanced NHE-1 activity *(45)*. In that study, basal and bradykinin-induced Ca^{2+} influx were found to be elevated on G$_{13}$ expression, similar to that caused by transfection with an activated form of G$_q$ *(45)*. Thus, the authors concluded that elevation of IP$_3$ and diacylglycerol and/or [Ca^{2+}] might be responsible for NHE stimulation by these G proteins. However, because attempts to demonstrate PIP$_2$-specific PLC-β activation by purified G$_{13}$ have been so far unsuccessful, it was proposed that G$_{13}$ might regulate the expression level of PLC-βs or activate distinct forms of PLCs. We can conclude that several lines of investigation suggest a role for G$_{12}$ and/or G$_{13}$ regulating the activity of NHE. However, the pathways mediating this effect, as well as whether that is an indirect consequence of a general metabolic stimulation by these transforming G proteins is still unclear.

c-Jun N-terminal Kinases

Critical molecules participating in the transduction of proliferative signals have just begun to be identified. One such an example is the family of extracellular signal-regulated kinases (ERKs) or MAP kinases (MAPKs). Their function is to convert extracellular stimuli to intracellular signals controlling the expression of genes essential for many cellular processes, including cell growth and differentiation. MAPKs have been classified in three subfamilies: ERKs, including ERK1 and ERK2, also known as p44^{mapk} and p42^{mapk}, respectively (referred to herein as MAPKs); stress-activated protein kinases (SAPKs), also termed JNKs; and p38 kinase *(46)*. Whereas Ras controls the activation of MAPK *(47)*, we and others have recently observed that two members of the Rho family of small GTP binding proteins, Rac1 and Cdc42, regulate the activity of JNKs *(48)*. Thus, the potent biological effect of the G$_{12}$ family of G proteins and the critical role of MAPKs in cell proliferation prompted several laboratories to explore whether MAPK or JNK are downstream components of the G$_{12}$ signaling pathways. Using transient expression of epitope-tagged MAPK and JNK in COS-7 cells as a model system, we observed that activated mutants of Gα_{12} and Gα_{13} do not elevate MAPK activity *(49)*, but induce an increase in the phosphorylating activity of JNK *(50)*. However, other laboratories have reported a remarkable increase in JNK in stably transfected NIH 3T3 cells and in transiently transfected COS cell lines, utilizing a Cdc42-dependent pathway *(51,52)*. These quantitative differences regarding the extent of activation of JNK in response to G$_{12}$ and G$_{13}$ might likely result from variations in experimental conditions utilized by each research group. Nevertheless, taken together, these studies strongly suggest that the G$_{12}$ family of G proteins can communicate, directly or indirectly, with small GTP binding proteins, thereby affecting the JNK biochemical route. More work will be necessary to identify those molecules connecting G$_{12}$ proteins to this novel MAPK signaling pathway.

Rho-Dependent Regulation of the Actin Cytoskeleton

G-protein-coupled receptors, such as those for lysophosphatidic acid (LPA) and thrombin, are known to regulate the polymerization of actin to produce stress fibers and the assembly of focal adhesions, and a large body of evidence suggests that the small GTP binding protein Rho mediates these effects *(53)*. Interestingly, pertussis toxin does not inhibit receptor-stimulated acting polymerization, and the combination of calcium ionophores and phorbol esters does not stimulate Rho-dependent responses *(54)*; thus suggesting that neither pertussis-toxin-sensitive G proteins, G$_o$ and G$_i$, nor G$_q$ proteins mediate these responses. In addition, the phenotypic appearance of G$_{12}$-induced foci in

NIH 3T3 cells resembles that caused by expression of activated RhoA (N. X. and J. S. G., recently published). Thus, it is conceivable that G_{12} proteins represent the missing link connecting G-protein-coupled receptors to Rho, thereby controlling the actin cytoskeleton. Supporting this hypothesis, in an elegant series of experiments involving microinjection of expression plasmids for activated heterotrimeric G proteins and small GTP binding proteins in Swiss 3T3 cells, Buhl et al. *(55)* demonstrated that activated $G\alpha_{12}$ and $G\alpha_{13}$, but not $G\alpha_{i2}$ and $G\alpha_q$ or different combinations of β- and γ-subunits, mimicked the effect of activated RhoA on stress fibers and focal adhesion assembly. Furthermore, with the use of botulinum C3 exoenzyme, which ADP-ribosylates and inactivates Rho, these investigators demonstrated that G_{12}-dependent effects on actin structures are strictly dependent on Rho functioning. Interestingly, recent studies have provided the first evidence that in addition to regulating the cytoskeleton, Rho proteins control signaling pathways connecting the membrane with the nuclear transcription factor SRF *(56)*. Also, preliminary results from our laboratory suggest that G_{12} mediates SRF activation by serum and G-protein-coupled receptors, utilizing a Rho-dependent pathway. Thus, taking these findings together, we can conclude that G_{12} proteins might link cell-surface receptors to Rho-related G proteins. Whether the proliferative effects of activated mutants of G_{12} and G_{13} are mediated by Rho is still unknown, and is under current investigation.

G PROTEINS AS ONCOGENES

As discussed, mutationally activated G proteins have been shown to transform fibroblasts in culture effectively. In these assays, established immortal fibroblasts lines, including NIH 3T3 and Rat 1 cells, are utilized because they display a number of properties common to normal, nontumorigenic cells, such as growth arrest on confluence; anchorage dependence for cell growth, reflected in inability to grow in soft agar; requirement of growth factors for proliferation; ability to form monolayers of "flat" appearance; and lack of tumorigenicity on injection in experimental animals. Most or all of these properties are affected by expression of tumor-inducing genes, collectively known as oncogenes. Thus, this experimental system has helped identify dominant-acting oncogenes expressed in naturally occurring tumors, as well as unveil novel pathways involved in growth control. Based on information generated in this biological model, we and others have proposed that the G_i, G_q, and G_{12} family of G proteins can harbor oncogenic potential.

Identification of Mutationally Activated G-Proteins in Tumors

THE *GSP* AND *GIP* ONCOGENES

Mutations diminishing the GTPase activity of α_s and α_{i2} have been reported in human endocrine tumors *(25,29–31,57–59)*. In particular, activating mutations in $G\alpha_s$ have been found in pituitary adenomas and thyroid tumors. In somatotrophs and thyrocytes, cAMP stimulates cell growth and hormone secretion *(60)*. Thus mutational activation of α_s and the consequent elevation in intracellular cAMP result in hyperplasia and enhanced secretion of GH and thyroid hormone in the pituitary and thyroid glands, respectively. Clinically, these activated forms of α_s, referred as the *gsp* oncogene *(30)*, in somatotrophs can lead to acromegaly and gigantism, whereas similar mutations in the thyroid causes hyperthyroidism. Mutational activation of $G\alpha_s$ has also been found in the McCune-Albright syndrome *(61)*, as described in Chapter 3. Activating mutations of $G\alpha_{i2}$ were identified in ovarian sex cord stromal tumors and adrenal cortical tumors, on amplification of Gα_{i2} coding exons by the PCR technique *(30)*. Although these findings have not been yet validated using DNA from fresh surgically resected human tumors, they nevertheless provide compelling evidence that this G-protein α-subunit might be implicated in cancer, and the activated form of Gα_{i2} has been referred to as the *gip2* oncogene *(30)*. Naturally occurring mutations in members of the α_q family of G-protein α-subunits, α_q, α_{11}, α_{14}, α_{15}, and α_{16}, have not been yet reported.

IS G$_{12}$ IMPLICATED IN HUMAN CANCER?

As discussed above, GTPase-deficient mutants of Gα_{12} and Gα_{13} behave as extremely potent transforming genes when expressed in a variety of cellular systems. Furthermore, overexpression of Gα_{12} is *per se* transforming, a feature unique compared with other G-protein α-subunits. Indeed, the human Gα_{12} cDNA was cloned by Chan and colleagues *(62)* as a transforming gene isolated from a soft tissue sarcoma-derived cell line, using an expression cDNA library approach. More recently, we have cloned the human Gα_{13} gene, and found that its overexpression is sufficient to transform NIH 3T3 cells (unpublished observation). Thus, the remarkable biological effect of both members of the Gα_{12} family of G proteins, α_{12} and α_{13}, suggests, that these proteins might be implicated in naturally occurring tumorigenesis. Although no activating mutations in these G-protein α-subunits have been so far described in human cancers, we have screened a collection of human tumor cell lines for α_{12} and α_{13} overexpression using an anti-serum specific for the G$_{12}$ G protein family *(36)*. Of interest, a number of breast, colon, and prostate adeno-carcinoma-derived cell lines were found to express high levels of G$_{12}$-G$_{13}$, even greater than that inducing malignant transformation of NIH 3T3 cells Table 4. Furthermore, immortal, nontumorigenic breast-derived cell lines express relatively low levels of G$_{12}$. Thus, G$_{12}$ is remarkably overexpressed in a fraction of tumor-derived cell lines. Whether that contributes to the neoplastic conversion of these cells is still unclear, and is currently being investigated by expression of wt and mutated forms of Gα_{12} in immortalized normal human cell lines, as well as in transgenic animal models.

CONCLUSION

The complete elucidation of the molecular mechanisms involved in mitogenic signaling is clearly one of the major challenges for the 1990s and for the new century ahead. Furthermore, the realization that subtle alteration of proteins involved in mitogenic signaling can cause profound aberrations in cell growth, including malignant transformation, lends support to the idea of exploring the molecular basis of cancer by studying biochemical pathways involved in growth promotion. Ectopic expression of G-protein-coupled receptors in fibroblasts has been used as a biologically relevant model for dissecting biochemical routes involved in mitogenic signaling through this class of cell-surface receptors. In this system, certain G-protein-linked receptors, such as the m1 subtype of mAChRs, can effectively activate proliferative pathways, and if persistently activated, these receptors can behave as potent dominant acting oncogenes. Accordingly, activated G-protein α-subunits were found to harbor transforming potential, and activating mutations for G proteins have been identified in naturally occurring human neoplasia. Using a variety of approaches, critical components responsible for their remarkable biological effects have just begun to be identified. One such an example is the partial elucidation of the pathways communicating cell-surface receptors and G proteins to the transcription machinery in the nucleus, thereby controlling genetic

Table 4
Expression of $G\alpha_{12}$-$G\alpha_{13}$ in Tumor-Derived Cell Lines[a]

Cell line	Origin	Relative G_{12} expression
NIH 3T3	Normal mouse fibroblasts	+
NIH 3T3/$G\alpha_{12}$ wt (36)	Transformed mouse fibroblasts	+++
MCF7	Breast adenocarcinoma	++++
MDA-MB231	Breast adenocarcinoma	+++
MDA-MB 415	Breast adenocarcinoma	++
MDA-MB 468	Breast adenocarcinoma	+
SK-BR-3	Breast adenocarcinoma	+
MDA-MB134 VI	Breast ductal carcinoma	+
MDA-MB 453	Breast carcinoma	+++
ZR-75-1	Breast carcinoma	+++
BT474	Breast ductal carcinoma	++++
BT20	Breast carcinoma	++
MCF10A	Mammary epithelial	+
H5578	Breast normal	+
colo 205	Colon adenocarcinoma	++
SW 48	Colon adenocarcinoma	++
HCT 15	Colon adenocarcinoma	+
SW948	Colon adenocarcinoma	+
HT 29	Colon adenocarcinoma	++
SW 1116	Colon adenocarcinoma	+++
W1 DR	Colon adenocarcinoma	++
T84	Colon carcinoma	+
HCT 116	Colon carcinoma	++
PC-3	Prostate adenocarcinoma	++++

[a] Lysates containing 40 μg of protein from the indicated cells, obtained from ATCC and grown in the appropriate culture medium, were subjected to Western blot analysis with antibodies against $G\alpha_{12}$-$G\alpha_{13}$ (36). Autoradiograms were quantitated, and relative expression with respect to untransfected NIH 3T3 cells was estimated.

programs involved in normal and aberrant cell growth. As discussed in other chapters in this book, an increasing number of diseases are being found to involve genetic changes in $G\alpha$ proteins and their linked receptors. Furthermore, because of the recently recognized importance of β- and γ-subunits in signaling from heterotrimeric G proteins to small GTP binding proteins of the Ras and Rho families (49,50,63), it can be predicted that mutations in these G-protein subunits will also be found in a number of disease states. In this regard, the recent availability of increasingly sophisticated detection techniques for biologically relevant alterations in G proteins, G-protein-coupled receptor, and their downstream signaling pathways will certainly allow investigators to define more readily the role of these molecules in cancer as well as in other human diseases.

REFERENCES

1. Yarden Y, Escobedo JA, Kuang WJ, Yang-Feng TL, Harkins RN, Francke U, Fried VA, Ullrich A, Williams LT. Structure of the receptor for platelet-derived growth factor helps define a family of closely related growth factor receptors. Nature 1986;323:226–232.

2. Downward J, Yarden Y, Mayes E, Scrace G, Totty N, Stockwell P, Ullrich A, Schlessinger J, Waterfield MD. Close similarity of epidermal growth factor receptor and v-erb-B oncogene protein sequences. Nature 1994;307:521–527.

3. Sherr CJ, Rettenmier CW, Sacca R, Roussel MF, Look AT, Stanley ER. The c-fms proto-oncogene product is related to the receptor for the mononuclear phagocyte growth factor CSF-1. Cell 1985; 41:665–676.

4. Jackson TR, Blair LA, Marshall J, Goedert M, Hanley MR. The *mas* oncogene encodes an angiotensin receptor. Nature 1988;335:437–440.

5. Doolitle RF, Hunkapiller MW, Hood L, Deware SG, Robbins KC, Aaronson SA, Antoniades HN. Simian sarcoma virus onc gene v-sis is derived from the gene or genes encoding a platelet-derived growth factor. Science 1983;221:275–277.

6. Ullrich A, Schlessinger J. Signal transduction by receptors with tyrosine kinase activity. Cell 1990;61: 203–212.

7. Dohlman HG, Caron MG, Lefkowitz RJ. A family of receptors coupled to guanine nucleotide regulatory proteins. Biochemistry 1987;26:2657–2664.

8. Rozengurt E. Early signals in the mitogenic response. Science 1986;234:161–166.

9. Young D, Waitches G, Birchmeier C, Fasano O, Wigler M. Isolation and characterization of a new cellular oncogene encoding a protein with multiple potential transmembrane domains. Cell 1986;45:711–719.

10. Seuwen K, Kahan C, Hartmann T, Pouyssegur J. Strong and persistent activation of inositol lipid breakdown induces early mitogenic events but not G$_0$ to S phase progression in hamsters fibroblasts. J Biol Chem 1990;265:22,292–22,299.

11. Seuwen K, Magnaldo I, Pouyssegur J. Serotonin stimulates DNA-synthesis in fibroblasts acting through 5-HT$_{1B}$ receptors coupled to G$_i$-protein. Nature 1988;335:254–256.

12. Seuwen K, Pouyssegur J. Serotonin as a growth factor. Biochem Pharmacol 1990;39:985–990.

13. van Corven EJ, Groenink A, Jalink K, Eichholtz T, Moolenaar WH. Lysophosphatidate-induced cell proliferation: identification and dissection of signaling pathways mediated by G proteins. Cell 1989;59:45–54.

14. Coughlin SR, Escobedo JA, Williams LT. Role of phosphatidylinositol kinase in PDGF receptor signal transduction. Science 1989;243:1191–1194.

15. Moolenar WH. G-protein-coupled receptors, phosphoinositide hydrolysis and cell proliferation. Cell Growth Differ 1991;2:359–364.

16. Bonner TI, Burkley NJ, Young AC, Brann MR. Identification of a family of muscarinic acetylcholine receptors genes. Science 1987;237:527–532.

17. Kubo T, Fukuda K, Mikami A, Maeda A, Takahashi H, Mishina M, Haga T, Haga K, Ichiyama A, Kangawa K, Kojima M, Matsuo H, Hirose T, Numa S. Cloning sequencing and expression of complementary DNA encodingthe muscarinic acetylcholine receptor. Nature 1986;323:411–416.

18. Peralta EG, Ashkenazi A, Winslow JW, Smith DH, Ramachandran J, Capon DJ. Distinct primary structures ligand-binding properties and tissue-specific expression of four human muscarinic acetylcholine receptors. EMBO J 1987;6:3923–3929.

19. Jones SVP, Barker JL, Burkley NJ, Bonner TI, Collins RM, Brann MR. Cloned muscarinic receptors subtypes expressed in A9 L cells differ in their coupling to electrical responses. Mol Pharmacol 1988;34:421–426.

20. Stephens EV, Kalinec G, Brann MR, Gutkind JS. Transforming G-protein-coupled receptors transduce potent mitogenic signals in NIH3T3 cells independent on cAMP inhibition or conventional protein kinases C. Oncogene 1993;8:19–26.

21. Gutkind JS, Novotny EA, Brann MR, Robbins KR. Muscarinic acetylcholine receptor subtypes as agonist dependent oncogenes. Proc Natl Acad Sci USA 1991;88:4703–4708.

22. Julius D, Livelli TJ, Jessell TM, Axel R. Ectopic expression of the serotonin 1c receptor and the triggering of malignat transformation. Science 1989;244:1057–1062.

23. Allen LF, Lefkowitz RJ, Caron MG, Cotecchia S. G-protein coupled receptor genes as protoonocogenes: constitutively activating mutation of the α_{1B}-adrenergic receptor enhances mitogenesis and tumorigenicity. Proc Natl Acad Sci USA 1991;88:11,354–11,358.

24. Bourne HR, Sanders DA, McCormick F. The GTPase superfamily: a conserved switch for diverse cell function. Nature 1991;349:117–127.

25. Landis CA, Masters SB, Spada A, Pace AM, Bourne HR, Vallar V. GTPase inhibiting mutations activate the alpha chain of G$_s$ and stimulate adenylyl cyclase in human pituitary tumours. Nature 1989;340: 692–696.

26. Barbacid M. *ras* genes. Annu Rev Biochem 1987;56:779–827.

27. Hermouet S, Merendino Jr JJ, Gutkind JS, Spiegel AM. Activating and inactivating mutations of the α subunit of G_{i2} protein have opposite effects on proliferation of NIH 3T3 cells. Proc Natl Acad Sci USA 1991;88:10,455–10,459.

28. Kalinec G, Nazarali AJ, Hermouet S, Xu N, Gutkind JS. Mutated α subunit of the G_q protein induces malignant transformation in NIH 3T3 cells. Mol Cell Biol 1992;12:4687–4693.

29. Pace AM, Wong YH, Bourne HR. A mutant α subunit of G_{i2} induces neoplastic transformation of Rat-1 cells. Proc Natl Acad Sci USA 1991;88:7031–7035.

30. Lyons J, Landis CA, Harsh G, Vallar L, Grunewald K, Feichtinger H, Duh Q-Y, Clark OH, Kawasaki E, Bourne HR, McCormick F. Two G protein oncogenes in human endocrine tumors. Science 1990;249:655–659.

31. Vallar L, Spada A, Giannasttasio G. Altered G_s and adenylate cyclase activity in human GH-secreting pituitary adenomas. Nature 1987;330:556–558.

32. Shenker A, Goldsmith P, Unson CG, Spiegel AM. The G protein coupled thromboxane A_2 receptor in human platelets is a member of the novel G_q family. J Biol Chem 1991;266:9309–9313.

33. Taylor SJ, Chae HZ, Rhee SG, Exton JH. Activation of the $β_1$ isozyme of phospholipase C by α subunits of the G_q class of G proteins. Nature 1991;350:516–518.

34. Strathmann MP, Simon MI. G alpha 12 and G aplha 13 subunits define a fourth class of G protein alpha subunits. Proc Natl Acad Sci USA 1991;88:5582–5586.

35. Parks S, Wieschaus E. The Drosophila gastrulation gene concertina encodes a G alpha-like protein. Cell 1991;64:447–58.

36. Xu N, Bradley L, Ambdukar I, Gutkind JS. A mutant α subunit of G_{i2} potentiates the eicosanoid pathway and is highly oncogenic in NIH 3T3 cells. Proc Natl Acad Sci USA 1993;90:6741–6745.

37. Xu N, Voyno-Yasenetskaya T, Gutkind JS. Potent transforming activity of the G_{13} α subunit defines a novel family of oncogenes. Biochem Biophys Res Commun 1994;201:603–609.

38. Jiang H, Wu D, Simon MI. The transforming activity of activated $Gα_{12}$ FEBS Lett 1993;3:319–322.

39. Wilkie TM, Gilbert DJ, Olsen AS, Chen X-N, Amatruda TT, Korenberg JR, Trask BJ, de Jong P, Reed RR, Simon MI, Jenkins NA, Copeland NG. Evolution of the mammalian G protein alpha subunit multigene family. Nature Genet 1992;1:85–89.

40. Offermanns S, Laugwitz KL, Spicher K, Schultz G. G proteins of the G_{12} family are activated via thromboxane A_2 and thrombin receptors in human platelets. Proc Natl Acad Sci USA 1994;91:504–508.

41. Aragay AM, Collins LR, Post GR, Watson AJ, Feramisco JR, Brown JH, Simon MI. G_{12} requirement for thrombin-stimulated gene expression and DNA synthesis in 1321N1 astrocytoma cells. J Biol Chem 1995;270:20,073–20,077.

42. Wilk-Blaszczak MA, Singer WD, Gutowski S, Sternweis PC, Belardetti F. The G protein G_{13} mediates inhibition of voltage-dependent calcium current by bradykinin. Neuron 1994;13:1215–1224.

43. Voyno-Yasenetskaya T, Conklin BR, Gilbert RL, Hooley R, Bourne HR, Barber DL. G alpha 13 stimulates Na-H exchange. J Biol Chem 1994;269:4721–4724.

44. Dhanasekaran N, Prasad MV, Wadsworth SJ, Dermott JM, van Rossum G. Protein kinase C-dependent and -independent activation of Na^+/H^+ exchanger by G alpha 12 class of G proteins. J Biol Chem 1994;269:11,802–11,806.

45. Kitamura K, Singer WD, Cano A, Miller RT. G alpha q and G alpha 13 regulate NHE-1 and intracellular calcium in epithelial cells. Am J Physiol 1995;268:C101–110.

46. Cano E, Mahadevan LC. Parallel signal processing among mammalian MAPKs. Trends Biochem Sci 1995;20:117–122.

47. Marshall CJ. Specificity of receptor tyrosine kinase signaling: transient versus sustained extracellular signal-regulated kinase activation. Cell 1995;80:179–185.

48. Coso OA, Chiariello M, Yu J-C, Teramoto H, Crespo P, Xu N, Miki T, Gutkind JS. The small GTP-binding protein rac1 and cdc42 regulate the activity of the JNK/SAPK signaling. Cell 1995;81:1137–1146.

49. Crespo P, Xu N, Simonds WF, Gutkind JS. Ras-dependent activation of MAP kinase pathway mediated by G-protein βγ subunits. Nature 1994;369:418–420.

50. Coso OA, Chiariello M, Kalinec G, Kyriakis JM, Woodgett J, Gutkind JS. Transforming G-protein-coupled receptors potently activate JNK (SAPK). Evidence for a divergence from the tyrosine kinase signaling pathway. J Biol Chem 1995;270:5620–5624.

51. Prasad MV, Dermott JM, Heasley LE, Johnson GL, Dhanasekaran N. Activation of Jun kinase/stress-activated protein kinase by GTPase-deficient mutants of $Gα_{12}$ and $Gα_{13}$. J Biol Chem 1995;270:18,655–18,659.

52. Collins LR, Minden A, Karin M, Brown JH. Gα$_{12}$ stimulates c-Jun NH$_2$-terminal kinase through the small G proteins Ras and Rac. J Biol Chem 1996;271:17,349–17,353.

53. Ridley A, Hall A. The small GTP-binding protein rho regulates the assembly of focal adhesions and acting stress fibers in response to growth factors. Cell 1992;70:389–399.

54. Ridley AJ, Hall A. Signal transduction pathways regulating Rho-mediated stress fibre formation: requirement for a tyrosine kinase. EMBO J 1994;13:2600–2610.

55. Buhl AM, Johnson NL, Dhanasekaran N, Johnson GL. Gα$_{12}$ and Gα$_{13}$ stimulate Rho-dependent stress fiber formation and focal adhesion assembly. J Biol Chem 1995;270:24,631–24,634.

56. Hill CS, Wynne J, Treisman R. The Rho family GTPases RhoA, Rac1, and CDC42Hs regulate transcriptional activation by SRF. Cell 1995;81:1159–1170.

57. Suarez HG, du Villard JA, Callou B, Schumberger M, Parmentier C, Monier R. *gsp* Mutations in human thyroid tumors. Oncogene 1991;6:677–679.

58. Climenti E, Malgaratti N, Meldolesi J, Toramelli R. A new constitutively activating mutation of G$_s$ protein α subunit-*gsp* oncogene is found in pituitary tumors. Oncogene 1990;5:1059–1061.

59. O'Sullivan C, Barton CM, Staddon SL, Brwn CL, Lemoine NR. Activating point mutations of the *gsp* oncogene in human thyroid adenomas. Mol Carcinog 1991;4:345–349.

60. Dumont JE, Jauniaux JC, Roger PP. The cyclic AMP-mediated stimulation of cell proliferation. Trends Biochem Sci 1989;14:67–71.

61. Weinstein LS, Shenker A, Gejman PV, Merino MJ, Friedman E, Spiegel AM. Activating mutations of the stimulatory G protein in the McCune-Albright syndrome. N Engl J Med 1991;325:1688–1695.

62. Chan AM-L, Fleming TP, McGovern ES, Chedid M, Miki T, Aaronson SA. Expression cDNA cloning of a transforming gene encoding the wild-type G alpha 12 gene product. Mol Cell Biol 1993;13:762–768.

63. Clapham DE, Neer EJ. New roles for G-protein beta gamma-dimers in transmembrane signalling. Nature 1993;365:403–406.

64. Zachary I, Masters SB, Bourne HR. Increased mitogenic responsiveness of Swiss 3T3 cells expressing constitutively activated G$_{sα}$ Biochem Biophys Res Commun 1990;168:1184–1193.

7

Hypo- and Hyperthyroidism Caused by Mutations of the TSH Receptor

Gilbert Vassart, MD, PhD

CONTENTS

INTRODUCTION

The main function of the thyroid gland is to synthesize, store, and secrete the thyroid hormones T_3 and T_4. Regulation of this function is achieved primarily through a positive control exerted by the pituitary hormone thyroid stimulating hormone (TSH) and a negative control exerted by iodine. In most physiological circumstances the maintenance of eumetabolism requires steady concentrations of circulating thyroid hormones. This is achieved by a classical chemostat that involves the feedback of thyroid hormones on TSH production. Compared with other endocrine organs, the control of thyroid function is subject to relatively slow changes. The main roles of the regulatory mechanisms are to ensure adequate use of the available iodine in the diet to maintain steady levels of circulating hormones and to protect the thyroid gland and the organism from the toxicity that can result from excessive availability of iodine. Regulation of thyroid function is thus mainly of a "tonic" nature, with virtually no physiological circumstances in which the gland should be put completely at rest. This chapter concentrates on the regulatory actions of thyrotropin via its receptor.

The regulatory actions of TSH are exerted on thyrocytes at three main levels: the expression of the differentiated phenotype, proliferation, and functional activity. In vitro and in vivo experiments have demonstrated that in the absence of TSH, thyrocytes

From: *Contemporary Endocrinology: G Proteins, Receptors, and Disease*
Edited by: A. M. Spiegel, Humana Press Inc., Totowa, NJ

decrease the expression of thyroid-specific genes (e.g., thyroglobulin, thyroperoxidase) *(1,2)*. However, this "dedifferentiation" is not complete; in particular, expression of the TSH receptor gene is maintained at a level compatible with restoration of the normal differentiated state on restimulation by TSH *(3)*. Whether TSH contributes with known (TTF1, TTF2, and Pax 8) *(4)* and unknown transcription factors to the differentiation program of thyrocytes is debated (see below).

It is well established that sustained stimulation by TSH of thyrocytes in vitro or of the whole gland in vivo leads to a proliferative response. With the exception of TSH receptor-dependent toxic thyroid hyperplasia (*see below*), the key role of TSH in the development of nonautoimmune goiters is generally accepted.

Acute experimental stimulation by TSH and TSH withdrawal modify the rate of thyroid hormone synthesis (organification of iodine and coupling of iodotyrosine) and release (secretion). As was mentioned, these effects of TSH on thyrocyte function are responsible under physiological conditions for the fine-tuning of the thyroid hormone chemostat but are not required for dramatic temporal changes in hormone production.

In the human thyroid, except for the iodination and coupling steps which are Ca^{2+}-dependent, all these effects of TSH can be reproduced by cyclic adenosine monophosphate (cAMP) agonists *(5–7)*. In particular and despite controversies, it is accepted that cAMP mediates both the functional activation of hormone secretion by TSH and its growth effects on thyrocytes *(7,8)* (Fig. 1). Whereas solid experimental arguments were obtained from cell culture experiments *(7)*, in vivo experiments in transgenic mice *(9)* and an understanding of the pathophysiology of the McCune-Albright syndrome *(10)* (*see Chapter 3*), toxic adenomas *(11,12)*, and toxic thyroid hyperplasia *(13)* contributed to the consolidation of this notion (*see below*).

For the sake of clarity, thyroid diseases can be subdivided into four broad categories:

1. Related to iodine deficiency;
2. Autoimmune;
3. Hereditary/congenital; and
4. Neoplastic.

Of course, this classification is artificial; there is much evidence for interactions between iodine availability, for instance, and both autoimmunity and neoplasia. The TSH receptor is implicated in virtually all disease categories as the target of its normal agonist TSH or autoantibodies or as a possible target for somatic or germline mutations.

THE TSH RECEPTOR

The TSH receptor belongs to the large family of G-protein-coupled receptors (GPCRs) *(2,6,14,15)*. More precisely, it is one of the three glycoprotein hormone receptors (LH/CGr, FSHr, and TSHr) that are structurally and evolutionary related by their serpentine portion to the large subfamily of opsin-related GPCRs. The primary structure of the receptor has been deduced from the sequence of the cDNA: It is composed of a serpentine C-terminal moiety typical of GPCRs that is encoded in a single exon (Nr 10) *(16)*. In contrast to other GPCRs but in common with LH/CGr and FSHr, the TSHr has a long (398 residues) N-terminal extracellular domain that is encoded in multiple exons (1 to 9 for TSHr) *(16)*. This domain has sequence similarity with proteins containing leucine repeats, the prototype of which is the ribonuclease inhibitor *(17,18)*.

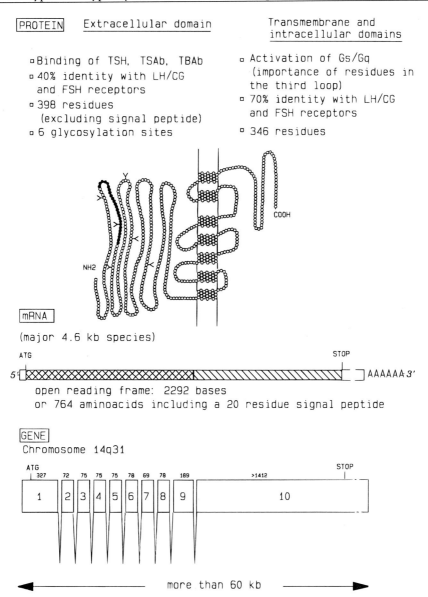

PROTEIN   Extracellular domain

Transmembrane and
intracellular domains

▫ Binding of TSH, TSAb, TBAb
▫ 40% identity with LH/CG
  and FSH receptors
▫ 398 residues
  (excluding signal peptide)
▫ 6 glycosylation sites

▫ Activation of Gs/Gq
  (importance of residues in
  the third loop)
▫ 70% identity with LH/CG
  and FSH receptors
▫ 346 residues

mRNA
(major 4.6 kb species)

open reading frame: 2292 bases
or 764 aminoacids including a 20 residue signal peptide

GENE
Chromosome 14q31

more than 60 kb

Fig. 1. Schematic representations of the TSH receptor protein, mRNA and gene.

The modular structure of the glycoprotein hormone receptors led to the early suggestion that their extracellular domains are responsible for high-affinity binding of the hormones, with the serpentine portion being the "effector" that transduces the binding signal to the G protein. Site-directed mutagenesis experiments and the construction of chimeric receptors *(15,19–22)* have validated this model, which provides an interesting approach to the understanding of GPCR activation. For GPCRs of the opsin family, ligand binding and activation of G proteins are carried out by the serpentine molecule itself. The binding domain for biogenic amines is within the slit between the seven transmembrane helices *(14,23)*; for (neuro)peptides, it seems to involve both the slit and the extracellular loops and the N-terminal segment *(24,25)*. For the glycoprotein hormone receptors, the observation that the N-terminal domain made of leucine repeats is sufficient to bind the hormone with high affinity *(22)* raises the question of how the binding signal is translated into a conformational change in the serpentine portion. We will see how spontaneous mutants of the TSHr may help answer this question.

The modular structure of the glycoprotein hormone receptors appeared very early in evolution. Receptors with a similar structure and highly significant sequence similarity have been cloned from cnidarians (*Anthopleura elegantissima*) *(26)* and *Drosophila* *(27)*. The cloning of the corresponding ligands in these species may help define a common mechanism of receptor activation.

The actual three-dimensional structure of the GPCRs is an open question. Models have been proposed that provide a basis for the design of site-directed mutagenesis experiments and an understanding of the phenotypes of spontaneous mutants. For the glycoprotein hormone receptors, models of the serpentine portion have been proposed *(28)* and are being tested (*see* Chapter 8). The recent availability of the three-dimensional structure of the porcine ribonuclease inhibitor *(18)* has provided a starting point to model the leucine repeat portion of the extracellular domain of TSHr *(29)*. This consists of a sector of a doughnut, with the concave and convex surfaces made of α-sheets and α-helices, respectively. Although they provide a potentially helpful basis for the interpretation of experimental observations, the future will indicate whether the current models are close to reality.

As was stated, the TSH receptor is coupled primarily to the adenylyl cyclase–cAMP regulatory cascade by interaction with Gs. In some species, including humans, the receptor is also capable of activating phospholipase C via Gq *(30)*. In both cultured thyrocytes and cells transfected with the human TSH receptor cDNA, stimulation of the inositol phosphate–diacylglycerol cascade requires higher concentrations of TSH than does activation of adenylyl cyclase *(30)*. Since stimulation of phospholipase C is not reproduced by cAMP agonists, it has been concluded that the same TSHr is coupled to both Gs and Gq, with its affinity for Gs being higher than that for Gq. In experiments in which direct interaction between the receptor and the G proteins was examined in human thyroid membranes, it was found that the TSH receptor was capable of interacting with all the G proteins present *(31,32)*. Whether this observation results from promiscuous interactions taking place in isolated membranes only or has a functional significance has not been established. From a physiopathological viewpoint it is safe to rely on the notion that in humans the TSHr is coupled mainly to Gs, with the potential to activate Gq when stimulated strongly (Fig. 2).

LOSS-OF-FUNCTION MUTATIONS

Expected Phenotypes

Loss-of-function mutations in the TSHr gene are expected to cause a syndrome of "resistance to TSH." The expected phenotype is likely to resemble that of patients with mutations in TSH itself. These mutations have been described because of the prior availability of the information on TSH α and β genes *(33–35)*. A mouse model of resistance to TSH is available in the *hyt/hyt* line. Homozygous *hyt/hyt* mice are hypothyroid secondary to a developmental anomaly of the thyroid, which remains hypoplastic *(36)*. The cause has been traced to a mutation of the TSH receptor gene (Pro556Leu) *(36,37)*. From this information one would expect patients with two mutated alleles to exhibit a

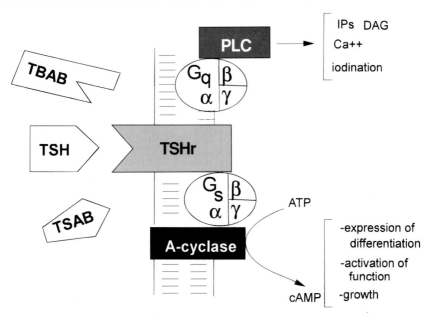

Fig. 2. Schematic representation of the regulation of thyroid cell physiology by the TSH receptor-dependent regulatory cascades. TSAB, thyroid-stimulating antibodies; TBAB, thyroid-blocking antibodies.

degree of hypothyroidism in relation to the extent of the loss of function. Heterozygous carriers are expected to be normal or to display a minimal increase in plasma TSH.

Clinical Cases with the Mutations Identified

A few patients with convincing resistance to TSH were described before molecular genetics allowed the identification of the mutations *(38,39)*. Another family was described more recently, but no mutation was found in the receptor gene *(40)*. The first patients described in molecular terms were euthyroid sibs with elevated TSH *(41)*. Sequencing of the TSH receptor gene identified a different mutation in each allele of the affected individuals, making them compound heterozygotes. The substitutions were in the extracellular amino-terminal portion of the receptor (maternal allele Pro162Ala, paternal allele Ile167Asn). The functional characteristics of the mutant receptors were studied by transient expression in COS cells: The paternal allele was virtually completely nonfunctional, while the maternal allele displayed an increase in EC_{50} for stimulation of cAMP production by TSH. Recent experiments have shown that the paternal allele is expressed in normal amounts in COS cells but remains trapped intracellularly and does not reach the cell surface. However, even when assayed on cell membranes, the paternal allele does not bind TSH, suggesting that the mutation has profound structural consequences that affect both the routing of the receptor to the plasma membrane and its ability to bind TSH (to be published).

When both mutations are displayed on a tentative model of the extracellular domain, their location is compatible with the observed phenotype: The Pro162Ala mutation affects a residue that has been predicted to be at the surface of the molecule, and this may explain its interference with the effects of TSH. The Ile167Asn mutation affects a residue protruding in the hydrophobic tunnel between the α-helices and the β-sheets of the doughnut-shaped model *(29)*. It is expected that a polar residue will be incompatible with that position and will result in severe misfolding of the whole extracellular domain. Coexpression in COS cells of the wild-type and mutated receptors did not show evidence of dominant negative effects of the mutants.

Recently, familial cases with loss-of-function mutations of the TSH receptor have been identified in screening programs for congenital hypothyroidism in Berlin *(42)* and Brussels *(87)*. The patients displayed the usual criteria for congenital hypothyroidism, including high TSH, low free T_4, and undetectable trapping of ^{99}Tc. The thyroids were small and normally located at ultrasonography. Surprisingly, plasma thyro-globulin levels were normal or high. In the Berlin study, the patient was a compound heterozygote for mutations situated in the extracellular domain (Cys390Trp and an insertion-deletion causing a frameshift, respectively). The functional characteristics have not been published. In the study from Brussels the patients were sibs born to consanguineous parents and were homozygous for a mutation in the transmembrane segment 4 (Ala553Thr), close to the *hyt* mutation of the mouse. When transiently expressed in COS cells, the mutants were barely expressed at the cell surface. However, the residual expression was compatible with some TSH binding and stimulation of cAMP production by TSH. When the phenotype of these cases are known in more detail, they will provide a means to understand the role of the receptor in thyroid organogenesis. Indeed, the difference in phenotype between people with mutations knocking out the hormone and those with mutations affecting the receptor will indicate whether the mere expression of a functional receptor (and of its constitutive activity on adenylyl cyclase stimulation; *see below*) plays a role in the development of a structurally normal thyroid. The relationship of any of these cases to the pathophysiology of *sporadic* athyreosis has not been established.

GAIN-OF-FUNCTION MUTATIONS

Expected Phenotypes

For a hormone receptor, "gain of function" may have two meanings: activation in the absence of ligand (constitutivity) or increased sensitivity to its normal agonist (for simplicity, we ignore modifications in specificity). When the receptor is part of a chemostat, as is the case for TSHr, the former situation is expected to lead to tissue "autonomy," whereas the latter situation is expected to cause adjustment of the agonist concentration to a lower value. If the mutation occurs in a cell that expresses the receptor normally (somatic mutation), it will become symptomatic only if the regulatory cascade controlled by the receptor is mitogenic in that particular cell type. Autonomous activity of the receptor will cause clonal expansion of the mutated cell. If the regulatory cascade also controls function positively, the resulting tumor will progressively take over the function of the normal tissue, leading ultimately to autonomous hyperfunction. If the mutation is present in all the cells of an organism (germline mutation), autonomy will be displayed by the whole tissue expressing the receptor. In cases where the regulatory cascade both is mitogenic and activates function, the expected result is hyperplasia associated with hyperfunction.

From what is known about thyroid cell physiology, it is easy to predict the phenotypes associated with gain of function of the cAMP-dependent regulatory cascade. Two observations provide pertinent models of this situation. Transgenic mice made to express the adenosine A2a receptor ectopically in the thyroid display severe hyper-thyroidism associated with thyroid hyperplasia *(9)*. As the A2a adenosine receptor is coupled to Gs and displays constitutive activity as a result of its continuous stimulation by ambient adenosine *(43)*, this model mimics closely the situation expected for a gain-of-function germline mutation of the TSH receptor. Patients with the McCune-Albright syndrome are mosaic for mutations in Gsα (Gsp mutations) leading to the constitutive stimulation of adenylyl cyclase *(10)* (Chapter 3). Hyperfunctioning thyroid adenomas develop in these patients from cells that harbor the mutation, making them a model for gain-of-function somatic mutations of the TSH receptor. A transgenic model in which Gsp mutations are targeted for expression in the mouse thyroid has been constructed *(44)*.

Somatic Mutations of the TSHr

These considerations made it a logical endeavor to look in hyperfunctioning thyroid adenomas (toxic, or "hot," nodules) for activating mutations in genes that are implicated in the cAMP regulatory cascade. Soon after mutations of Gsα were found in adenomas of the pituitary somatotrophs *(10)*, similar Gsp mutations were found in some toxic adenomas and follicular carcinomas *(45–48)*.

The demonstration by site-directed mutagenesis that GPCRs can be constitutively activated by amino acid substitutions in the third cytoplasmic loop *(49–51)* led to a search for similar mutations in the TSH receptor *(11,52)*. It was soon realized that toxic adenoma is a fruitful source of somatic mutations of TSHr. Initially, most of the mutations were found in the third cytoplasmic loop or in the adjacent sixth transmembrane segment. This clustering reflects both the existence of a real hot spot of activating mutations (*see below*) and a sampling bias resulting from the inference that the mutations should affect the same region identified in the adrenergic receptors. However, amino acid substitutions were subsequently found over most of the serpentine portion of the receptor *(11,52–55)* and even in the extracellular amino-terminal domain *(56)*.

When analyzed by transient expression in COS cells, all these mutant receptors exhibited an increase in constitutive activity (*see below*). A total of 10 different residues (15 if the germline mutations are included) have been identified in TSHr, the mutation of which leads to receptor activation. In 33 adenomas found in 37 patients (2 patients had 2 autonomous adenomas in the thyroid) the coding portion of the TSH receptor gene was completely sequenced together with the hot spots for Gsα mutations. Twenty-seven mutations were identified in the TSHr gene, and only two in GSα. Despite some dispute about this prevalence, which may be due to the different origins of the patients *(57,58)*, different sensitivities of mutation detection, or the fact that in some studies only segments of the TSHr gene were analyzed, we conclude that in a country, like Belgium, with a moderate shortage of iodine, activating mutations of the TSH receptor are the major cause of solitary toxic adenomas.

In one patient with a multinodular goiter and two zones of autonomy at scintigraphy, a different mutation of the TSH receptor was identified in each nodule *(56)*; a similar observation has been made independently *(42)*. This indicates that the pathophysiological mechanism responsible for solitary toxic adenomas can be at work on a background of multinodular goiter and may be responsible for some of the autonomous zones that appear late in the evolution in these patients. The independent occurrence of two activating mutations in a patient may seem highly improbable, but the multiplicity of the possible targets for activating mutations within the TSH receptor (at least 15 different residues) makes this occurrence less unlikely. It is also possible that a mutagenic environment is created in the gland by chronic stimulation. In this respect, it will be interesting to explore whether the TSH receptor gene in the thyroids of patients in an endemic goiter area becomes hyperthyroid after iodine supplementation *(59)*.

Finally, the possible involvement of TSH receptor mutations in thyroid cancers has been considered. After initially negative results, recent studies have suggested that activating mutations of the TSH receptor gene may be implicated in a limited proportion of follicular thyroid carcinomas selected for their high basal activity of adenyl cyclase *(60 and unpublished observations)*.

Germline Mutations

HEREDITARY TOXIC THYROID HYPERPLASIA

The major cause of hyperthyroidism is Graves' disease, in which an autoimmune reaction is mounted against the thyroid gland and autoantibodies are produced that recognize and stimulate the TSH receptor. The mechanisms that lead to autoimmune thyroid diseases are unknown, but genetic factors certainly are involved, since familial clustering is observed frequently. This may explain why the initial description by Thomas et al. *(61)* of a family showing segregation of thyrotoxicosis as an autosomal dominant trait in the absence of signs of autoimmunity was met with skepticism. Reinvestigation of this family together with another family from Reims identified two mutations of the TSH receptor gene that segregated in perfect linkage with the disease *(13)*. Three additional families have been studied since that time, and surprisingly, each showed a different mutation of the TSHr gene *(62)*. The functional characteristics of these mutant receptors confirm the idea that they are constitutively stimulated *(see below)*. This new nosological entity, which we propose calling Leclère's disease or hereditary toxic thyroid hyperplasia (HTTH), is characterized by the following clinical characteristics: autosomal dominant transmission, hyperthyroidism with a variable age of onset (from infancy to adulthood) even in a given family, hyperplastic goiter of variable size but with steady growth, and absence of the clinical or biological stigmata of autoimmunity. An observation common to the cases decribed to date is the need for drastic ablative therapy (surgery or radioiodine) to control the disease once the patient has become hyperthyroid. The autonomous nature of the thyroid tissue from these patients has been elegantly demonstrated by grafting in nude mice *(63)*. Unlike tissue from Graves' disease patients, HTTH cells continue to grow in the absence of stimulation by TSH or thyroid-stimulating antibody (TSAb).

The prevalence of HTTH is difficult to estimate at present. It is likely that many cases have been, and still are, mistaken for Graves' disease. This may be explained by the relative insensitivity and lack of specificity of thyroid-stimulating antibody assays, together with the high frequency of the other thyroid autoantibodies (antithyroglobulin, antithyroperoxidase) in the general population. It is expected that wider knowledge of the existence of the disease will lead to better diagnosis. This is not a purely academic problem, since presymptomatic diagnosis in children from affected families may prevent the developmental or psychological complications associated with infantile or juvenile hyperthyroidism.

SPORADIC TOXIC THYROID HYPERPLASIA

Three cases of toxic thyroid hyperplasia have been described in children born of unaffected parents *(55,64,65)*. Conspicuously, congenital hyperthyroidism was present in these three patients and required aggressive treatment. Mutations of one TSH receptor allele were identified in these children but were absent in their parents. As paternity was confirmed by mini- or microsatellite testing, these cases qualify as true neomutations. In comparing the amino acid substitutions implicated in hereditary and sporadic cases, it is surprising at first that they do not overlap (Fig. 3). Whereas the sporadic cases harbor mutations that also are found in toxic adenomas, the hereditary cases up to now have "private" mutations. The analysis of the functional characteristics of the individual mutant receptors in COS cells and the clinical course of individual patients suggest an explanation for this observation: "Sporadic" mutations seem to have a much stronger activating effect than do "hereditary" mutations. From their severe phenotype, it is likely that newborns with the neomutations that have been described would not have survived in the recent past. On the contrary, from inspection of the available pedigrees, it seems that the milder phenotype of patients with hereditary mutations has only a limited effect on reproductive fitness. The fact that hereditary mutations have not been observed in toxic adenomas is compatible with the suggestion that they cause extremely slow tissue growth and accordingly rarely cause thyrotoxicosis. If this explanation holds true, it can be predicted that mutations of the hereditary type will be found in the older patients with toxic adenoma.

FUNCTIONAL CHARACTERISTICS OF MUTANT RECEPTORS

All the mutations illustrated in Fig. 3 have been tested by transient transfection in COS cells. Before analyzing their phenotype, it is appropriate to describe the advantages and limitations of this system. Transfection of an expression plasmid containing the origin of replication of SV40 in COS cells leads within a couple of days to a replicative amplification that yields approx 10^5 copies/cell. The final number of copies per cell is quite independent of the number of plasmids that entered the cell initially. An important consequence of this is that under most experimental conditions, the level of expression of a given construct in COS cells is close to an all-or-none phenomenon at the level of the individual cell. Another consequence of this amplification process is that the level of expression of the protein encoded in the expression construct is extremely high. While TSH receptors at the surface of thyrocytes are in the range of 10^3/cell, this can reach 10^5 to 10^6 at the surface of COS cells, not counting the large amount of protein that remains trapped in the endoplasmic reticulum and Golgi apparatus.

The advantage of these characteristics is that they increase the sensitivity of the system. However, by modifying the stoichiometry of the interacting molecules, they may constitute a caricature of the situation in thyrocytes. The power of transfection studies resides in the possibility of studying the characteristics of one component, in this case TSHr, on a nonthyroid background, thus avoiding the confounding effects of other thyroid-specific gene products. Again, this has a drawback, since it does not necessarily allow analysis of the mutated receptors as they interact with their normal partners.

Despite these limitations and perhaps because of some of them, the COS cell system makes it possible to detect even slight increases in the constitutive activity of the TSH receptor. An important observation in the early studies *(13,66)* was that the wild-type receptor displays significant constitutive activity in the COS cell system (and, as we know now, in other cell types as well). This characteristic is not unique to the TSH receptor *(67–69)* but interestingly, it is not shared by its close relative, the LH/CG receptor *(67–69)* (*see* Chapter 8). The effect of activating-mutations must accordingly be interpreted in terms of the "increase in constitutive activity." An important corollary is that to assay

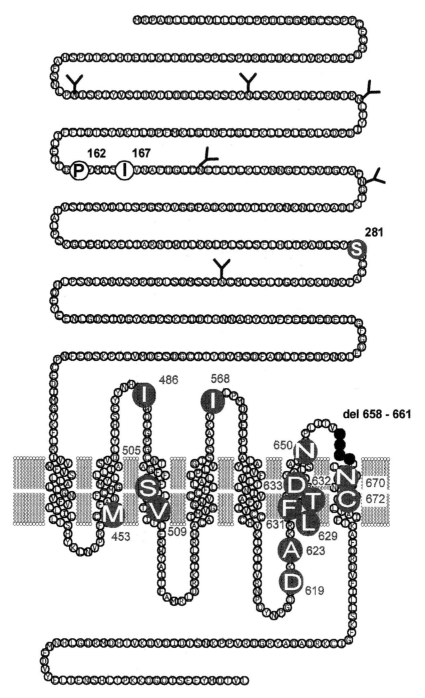

Fig. 3. Table of spontaneous mutations affecting the function of the TSH receptor, with the schematic indication of their locations within the protein structure. NT, not tested; Somatic, mutations found in toxic adenomas; Germline, mutations transmitted through the germline in hereditary (familial) or sporadic (neomut.) toxic thyroid hyperplasia.

Loss-of-function mutations.

Residue	Mutation	Function	Expression
162	Pro-Ala	higher EC$_{50}$ for TSH	present on cell surface
167	Ile-Asn	non functional	trapped in the cell

Gain-of-function mutations.

Residue	Mutation	Somatic	Germline (neomut)	Germline (familial)	cAMP	IP
281	Ser-Asn Ser-Thr	X X			+	-
453	Met-Thr	X	X		+	NT
486	Ile-Met Ile-Phe	X X			+ +	+ +
505	Ser-Asn			Lausanne	+	-
509	Val-Ala			Nancy	+	-
568	Ile-Thr	X			+	±
619	Asp-Gly	X			+	-
623	Ala-Ile	X			+	±
629	Leu-Phe	X			+	NT
631	Phe-Leu	X	X		+	-
632	Thr-Ile	X			+	-
633	Asp-Glu Asp-Tyr	X X			+ +	-
650	Asn-Tyr			Belfort	+	-
658-661	deletion	X			+	NT
670	Asn-Ser			Reims II	+	-
672	Cys-Tyr			Reims I	+	-

Fig. 3. *(Continued)*

mutant receptors properly it is mandatory to have a measure of the number of receptors expressed at the cell surface. This is usually achieved by ^{125}I TSH-binding experiments, but it also is safe to rely on independent measurments such as flow immunofluorometry.

Most amino acid substitutions found in toxic adenomas and/or toxic thyroid hyperplasia (Fig. 3) share common characteristics:

1. They increase the constitutive activity of the receptor toward stimulation of adenylyl cyclase;
2. With a few notable exceptions *(54)*, they do not display constitutive activity toward the inositol phosphate–diacylglycerol pathway;
3. Their expression at the cell surface is decreased (from slightly to severely);
4. Most but not all of them keep responding to TSH for stimulation of cAMP and inositol phosphate generation, with a tendency to do so with a decreased EC$_{50}$; and
5. They bind 125I bovine TSH with an apparent affinity higher than that of the wild-type receptor.

There is not a simple relationship between the position of the mutations or the nature of the amino acid substitution and their functional characteristics. Mutations found in transmembrane segments 2, 3, 5, and 7 and the third cytoplasmic loop all have similar phenotypes; they involve amino acids belonging to all classes (charged, polar, and hydrophobic), with substitutions that do not necessarily involve a shift to another class (*see* Fig. 3). Mutations involving Ile486 and Ile568 in the first and second extracellular loops, respectively, are exceptional in that in addition to stimulating adenylyl cyclase, they cause constitutive activation of the inositol phosphate pathway *(54)*. Two additional mutations deserve special mention because of their unexpected nature or location: the four amino acid deletion (residues 658–661) in the third extracellular loop and the substitutions at serine 281 in the amino-terminal extracellular domain (Fig. 3). The possible significance of these mutations are discussed later. Their functional characteristics are being studied in detail.

Although it has not been studied systematically for all mutants, the level of expression of individual mutated receptors varies over a wide range. Interestingly, there is not a direct relationship between the level of cAMP achieved by different mutants in transfected COS cells and their level of expression at the cell membrane *(70)*. This means that individual mutants have widely different "specific constitutive activity" (measured as the stimulation of cAMP accumulation divided by receptor number at the cell surface). Although this specific activity may indicate something about the mechanisms of receptor activation, it is not a measure of the actual phenotypic effect of the mutation in vivo. Indeed, one of the relatively mild mutations, which had been observed up to now only in an HTTH family (Cys672Tyr), is among the strongest according to this criterion. It would be logical to expect the best correlation to be found between the phenotype and the actual level of cAMP achieved regardless of the level of receptor expression. As was stated, however, possible differences between the effects of the mutants in COS cells and thyrocytes in vivo may render making these correlations a difficult exercise.

According to a current model for GPCR activation, the receptor would exist under at least two interconverting conformations: R (silent conformation) and R* (the active forms) *(50)*. The unliganded receptor would shuttle between both forms, with the equilibrium being in favor of R. Binding of the ligand, to the slit between the transmembrane segments (for biogenic amines) and/or residues of the N-terminal segment or extracellular loops (for neuropeptides) is believed to stabilize the R* conformation. The resulting R to R* transistion is supposed to involve a conformational change that modifies the relative positions of transmembrane helices. In turn, this would translate into conformational changes of the cytoplasmic domains interacting with trimeric G proteins.

In seminal studies with the adrenergic receptor α1b, a variety of amino acid substitutions in the C-terminal portion of the third intracellular loop led to their constitutive activation *(49)*. The observation that all amino acid substitutions at Ala293 were effective in activating the receptor led to the concept that the silent form of GPCRs would be submitted to a structural constraint, requiring the wild-type primary structure of the third intracellular loop. This constraint could be released by a wide spectrum of amino acid substitutions in this segment *(49,50,71,72)*.

The observation that amino acid substitutions in a large number of residues scattered over the serpentine portion of the TSH receptor cause an increase in its constitutive activity is fully compatible with this model and provides arguments for its extension. One of the first residues we found mutated in a toxic adenoma (Ala623) was the exact homolog of Ala293 in the α_{1b}-adrenergic receptor *(11)*. The fact that mutations in residues distributed over most of the serpentine portion of the receptor are equally effective in activating it (which does not seem to be a general characteristic of all GPCRs) suggests that the unliganded TSH receptor may be less constrained than others are. The readily measurable constitutive activity of the wild-type receptor is compatible with this contention. Since it already is "noisy," the TSHr would be more prone to further destabilization by a variety of mutations.

The precise effects of individual mutations in structural terms are difficult to predict: The sixth transmembrane segment, along with its continuation in the C-terminal portion of the third cytoplasmic loop, is clearly a hot spot (Fig. 3), with at least four residues potentially implicated in keeping the receptor inactive. The fact that consecutive residues in transmembrane helix 6 are implicated (residues 631, 632, and 633) argues against a simple model in which activation simply results from the rupture of an interaction with specific residues in another transmembrane helix (e.g., TM 3). Nevertheless, it is likely that the common consequence of activating mutations is the stabilization of a conformation of the serpentine with individual helices in a different relative position. The identification of activating amino acid substitutions in TM 2, 3, and 7 also fits well with this notion.

The activating mutations identified in the extracellular loops are more difficult to include in the model. Interestingly, these are among the strongest mutations when normalized for the level of receptor expression and display constitutive activity toward both cAMP and inositol phosphate generation (Fig. 3). Although it is possible that amino acid substitutions or deletions in the extracellular loops activate the receptor by affecting the position of the nearby transmembrane helices directly, two observations led us to hypothesize that a different mechanism may operate involving the extracellular aminoterminal domain: Binding experiments with bovine ^{125}I TSH showed that constitutively activated mutants display a higher apparent affinity than does the wild-type receptor *(70)*, and exposure of cells expressing the wild-type receptor to low concentrations of trypsin results in its constitutive activation while it simultaneously destroys an epitope of the amino-terminal domain *(73)*.

These observations are compatible with a model in which the unliganded amino-terminal domain would contribute to the silencing of the serpentine portion. The receptor would thus exist in an equilibrium between an open (active) conformation and a closed (inactive) conformation (Fig. 4). According to this model, activation would result from the release of the silencing interaction between the extracellular loops and the amino-terminal domain. This could be achieved by mutations in the extracellular loops, by proteolytic digestion of segments of the amino-terminal domain, or physiologically by stabilization of the "open" conformation by TSH binding to the amino-terminal domain.

The model predicts that activating mutations also should exist in the amino-terminal extracellular domain whose effects would be to destroy or reduce its interactions with the serpentine portion and constructs of the TSH receptor devoid of the amino-terminal domain should display constitutive activity. The first prediction was borne out by our recent identification of activating mutations involving serine at position 281 in the amino-terminal domain *(56)* (Fig. 3). Deletion by site-directed mutagenesis of a segment of the amino-terminal domain also was shown to produce an increase in constitutive activity *(74)*. The second prediction could not be tested properly, since it has not been possible to obtain convincing expression of the serpentine portion of the TSH receptor alone at the cell surface *(75)*.

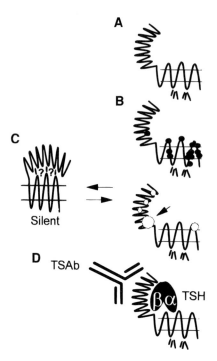

Fig. 4. Hypothetical mechanistic model for the activation of the TSH receptor. **(A) Spontaneous isomerization** (basal activity)—functional significance? **(B) Mutations:** evidence for the *release of an inhibitory constraint* exerted—in the serpentine (at least 14 residues involved) and/or with contribution of the amino terminus (at least one residue, Ser281). **(C) Trypsin**—*release of an inhibitory constraint* exerted in part by the extracellular domain and/or unmasking of a tethered ligand? **(D) TSH or TSAb**—activating interaction of TSH with the serpentine, *release of inhibitory constraint* exerted by the extracellular domain, both, or unmasking of a tethered ligand?

For the LH receptor, a widely quoted study found that the serpentine portion expressed alone was capable of low-affinity binding of human chorionic gonadotropin (hCG) and (minimal) hormone-dependent stimulation of cAMP accumulation *(76)*. This suggested that direct interaction of hCG with the serpentine portion of the receptor is implicated in activation. Despite the importance of this conclusion, this study has not been replicated and no independent evidence of expression of the truncated receptor at the cell surface was provided. Nevertheless, the model we have proposed is fully compatible with a dual participation of TSH in the activation mechanism. By binding with high affinity to the amino-terminal domain, the hormone would stabilize an "open" conformation of the receptor with constitutive activity; interaction of specific residues of the hormone with amino acids of the extracellular loops of the serpentine domain could further stabilize the active conformation. Arguments exist for a direct interaction of residues of the α-subunit of glycoprotein hormones with the extracellular loops of the corresponding receptors *(77–80)*. Also, carbohydrates of the glycoprotein hormones could play a role in providing additional interactions with the serpentine segment that is important for full activation *(81–83)*.

The "open-closed" model is certainly a gross oversimplification of reality. Nevertheless, we believe that it has heuristic value, as it provides an explanation for the activation of the receptor by proteolysis and suggests an appealing explanation for the activation by autoantibodies in patients with Graves' disease. A variety of TSAb recognizing different epitopes of the receptor would be able to stabilize the open conformation by interfering with the interaction between the amino terminus and the extracellular loops. Some recently described monoclonal antibodies with a TSBAb (blocking effect on TSH-induced cAMP accumulation) effect would similarly stabilize the closed conformation of the receptor, thus providing an explanation for the effect of these monoclonals on the basal (constitutive) activity of the TSH receptor (84).

The functional characteristics of some of the mutants with a differential effect on cAMP and inositol phosphate generation may provide additional information on the mechanism of activation of these two regulatory cascades. Mutants with a similar effect on basal cAMP (and not involving residues in the intracellular loops) may have very different effects on basal inositol phosphate accumulation (54). In agreement with recent studies of other GPCRs (85), this is compatible with a model involving more than one activated state of the receptor (R_1^*, R_2^*, R_3^*, etc.), with each one being endowed potentially with a different spectrum of affinities for the various G proteins.

CONCLUSION AND PERSPECTIVES

The study of spontaneous mutations of the TSH receptor in human diseases has been a rewarding experience. It has provided a new and satisfactory pathophysiological explanation for a variety of clinical situations and has led to the identification of a new nosological entity. The high frequency of occurrence of autonomous toxic nodules in our population has provided a host of different activating mutations, and this has allowed for an extensive exploration of the structure–function characteristics of the TSH receptor. Together with information from previous site-directed mutagenesis experiments, this led to the elaboration of a model for TSH receptor activation that is compatible with many experimental and clinical observations.

The analysis of spontaneous mutants has obvious limitations: One observes only the mutations that are statistically likely to occur given the structure of the genetic code. The logical next step is to use the data from the available mutations to elaborate a molecular model of receptor activation with resolution at the atomic scale. This model could then be used to make predictions regarding additional gain-of-function mutations, which for purely genetic reasons would be less likely to occur spontaneously. A nice example of this strategy has been provided by further studies of the α_{1b}-adrenergic receptor (86). Of course, what is really missing is an experimentally determined three-dimensional structure of both the serpentine and extracellular amino-terminal domains of the TSH receptor. Only then will it be possible to link the hormone realistically to its receptor and understand the structural and functional consequences in molecular terms.

ACKNOWLEDGMENTS

This text provides an occasion to thank the many people from our laboratory and abroad who contributed to the identification and analyses of TSH receptor mutants. Jacques Dumont and Jacqueline Van Sande opened the field with their biochemical studies of hot nodules. Jacques Dumont and Pierre Roger provided the rationale for the search for constitutive activation of the cAMP pathway. Jasmine Parma, Jacqueline Van Sande, Laurence Duprez, Massimo Tonacchera, Sabine Costagliola, Filomena Cetani,

Patrice Rodien, Isabelle Migeotte, Marc Abramowicz, and Ralf Paschke contributed to the study of the various mutations. Jean Mockel, Jacques Hermans, Pierre Rocmans, Guy Andry, Jacques Leclère, Jacques Orgiazzi, Claire Schvartz, Peter Kopp, Marc Decoulx, Marie-Joëlle Delisle, Luc Portmann, Jean-Louis Wemeau, P. Winiszewski, Nelly Mirkine, and Claudine Heinrich provided the patients. This study was supported by the Belgian Programme on University Poles of Attraction initiated by the Belgian State, Prime Minister's Office, Service for Sciences, Technology and Culture. The scientific responsibility is assumed by the author. Also supported by grants from the Fonds de la Recherche Scientifique Médicale, the FNRS, Télévie, the European Union (Biomed), Association Belge contre le Cancer, and Association de Recherche Biomédicale et de Diagnostic.

REFERENCES

1. Dumont JE, Vassart G, Refetoff S. Thyroid disorders. In: Scriver CR, ed. The Metabolic Basis of Inherited Diseases. McGraw-Hill, 1989, pp. 1843–1879.
2. Vassart G, Dumont JE. The thyrotropin receptor and the regulation of thyrocyte function and growth. Endocr Rev 1992;13:596–611.
3. Maenhaut C, Brabant G, Vassart G, Dumont JE. In vitro and in vivo regulation of thyrotropin receptor mRNA levels in dog and human thyroid cells. J Biol Chem 1992;15:3000–3007.
4. Damante G, Di Lauro, R. Thyroid-specific gene expression. Biochim Biophys Acta 1994;1218: 255–266.
5. Dumont JE, Lamy F, Roger P, Maenhaut C. Physiological and pathological regulation of thyroid cell proliferation and differentiation by thyrotropin and other factors. Physiol. Rev 1992;72:667–697.
6. Vassart G, Parma J, Van Sande J, Dumont J. The thyrotropin receptor and the regulation of thyrocyte function and growth: update 1994. Endocr Rev 1994;3:77–80.
7. Roger P, Reuse S, Maenhaut C, Dumont JE. Multiple facets of the modulation of growth by cAMP. Vitam Horm 1995;51:59–191.
8. Dumont JE, Jauniaux JC, Roger PP. The cyclic AMP-mediated stimulation of cell proliferation. Trends Biochem Sci 1989;14:67–71.
9. Ledent, C., Dumont JE, Vassart G, Parmentier M. Thyroid expression of an A2 adenosine receptor transgene induces thyroid hyperplasia and hyperthyroidism. EMBO J 1992;11:537–542.
10. Weinstein LS, Shenker A, Gejman PV, Merino MJ, Friedman E, Spiegel AM. Activating mutations of the stimulatory G protein in the McCune-Albright syndrome. N Engl J Med 1991;325:1688–1695.
11. Parma J, Duprez L, Van Sande J, Cochaux P, Gervy C, Mockel J, Dumont JE, Vassart G. Somatic mutations in the thyrotropin receptor gene cause hyperfunctioning thyroid adenomas. Nature 1993;365:649–651.
12. Van Sande J, Parma J, Tonacchera M, Swillens S, Dumont J, Vassart G. Somatic and germline mutations of the TSH receptor gene in thyroid diseases. J Clin Endocrinol Metab 1995;80:2577–2585.
13. Duprez L, Parma J, Van Sande J, Allegeier A, Leclère J, Schvartz C, Delisle M, Decoulx M, Orgiazzi J, Dumont J, Vassart G. Germline mutations in the thyrotropin receptor gene cause nonautoimmune autosomal dominant hyperthyroidism. Nat Genet 1994;7:396–401.
14. Strader CD, Fong TM, Tota MR, Underwood D. Structure and function of G protein-coupled receptors. Annu Rev Biochem 1994;63:101–132.
15. Nagayama Y, Rapoport B. The thyrotropin receptor 25 years after its discovery: new insight after its molecular cloning. Mol Endocrinol 1992;6:145–156.
16. Gross B, Misrahi M, Sar S, Milgrom E. Composite structure of the human thyrotropin receptor gene. Biochem Biophys Res Commun 1991;177:679–687.
17. Kobe B, Deisenhofer J. A structural basis of the interactions between leucine-rich repeats and protein ligands. Nature 1995;374:183–186.
18. Kobe B, Deisenhofer J. The leucine-rich repeat: a versatile binding motif. Trends Biochem Sci 1994; 19:415–421.
19. Nagayama Y, Russo D, Wadsworth HL, Chazenbalk GD, and Rapoport B. Eleven amino acids (Lys-201 to Lys-211) and 9 amino acids (Gly-222 to Leu-230) in the human thyrotropin receptor are involved in ligand binding. J Biol Chem 1991;266:14,926–14,930.

20. Nagayama Y, Wadsworth HL, Chazenbalk GD, Russo D, Seto P, Rapoport B. Thyrotropin-luteinizing hormone/chorionic gonadotropin receptor extracellular domain chimeras as probes for thyrotropin receptor function. Proc Natl Acad Sci USA 1991;88:902–905.

21. Braun T, Schofield PR, Sprengel R. Amino-terminal leucine-rich repeats in gonadotropin receptors determine hormone selectivity. EMBO J 1991;10:1885–1890.

22. Segaloff DL, and Ascoli M. The lutropin/choriogonadotropin receptor . . . 4 years later. Endocr Rev 1993;14:324–347.

23. Lefkowitz RJ, Cotecchia S, Kjelsberg MA, Pitcher J, Koch WJ, Inglese J, and Caron MG. Adrenergic receptors: recent insights into their mechanism of activation and desensitization. Adv Second Messenger Phosphoprotein Res 1993;28:1–9.

24. Gether U, Johansen TE, and Schwartz TW. Chimeric NK1 (substance P)/NK3 (neurokinin B) receptors: identification of domains determining the binding specificity of tachykinin agonists. J Biol Chem 1993;268:7893–7898.

25. Yokota Y, Akazawa C, Ohkubo H, and Nakanishi S. Delineation of structural domains involved in the subtype specificity of tachykinin receptors through chimeric formation of substance P/substance K receptors. EMBO J 1992;11:3585–3591.

26. Nothacker HP, Grimmelikhuijzen CJ. Molecular cloning of a novel, putative G protein-coupled receptor from sea anemones structurally related to members of the FSH, TSH, LH/CG receptor family from mammals. Biochem Biophys Res Commun 1993;197:1062–1069.

27. Hauser F, Nothacker H, Grimmelikhuizen C. Molecular cloning, genomic organization and developmental regulation of a novel receptor from Drosophila melanogaster structurally related to members of the TSH, FSH, LH/CG receptor family from mammals. J Biol Chem, 1996; in press.

28. Hoflack J, Hibert MF, Trumpp Kallmeyer S, and Bidart JM. Three-dimensional models of gonado-thyrotropin hormone receptor transmembrane domain. Drug Des Discov 1993;10:157–171.

29. Kajava AV, Vassart G, and Wodak SJ. Modeling of the three-dimensional structure of proteins with the typical leucine-rich repeats. Structure 1995;3:867–877.

30. Laurent E, Mockel J, Van Sande J, Graff I, Dumont JE. Dual activation by thyrotropin of the phospholipase C and cyclic AMP cascades in human thyroid. Mol Cell Endocrinol 1987;52:273–278.

31. Laugwitz KL, Allgeier A, Offermanns S, Spicher K, Van Sande J, Dumont JE, Schultz G. The human thyrotropin receptor: a heptahelical receptor capable of stimulating members of all four G protein families. Proc Natl Acad Sci USA 1996;93:116–120.

32. Allgeier A, Offermanns S, Van Sande J, Spicher K, Schultz G, Dumont JE. The human thyrotropin receptor activates G-proteins Gs and Gq/11. J Biol Chem 1994;269:13,733–13,735.

33. Miyai K, Azukizawa M, and Kumahara Y. Familial isolated thyrotropin deficiency with cretinism. N Engl J Med 1971;285:1043–1048.

34. Hayashizaki Y, Hiraoka Y, Endo Y, Miyai K, and Matsubara K. Thyroid-stimulating hormone (TSH) deficiency caused by a single base substitution in the CAGYC region of the beta-subunit [published erratum, EMBO J 1989;8:3542]. EMBO J 1989;8:2291–2296.

35. Hayashizaki Y, Hiraoka Y, Tatsumi K, Hashimoto T, Furuyama J, Miyai K, Nishijo K, Matsuura M, Kohno H, Labbe A, et al.. Deoxyribonucleic acid analyses of five families with familial inherited thyroid stimulating hormone deficiency [see comments]. J Clin Endocrinol Metab 1990;71: 792–796.

36. Stein SA, Shanklin DR, Krulich L, Roth MG, Chubb M, and Adams PM. Evaluation and characterization of the hyt/hyt hypothyroid mouse: II. Abnormalities of TSH and the thyroid gland. Neuroendocrinology 1989;49:509–519.

37. Stein S, Oates E, Hall C, Grumbles R, Fernandez L, Taylor N, Puett D, and Jin S. Identification of a point mutation in the thyrotropin receptor of the hyt/hyt hypothyroid mouse. Mol Endocrinol 1994;8:129–138.

38. Stanbury JB, Rocmans P, Buhler UK, and Ochi Y. Congenital hypothyroidism with impaired thyroid response to thyrotropin. N Engl J Med 1968;279:1132–1136.

39. Codaccioni JL, Carayon P, Michel Bechet M, Foucault F, Lefort G, and Pierron H. Congenital hypothyroidism associated with thyrotropin unresponsiveness and thyroid cell membrane alterations. J Clin Endocrinol Metab 1980;50:932–937.

40. Takeshita A, Nagayama Y, Yamashita S, Takamatsu J, Oshawa N, Maesaka H, Tachibana K, Tokuhiro E, Ashizawa K, Yokoyama N, and Nagataki S. Sequence analysis of the TSH receptor gene in congenital primary hypothyroidism associated with TSH unresponsiveness. Thyroid 1994;4:255–259.

41. Sunthornthepvarakul T, Gottschalk M, Hayashi Y, and Refetoff S. Resistance to thyrotropin caused by mutations in the thyrotropin-receptor gene. N Engl J Med 1995;332:155–160.

42. Biebermann H, Krude H, Thiede C, Kotulla D, Gruters A. Sporadic congenital hypothyroidism due to compound heterozygosity for two mutations of the coding sequence of the TSH receptor gene. Int Congress of Endocrinol. San Francisco, 1996, Abs 1996;1:P2–954

43. Maenhaut C, Van Sande J, Libert F, Abramowicz M, Parmentier M, Vanderhaegen JJ, Dumont JE, Vassart G, Schiffmann S. RDC8 codes for an adenosine A2 receptor with physiological constitutive activity. Biochem Biophys Res Commun 1990;173:1169–1178.

44. Michiels FM, Caillou B, Talbot M, Dessarps Freichey F, Maunoury MT, Schlumberger M, Mercken L, Monier R, Feunteun J. Oncogenic potential of guanine nucleotide stimulatory factor alpha subunit in thyroid glands of transgenic mice. Proc Natl Acad Sci USA 1994;91:10,488–10,492.

45. Lyons J, Landis CA, Harsh G, Vallar L, Grunewald K, Feichtinger H, Duh QY, Clark OH, Kawasaki E, Bourne HR, et al. Two G protein oncogenes in human endocrine tumors. Science 1990;249:655–659.

46. Goretzki PE, Lyons J, Stacy Phipps S, Rosenau W, Demeure M, Clark OH, McCormick F, Roher HD, Bourne HR. Mutational activation of RAS and GSP oncogenes in differentiated thyroid cancer and their biological implications. World J Surg 1992;16:576–581.

47. Suarez HG, du Villard JA, Caillou B, Schlumberger M, Parmentier C, Monier R. gsp mutations in human thyroid tumours. Oncogene 1991;6:677–679.

48. O'Sullivan C, Barton CM, Staddon SL, Brown CL, Lemoine NR. Activating point mutations of the gsp oncogene in human thyroid adenomas. Mol Carcinog 1991;4:345–349.

49. Kjelsberg MA, Cotecchia S, Ostrowski J, Caron MG, Lefkowitz RJ. Constitutive activation of the alpha 1B-adrenergic receptor by all amino acid substitutions at a single site: evidence for a region which constrains receptor activation. J Biol Chem 1992;267:1430–1433.

50. Samama P, Cotecchia S, Costa T, Lefkowitz RJ. A mutation-induced activated state of the beta 2-adrenergic receptor: extending the ternary complex model. J Biol Chem 1993;268:4625–4636.

51. Cotecchia S, Exum S, Caron MG, Lefkowitz RJ. Regions of the alpha 1-adrenergic receptor involved in coupling to phosphatidylinositol hydrolysis and enhanced sensitivity of biological function. Proc Natl Acad Sci USA 1990;87:2896–2900.

52. Porcellini A, Ciullo I, Laviola L, Amabile A, Fenzi G, Avvedimento V. Novel mutations of thyrotropin receptor gene in thyroid hyperfunctioning adenomas. J Clin Endocrinol Metab 1994;79:657–661.

53. Paschke R, Tonacchera M, Van Sande J, Parma J, Vassart G. 1994. Identification and functional characterization of two new somatic mutations causing constitutive activation of the TSH receptor in hyperfunctioning autonomous adenomas of the thyroid. J Clin Endocrinol Metab, 1994;79:1785–1789.

54. Parma J, Van Sande J, Swillens S, Tonacchera M, Dumont JE, Vassart G. Somatic mutations causing constitutive activity of the TSH receptor are the major cause of hyperfunctional thyroid adenomas: identification of additional mutations activating both the cAMP and inisitolphosphate-Ca++ cascades. Mol Endocrinol 1995;9:725–733.

55. DE Roux N, Polak M, Couet J, Leger J, Czernichow P, Milgrom E, Misrahi M. A neomutation of the TSH receptor in a severe neonatal hyperthyroidism. J Clin Endocrinol Metab 1996;81:2023–2026.

56. Parma J, Duprez L, Van Sande J, Hermans J, Rocmans P, Van Vliet G, Costagliola S, Rodien P, Dumont JE, Vassart G. Diversity and prevalence of somatic mutations in the TSH receptor and Gs alfa genes as a cause of toxic thyroid adenomas. J Clin Endocrinol Metab 1997;82(8):2695–2701.

57. Takeshita A, Nagayama Y, Yokoyama N, Ishikawa N, Ito K, Yamashita T, Obara T, Murakami Y, Kuma K, Takamatsu J, et al. Rarity of oncogenic mutations in the thyrotropin receptor of autonomously functioning thyroid nodules in Japan. J Clin Endocrinol Metab 1995;80:2607–2611.

58. Russo D, Arturi F, Wicker R, Chazenbalk G D, Schlumberger M, DuVillard JA, Caillou B, Monier R, Rapoport B, Filetti S, et al. Genetic alterations in thyroid hyperfunctioning adenomas. J Clin Endocrinol Metab 1995;80:1347–1351.

59. Delange F. Correction of iodine deficiency: benefits and possible side effects. Eur J Endocrinol 1995;132:542–543 (comment).

60. Russo D, Arturi F, Schlumberger M, Caillou B, Filetti S, Suarez HG. Activating mutations of the TSH receptor in differentiated thyroid carcinomas. Oncogene 1995;11:1907–1911.

61. Thomas JS, Leclère J, Hartemann P, Duheille J, Orgiazzi J, Petersen M, Janot C, Guedenet JC. Familial hyperthyroidism without evidence of autoimmunity. Acta Endocrinol (Copenh) 1982;100:512–518.

62. Tonacchera M, Van Sande J, Cetani F, Swillens S, Schvartz C, Winiszewski L, Portmann L, Dumont JE, Vassart G, Parma J. Functional characteristics of three new germline mutations of the thyrotropin receptor gene causing autosomal dominant toxic thyroid hyperplasia. J Clin Endocrinol Metab 1996;81:547–554.

63. Leclere J, Béné M, Duprez A, Faure G, Thomas J, Vignau M, Burlet C. Behavior of thyroid tissue from patients with Graves' disease in nude mice. J Clin Endocrinol Metab 1984;59:175–177.
64. Kopp P, Van Sande J, Parma J, Duprez L, Zuppinger K, Jameson JL, Vassart G. Congenital non-autoimmune hyperthyroidism caused by a neomutation in the thyrotropin receptor gene. N Engl J Med 1995;332:150–154.
65. Kohler B, Biebermann H, Krohn HP, Dralle D, Finke R, Gruters A. A novel germline mutation in the TSH receptor gene causing nonautoimmune congenital hyperthyroidism. Int Congress Endocrinol, San Francisco, 1996, Abst 1996;1:P-946.
66. Kosugi S, Okajima F, Ban T, Hidaka A, Shenker A, Kohn L. Mutation of Alanine 623 in the third cytoplasmic loop of the rat TSH receptor results in a loss in the phosphoinositide but not cAMP signal induced by TSH and receptor autoantibodies. J Biol Chem 1992;267:24,153–24,156.
67. Eggerickx D, Denef JF, Labbe O, Hayashi Y, Refetoff S, Vassart G, Parmentier M, Libert F. Molecular cloning of an orphan G-protein-coupled receptor that constitutively activates adenylate cyclase. Biochem J 1995;309:837–843.
68. Westphal RS, Backstrom JR, Sanders Bush E. Increased basal phosphorylation of the constitutively active serotonin 2C receptor accompanies agonist-mediated desensitization. Mol Pharmacol 1995;48:200–205.
69. Tiberi M, Caron MG. High agonist-independent activity is a distinguishing feature of the dopamine D1B receptor subtype. J Biol Chem 1994;269:27,925–27,931.
70. Chazenbalk GD, Rapoport B. Expression of the extracellular domain of the thyrotropin receptor in the baculovirus system using a promoter active earlier than the polyhedrin promoter: implications for the expression of functional highly glycosylated proteins. J Biol Chem 1995;270:1543–1549.
71. Ren Q, Kurose H, Lefkowitz RJ, Cotecchia S. Constitutively active mutants of the α2-adrenergic receptor. J Biol Chem 1993;268:16,483–16,487.
72. Lefkowitz RJ, Cotecchia S, Samama P, and Costa T. Constitutive activity of receptors coupled to guanine nucleotide regulatory proteins. Trends Pharmacol Sci 1994;14:303–307.
73. Van Sande J, Massart C, Costagliola S, Alleier A, Cetani F, Vassart G, and Dumont JE. Specific activation of the thyrotropin receptor by trypsin. Mol Cell Endocrinol 1996;119:161–168.
74. Zhang ML, Sugawa H, Kosugi S, and Mori T. Constitutive activation of the thyrotropin receptor by deletion of a portion of the extracellular domain. Biochem Biophys Res Commun 1995;211: 205–210.
75. Paschke R, Parmentier M, and Vassart G. Importance of the extracellular domain of the human thyrotrophin receptor for activation of cyclic AMP production. J Mol Endocrinol 1994;13:199–207.
76. Ji I, Ji T. Human choriogonadotrophin binds to a lutropin receptor with essentially no N-terminal extension and stimulates cAMP synthesis. J Biol Chem 1991;266:1306–1309.
77. Zeng H, Ji I, and Ji TH. Lys91 and His90 of the alpha-subunit are crucial for receptor binding and hormone action of follicle-stimulating hormone (FSH) and play hormone-specific roles in FSH and human chorionic gonadotropin. Endocrinology 1995;136:2948–2953.
78. Ji I, Zeng H, and Ji TH. Receptor activation of and signal generation by the lutropin/choriogonadotropin receptor: cooperation of Asp397 of the receptor and alpha Lys91 of the hormone. J Biol Chem 1993;268:22,971–22,974.
79. Yoo J, Zeng H, Ji I, Murdoch WJ, and Ji TH. COOH-terminal amino acids of the alpha subunit play common and different roles in human choriogonadotropin and follitropin. J Biol Chem 1993;268: 13,034–13,042.
80. Ji I, and JI T. Receptor activation is distinct from hormone binding in intact lutropion-choriogonadotropin receptors and Asp397 is important for receptor activation. J Biol Chem 1995;268:20,851–20,854.
81. Amr S, Shimohigashi Y, Carayon P, Chen HC, and Nisula B. Role of the carbohydrate moiety of human choriogonadotropin in its thyrotropic activity. Arch Biochem Biophys 1984;229:170–176.
82. Thotakura NR, Weintraub BD, and Bahl OP. The role of carbohydrate in human choriogonadotropin (hCG) action: effects of N-linked carbohydrate chains from hCG and other glycoproteins on hormonal activity. Mol Cell Endocrinol 1990;70:263–272.
83. Thotakura NR, LiCalzi L, and Weintraub BD. The role of carbohydrate in thyrotropin action assessed by a novel approach using enzymatic deglycosylation. J Biol Chem 1990;265:11,527–11,534.
84. Dallas JS, Cunningham SJ, Patibandla SA, Seetharamaiah GS, Morris JC, Tahara K, Kohn LD, and Prabhakar BS. TSH receptor antibodies can inhibit TSH-mediated cAMP production in thyroid cells by either blocking TSH binding or affecting a step subsequent to TSH binding. Endocrinology 1996;137:3329–3339.

85. Perez DM, DeYoung MB, Graham RM. Coupling of expressed alpha 1B- and alpha 1D-adrenergic receptor to multiple signaling pathways is both G protein and cell type specific. Mol Pharmacol 1993;44:784–795.
86. Scheer A, Fanelli F, Costa T, De Benedetti PG, and Cotecchia S. Constitutively active mutants of the alpha1b-adrenergic receptor: role of highly conserved polar amino acids in receptor activation. EMBO J 1996;15:3566–3578.
87. Abramowicz M, Duprez L, Parma J, Vassart G, and Heinrichs C. Familial congenital hypothyroidism due to inactivating mutation of the thyrotropin receptor causing profound hypoplasia of the thyroid gland. J Clin Invest 1997;99(12):3018–3024.

8

Disorders Caused by Mutations of the Lutropin/ Choriogonadotropin Receptor Gene

Andrew Shenker, MD, PhD

CONTENTS

THE LUTROPIN/CHORIOGONADOTROPIN RECEPTOR

Structure and Function

The human receptor for lutropin and chorionic gonadotropin (LHR) plays a key role in normal and abnormal reproductive physiology *(1–3)*. In males lutropin luteinizing hormone (LH) regulates the development and function of Leydig cells. Testosterone secreted by the Leydig cells is obligatory for the development of male internal and external genitalia, and for the establishment of secondary sexual characteristics during puberty. In women, LH acts on the theca cells to produce androgen precursors necessary for estrogen synthesis, and on the ovarian follicles to promote ovulation, subsequent corpus luteum formation, and progesterone secretion. Chorionic gonadotropin produced by the placenta acts on the corpus luteum and promotes development of the fetal testes in the first trimester of pregnancy.

The human LHR is a G-protein-coupled receptor (GPCR) encoded by a single gene consisting of 11 exons. Like the other members of the GPCR subfamily whose agonists are glycoprotein hormones (FSH, TSH), the LHR is characterized by a large, glycosylated N-terminal extracellular (EC) domain that independently determines hormone binding affinity and specificity *(2)*. The EC domain is encoded by the first 10 exons, and

From: *Contemporary Endocrinology: G Proteins, Receptors, and Disease*
Edited by: A. M. Spiegel, Humana Press Inc., Totowa, NJ

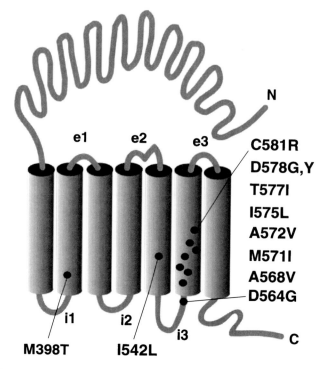

Fig. 1. Location of activating human LHR mutations identified in testotoxicosis.

contains imperfect leucine-rich repeats of approx 25 residues each *(4–7)*. These repeats are believed to be arranged in the shape of a horseshoe, with the parallel β-strands and loops comprising an inner circumference that provides important contact sites for hormone binding. Exon 11 encodes the transmembrane (TM) domain, seven membrane-spanning α-helical segments (TM1-7) that are connected by alternating EC (e1, e2, e3) and intracellular (i1, i2, i3) loops (Fig. 1). As with other GPCRs, the helical segments are predicted to be arranged in a compact bundle with a central hydrophilic pocket *(8)*. Portions of the intracellular loops, especially i3, are thought to be important for G-protein coupling.

The mechanism by which hormone binding to the EC domain relays a conformational change to the cytoplasmic surface of the transmembrane bundle remains mysterious, and several scenarios have been proposed *(4,5,9)*. The effect may be indirect or may involve a portion of the hormone directly contacting EC loops or actually penetrating into the hydrophilic cleft. For the TSHR, it has been suggested that contacts between the EC domain and the EC loops normally help maintain the receptor in its inactive state, and that hormone binding serves to relieve this constraint *(10,11)*. Although rearrangement of side chains buried within the transmembrane core appears to be the primary trigger for receptor activation in rhodopsin and in monoamine GPCRs, there is no reason to suppose that all GPCRs have the same triggering mechanism *(12)*. In fact, the external location of several charged residues whose replacement allows normal hormone binding, but impairs signal transduction *(13–16)* suggests that glycoprotein receptors might be activated primarily by forces exerted on the extracellular surface of the receptor.

The TM bundle of glycoprotein hormone receptors has many of the common residues and features found in other GPCRs, including a conserved Asp residue in the middle of TM2 and the Glu-Arg motif at the cytoplasmic end of TM3 *(8,17,18)*, but there are also some salient differences. Sequence comparison reveals that glycoprotein hormone receptors lack a conserved Pro residue found in TM5 in other GPCRs, but that they share an extra Pro in TM7 *(9,17)*. Kinks caused by Pro residues have the potential to influence interhelical packing and to participate in agonist-induced conformational transitions *(19,20)*, and in the case of TM7, the additional Pro is predicted to increase the helix bending angle significantly *(21)*. Furthermore, several conserved aromatic side chains predicted to stack in the GPCR central cavity and play a role in signal transduction *(19)* are replaced with smaller side chains in the glycoprotein hormone receptor subfamily *(9,21)*. It is plausible that the distinctive structural features of the TM bundle in this subfamily have evolved in conjunction with the large EC domain, and reflect a key difference in the mechanism by which this group of receptors undergoes agonist-induced activation.

Second Messenger Pathways

Activation of the LHR stimulates G_s, the G protein coupled to adenylyl cyclase, and leads to increased intracellular cAMP. Many of the downstream effects of LH and hCG, including induction of steroidogenic enzymes, can be related to the cAMP-protein kinase A signaling pathway. At higher concentrations, however, LH and hCG can also stimulate production of inositol phosphates by phospholipase C (PLC). Coupling to this pathway is considerably less efficient than to adenylyl cyclase, is more dependent on receptor density, and is apparently mediated by a different G protein *(22,23)*. In females, it is plausible that the serum LH concentration and LHR density are both sufficiently high at the time of ovulation to stimulate PLC as well as adenylyl cyclase, but the physiological significance of the secondary PLC pathway in males remains unclear.

ACTIVATING LHR MUTATIONS IN TESTOTOXICOSIS

Clinical Features

In 1852 Robert King Stone presented the following case *(24)*:

> *Mr. Charles S . . . brought his son, Theodore, to my house . . . for my inspection and opinion; stating that on that day he was four years old. I at once declared my incredulity, for his height and robust development seemed those of a child at least six years older than the age he mentioned . . . If the child's face is concealed, the examiner would declare his figure to be that of miniature man, perfectly developed and at least 21 years of age . . . In terminating this simple statement, I may observe that the father presented extreme precocity, having experienced his first sexual indulgence at the age of 8 years.*

Stone was describing the condition now known as familial male precocious puberty, or testotoxicosis *(25,26)*. It is a gonadotropin-independent disorder that is inherited in an autosomal dominant, male-limited pattern. Testosterone secretion and Leydig cell hyperplasia occur in the context of prepubertal levels of LH, and the onset of puberty in affected boys, including virilization, rapid growth, and behavioral changes, usually occurs by age four. Premature epiphyseal fusion results in short adult stature in affected males. Female carriers are apparently unaffected. Drugs that have been used to treat

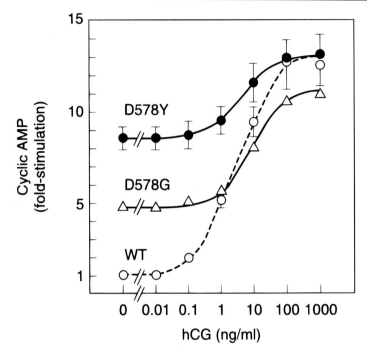

Fig. 2. Basal and hCG-stimulated cAMP production in COS-7 cells transfected with wild-type LHR cDNA (WT), or LHR cDNA encoding the D578Y or D578G mutations. Basal cAMP production in WT-transfected cells is the same as that in cells transfected with empty vector. Data are adapted from ref. *46.*

testotoxicosis include cyproterone acetate (antiandrogen), ketoconazole (inhibitor of steroidogenesis), and a combination of spironolactone (antiandrogen) and testolactone (aromatase inhibitor) *(26,27)*. Primary therapy with GnRH analogs is ineffective, but may be a useful adjunct when maturation of the hypothalamic–pituitary axis becomes superimposed.

The D578G Mutation

The existence of a circulating factor in the plasma of patients that could stimulate testosterone production in monkeys was reported in 1991 *(28)*, but the nature of this factor was not further characterized. Galvanized by the discovery that site-directed mutagenesis of an Ala residue at the junction of i3 and TM6 could be used to generate an α_{1b}-adrenergic receptor that became activated in the absence of agonist *(29)*, and that activating point mutations of other GPCRs could cause hyperpigmentation in mice *(30)* and retinitis pigmentosa in humans *(31)*, investigators postulated that an analogous, naturally occurring mutation of the LHR gene might be the basis of testotoxicosis.

Initial studies focusing on a segment of the LHR gene encompassing i3 and TM6 revealed a heterozygous mutation that results in substitution of Asp[578] in TM6 with Gly (D578G) in affected individuals from nine different kindreds *(32,33)*. Restriction digest analysis demonstrated linkage of the mutation to the disease phenotype.

To assess the functional effect of the D578G mutation, wild-type and mutated human LHR were transiently expressed in COS-7 cells *(32)*. In contrast to the silent wild-type LHR, the mutant LHR produces a 4.5-fold increase in basal cAMP production in COS-7 cells, indicating that it is constitutively active (Fig. 2). Agonist-independent stimulation of cAMP production represents about 40% of the maximal stimulation produced by the agonist hCG, and is not simply a result of increased receptor expression *(34,35)*. The mutant receptor is also capable of responding to increasing concentrations of hCG, with an EC_{50} and maximal hCG-stimulated cAMP production similar to that of the wild-type receptor (Fig. 2). The mutation has no effect on agonist binding affinity and does not cause constitutive activation of inositol phosphate production *(34,35)*. When transfected into MA10 mouse tumor cells, the D578G LHR causes constitutive production of cAMP and steroids *(3)*.

Other Activating Mutations

The D578G LHR mutation is the most common cause of familial and sporadic testotoxicosis *(32–34,36–38)*, but different mutations of the LHR have been found in other patients: M398T *(39–41)*, I542L *(36)*, D564G *(36)*, A568V *(42)*, M571I *(33,35)*, A572V *(43)*, I575L *(44)*, T577I *(35)*, D578Y *(36,45)*, and C581R *(36)*. The location of the 10 affected residues, mostly clustered in TM 6, is shown in Fig. 1. Most activating LHR mutations produce biochemical phenotypes similar to that of the D578G substitution, but several do not. For example, the I542L and C581R mutants are reported to have diminished agonist-stimulated signaling *(36)*, and the D578Y mutant promotes almost twice as much basal cAMP accumulation in transfected cells as the other activating mutations *(36,46)* (Fig. 2). The D578Y mutant is also unique in causing twofold activation of the PLC pathway *(46)*.

Most of the affected amino acid residues are conserved in other glycoprotein hormone receptors and in homologous invertebrate GPCRs *(47,48)*, indicating that these residues normally serve an important functional role. Many of the corresponding residues in the TSHR have also been found to be sites of activating mutations in thyroid adenomas or hereditary thyroid hyperplasia, but other TSHR mutations are more widely distributed, including residues in e1, e2, TM3, and TM7 *(10,49)*. The differences in distribution may reflect differences in sampling or mutation rate, but may also be related to data indicating that the structure of the inactive TSHR is inherently less constrained than that of the LHR, i.e., more susceptible to the effect of mutations *(10,50)*.

Pathophysiology

Dominant mutations that lead to constitutive activation of the LHR-mediated cAMP signaling pathway can explain the pathophysiology of gonadotropin-independent precocious puberty in males. LHR-mediated effects, including testosterone production, are known to involve increased production of cellular cAMP *(1,2)*. Intracellular cAMP accumulation triggered by unoccupied mutant receptors appears sufficient to cause Leydig cell hyperfunction and hyperplasia, although the appearance of the phenotype must be dependent on other developmental events in the cell. The significance of increased basal inositol phosphate accumulation in the D578Y mutant remains to be determined. The reason why desensitization mechanisms are unable to compensate for LHR activation in the Leydig cell is unknown; this question pertains to all diseases caused by activated GPCRs. Another aim for future research is to define the mechanism by which cAMP stimulates proliferation in these cells.

Because LH alone is adequate to trigger steroidogenesis in Leydig cells, but both LH and FSH are required to activate ovarian steroidogenesis, inappropriate activation of

LHR alone would not be expected to cause precocious puberty in females. For example, hCG-secreting germ-cell tumors cause sexual precocity in males, but not females (51). Nevertheless, one might expect that adult females with an activated ovarian LHR would demonstrate menstrual irregularities or hyperandrogenism. The reproductive endocrine status of one female who carries the D578G mutation has recently been studied, but no evidence of subclinical ovarian hyperandrogenism was found (38).

There are several reasons why adult carrier females might exhibit no manifestations. One possibility is that compared to the Leydig cell, ovarian cells express little or none of the mutant LHR protein. Another is that the ovarian cells are better able to compensate for low levels of constitutive cAMP production, either through receptor desensitization or other counterregulatory mechanisms.

Allelic Heterogeneity and Phenotype

As shown in Fig. 2, an LHR containing the D578Y mutation causes much higher basal cAMP accumulation than that produced by the original D578G mutation. The D578Y mutation has been found in three unrelated boys with unusually early (<1 yr old) and severe presentations of nonfamilial testotoxicosis, suggesting that their clinical phenotype is related to the strongly activating nature of the D578Y substitution (36,45,46,52). It remains to be seen whether the D578Y mutation exists in familial cases of testotoxi-cosis, and whether all cases of early testotoxicosis are a result of the D578Y mutation.

Mutations that affect signaling by GPCRs have only recently been recognized as a cause of human disease, and little is known about the dependence of phenotype on allelic heterogeneity. In the case of rhodopsin, patients with missense mutations of a Pro residue in the C-terminal tail tend to have more severe retinal disease than patients bearing different alleles, and certain mildly activating mutations are associated with the less severe night blindness phenotype (53–55). Although no clear association has yet been made between allelic heterogenity and severity of thyroid hyperplasia or hyperfunction, somatic TSHR mutations tend to be more activating than those found in cases of hereditary toxic thyroid hyperplasia (10,49).

The penetrance of an activating mutant LHR allele in males was thought to be 100%, but one 12-yr-old prepubertal boy harboring the M398T mutation has recently been described (40). It is important to note that age of presentation can vary among affected males with the same mutation and even among those within the same family.

Insights into LHR Mechanism of Activation

Activating LHR mutations can provide novel insights into the structural features involved in GPCR activation. The best studied GPCR is rhodopsin, whose inactive state is characterized by a salt bridge between charged residues in TM3 and TM7. Light-induced isomerization of retinal disrupts this bridge and triggers a series of changes, including protonation of a highly conserved Glu residue at the cytoplasmic end of TM3, that allow rhodopsin to assume an activated conformation and couple to its G protein (17). The effect of agonists on other GPCRs is also believed to involve disruption of interhelical constraints that stabilize the inactive state (29,56) However, the nature of these constraints has not been well defined. Studying the properties of activating mutations that mimic the effect of agonist occupancy is one way to address this issue (57,58).

The 3-D structure of the LHR is unknown, but models of the TM domain have been constructed based on GPCR sequence alignment, the arrangement of conserved residues, and structural information available on bacteriorhodopsin (a topologically similar, bacterial membrane proton pump) *(9)* or rhodopsin *(8,21)*. Such models can be used to develop hypotheses about the normal role of residues found to be mutated in testotoxicosis and to design site-directed mutagenesis experiments to test them. The rhodopsin-based LHR model places Asp[578] near the middle of TM6, oriented toward TM7 and the internal cleft. Asp[578] is conserved in all glycoprotein hormone receptors, but is not found in other GPCRs *(18)*. The corresponding residue in opsins and many other GPCRs is a Phe that lies in proximity to the retinal or agonist binding pocket *(19,59)*. An artificial mutation of this residue in rhodopsin has recently been shown to promote mild constitutive activity *(60)*.

Just as disruption of a critical electrostatic interaction between TM3 and TM7 appears to explain constitutive activation of certain mutant rhodopsin molecules *(31)*, the activating effect of mutations in the LHR may be attributed to the loss of stabilizing interhelical bonds *(9,46)*. Substitution of Asp[578] with polar residues that have shorter (Ser) or longer (Glu, Tyr) side chains, or with a similarly sized hydrophobic residue (Leu), produces constitutive activation of the LHR, but substitution with an uncharged, isomorphous Asn does not *(46)*. These results indicate that it is the ability of Asp[578] to serve as a properly positioned H-bond acceptor, rather than its negative charge, that is important for stabilizing the inactive state.

The rhodopsin-based LHR model suggests that Asp[578] and Thr[577] form H-bonds with two conserved Asn residues on TM7 *(21)*. It is possible that the strongly activating effect of the bulky Tyr substituent at position 578 results from additional disruption of packing between TM6 and TM7, a notion that is supported by data showing that a Phe substituent is equally activating *(46)*. The activating effect of an Arg substitution at Cys[581] may be caused by the introduction of a long, positively charged side chain that is capable of competing for interaction with the neighboring Asp[578] residue *(21)*. This mechanism would be analogous to that described for activating rhodopsin mutants in congenital night blindness *(54,55)*.

In addition to polar interactions between TM6 and TM7, the LHR model predicts the existence of tight contacts between hydrophobic side chains from the cytoplasmic ends of TM5 and TM6. Half of the residues found to be mutated in testotoxicosis (I542L, A568V, M571I, A572V, I575L) are located here. Although the activating substitutions in this region are conservative, local side chain adjustment may not be able to compensate for steric overlap or diminished van der Waals packing, and rigid body motion of TM5, TM6, or both may result. Studies of other α-helical TM proteins have revealed the importance of hydrophobic interactions in determining the specificity of helix–helix interactions, and demonstrated that even minor alterations in the nature of certain hydrophobic side chains can have a disruptive effect on helix packing *(61)*. As with activating mutations of the bacterial chemoreceptor Trg *(62)*, the distribution of LHR mutations on TM6 appears to define a detailed packing surface that is important for stabilizing the inactive receptor conformation. Although changes in secondary structure have been proposed to underlie the activating effects of TM6 mutations in the LHR *(43)*, it seems more likely that changes in tertiary structure are responsible. The concept that the flexibility of the TM5-TM6 packing arrangement plays a key role in determining the activated state of glycoprotein hormone receptors receives support from recent studies of chimeric LHR/FSHR constructs *(63)*.

If one assumes that the N- and C-terminal portions of the LHR i3 exist as cytoplasmic α-helical extensions of TM5 and TM6, respectively *(64)*, then the conserved acidic residue Asp[564] is located one turn below Ala[568], facing TM3 and N-i3 at the cytoplasmic opening of the cleft. It is possible that the activating effect of D564G results from the loss of a negative charge at this site. Met[398] is located near the cytoplasmic end of TM2, also oriented toward the interior of the bundle *(8,21)*. Additional site directed mutagenesis studies are needed to define the reasons why D564G and M398T are activating in the LHR.

Although the trigger for glycoprotein hormone receptor activation may differ from that of other GPCRs, changes at the cytoplasmic face are likely to be similar. There is extensive evidence that residues at the junctions of i3 with TM5 and TM6 are involved in G-protein coupling throughout the GPCR family *(17,18)* and it is easy to visualize how an alteration in the TM5-TM6 interface, as the result of agonist binding or a mutation, might increase the accessibility of these residues. Activating mutations in TM6 or at the i3-TM6 junction have now been found in a variety of GPCRs, including muscarinic receptors *(65–68)*, the PAF receptor *(69)*, the D_1-dopamine receptor *(70)*, the PTH receptor *(71)*, and yeast pheromone receptors *(72,73)*.

The results of mutational and modeling studies are consistent with the concept that rigid body movement of TM6 is involved in the activation mechanism of the LHR. Movement of TM6 has been observed in molecular dynamics simulations of receptor activation *(20,57)*, and experimental evidence of TM6 tilting has been obtained for light-activated bacteriorhodopsin *(74,75)* and rhodopsin *(64,76)*. For both proteins, it appears that the cytoplasmic end of TM6 tilts away from the central pore. In the case of bacteriorhodopsin, this "relaxed" conformation allows the influx of water and subsequent proton transfer. For a GPCR, it may permit key domains, including the N- and C-terminal ends of i3, to bind and activate G proteins. Interestingly, one of the rhodopsin residues that appears to move during activation (Thr[251]) corresponds to Ala[568] in the LHR and to Ala[293] in the $α_{1b}$-adrenergic receptor *(29,57)*, the site of the "original" activating GPCR mutation.

Although most activating GPCR mutations are thought to act primarily by increasing the proportion of receptors in the active conformation, it is possible that some will also be shown to increase the affinity of the isomerized receptor for G protein or by interfering with normal desensitization mechanisms *(8,56)*.

LEYDIG CELL AND OVARIAN LH-RESISTANCE CAUSED BY INACTIVATING LHR MUTATIONS

Clinical Features

Male pseudohermaphroditism resulting from Leydig cell unresponsiveness to hCG/LH is a rare, autosomal-recessive condition characterized by Leydig cell agenesis or hypoplasia in a 46, XY individual. Phenotypically, patients may present with normal-appearing female external genitalia and primary amenorrhea, or as males with hypergonadotropic hypogonadism and micropenis. Testes contain normal Sertoli cells with no mature Leydig cells. Because normal masculinization of the genitalia during late fetal life (including most of penile growth) depends on production of testosterone by fetal Leydig cells, it was postulated that this disorder was the result of an inherited defect in the LHR, with resultant testosterone deficiency *(77)*. Some genetically female members of kindreds with Leydig cell hypoplasia were noted to have primary amenorrhea.

Inactivating Mutations

A homozygous missense mutation of the LHR (A593P) at the junction of TM7 and e3 has been described in two 46, XY siblings with female genitalia and primary amenorrhea, and in their 46, XX amenorrheic, anovulatory sister *(78,79)*. The parents were first cousins. Signaling through the mutant LHR is absent in transfected cells, but the defect cannot be entirely attributed to diminished surface expression; it appears that the low number of receptors that do reach the surface bind hCG with normal affinity, but are incapable of triggering cAMP production *(78,79)*.

XY sisters from another family were shown to be heterozygous for an LHR gene mutation encoding a premature stop codon, C545Stop *(80)*. A homozygous R554Stop mutation has been found in XY and XX individuals in a third affected kindred, and a homozygous mutation encoding S616Y in the middle of TM7 has been detected in a boy with micropenis and hCG-resistance *(81)*. The same S616Y mutation is found in association with an allele lacking exon 8 in another boy with micropenis and cryptorchidism *(82)*. Cells transfected with a mutant receptor construct bearing the S616Y substitution show drastically reduced hCG binding and responsiveness *(81,82)*.

The fact that affected XY individuals have a vas deferens and epididymis, and in some cases, a micropenis suggests that there is some small, variable amount of androgen synthesis by Leydig cells during the first trimester of pregnancy. The phenotype of XX females expressing no functional LHR indicates that LH does not play a significant role in female sexual differentiation, pubertal development, or follicular maturation, but is essential for ovulation and subsequent corpus luteum formation. Lack of LHR seems to produce a less severe ovarian phenotype than lack of FSHR *(79,83)*. Individuals who have one defective LHR allele have no clinical abnormalities. The locations of the defined mutations responsible for LH resistance are shown in Fig. 3.

Insights into LHR Structure and Function

Naturally occuring gene mutations that create premature stop codons or large deletions in GPCR genes are generally less informative than missense mutations. Even if the truncated receptors encoded by C545Stop and R554Stop were to be expressed, they would be unable to couple to G_s. Both the A593P and S616Y substitutions have detrimental effects on LHR expression and function, and methods utilizing antibodies to detect receptor protein in transfected cells may be helpful in differentiating defects in folding, trafficking, and membrane insertion. It is possible that a bulky residue at position 616 interferes with proper packing of TM7. Ser^{616} is predicted to lie on the same inner helical face of TM7 as several other residues shown to be important for LHR function *(84)*, and site-directed mutagenesis could be used to determine if other substitutions at this position are permitted. It is possible that LHR mutations that lead to only partial loss of function will be detected in other patients with milder phenotypes.

CONCLUSIONS

Equipped with the crystal structure of hCG, 3-D models of the EC and TM domains of the LHR, and an abundance of biochemical, immunochemical, and mutational data, inves-

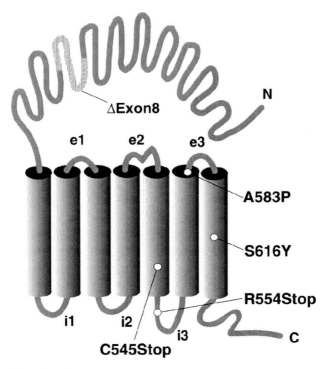

Fig. 3. Location of inactivating human LHR mutations identified in Leydig cell and ovarian LH resistance.

tigators are poised to make progress in understanding how conformational signaling occurs in glycoprotein hormone receptors. Defining the binding surface between the EC domain and hormone will allow better predictions concerning how this complex interacts with the membrane-embedded portion of the LHR. Analysis of natural and artificially generated mutations can be used to gain insight into the changes in helical packing or charge distribution that might normally be triggered by hormone binding. Basic research on the mechanisms by which the LHR becomes desensitized and causes cellular proliferation may provide a deeper understanding of the molecular pathogenesis of testotoxicosis.

It is becoming clear that even closely related glycoprotein hormone receptors exhibit important differences in signaling. Despite their high degree of sequence homology, the normal human TSHR differs from the LHR and FSHR in the ease with which it undergoes isomerization to the active state in the absence of agonist, as evidenced by its ability to stimulate basal cAMP production in transfected cells *(50)*. In addition, naturally occurring mutations that cause constitutive activation in the LHR and TSHR are without effect in the human FSHR *(63)*, and the FSHR couples only weakly to the PLC pathway *(85)*. Identification of the structural features that are responsible for these differences will increase our understanding of conformational signaling in glycoprotein hormone receptors.

ACKNOWLEDGMENTS

I thank my collaborators, Shinji Kosugi, Toru Mori, Zhaolan Lin, and Bob Pearlstein for their contributions.

REFERENCES

1. Leung P, Steele GL. Intracellular signaling in the gonads. Endocr Rev 1992;13:476–498.
2. Segaloff DL, Ascoli M. The lutropin/choriogonadotropin receptor . . . 4 years later. Endocr Rev 1993;14:324–347.
3. Themmen APN, Brunner HG. Luteinizing hormone receptor mutations and sex differentiation. Eur J Endocrinol 1996;134:533–540.
4. Moyle WR, Campbell RK, Rao SNV, et al. Model of human chorionic gonadotropin and lutropin receptor interaction that explains signal transduction of the glycoprotein hormones. J Biol Chem 1995;270:20,020–20,032.
5. Jiang X, Dreano M, Buckler DR, et al. Structural predictions for the ligand-binding region of glycoprotein hormone receptors and the nature of hormone–receptor interactions. Structure 1995;3:1341–1353.
6. Bhowmick N, Huang J, Puett D, Isaacs NW, Lapthorn AJ. Determination of residues important in hormone binding to the extracellular domain of the luteinizing hormone/chorionic gonadotropin receptor by site-directed mutagenesis and modeling. Mol Endocrinol 1996;10:1147–1159.
7. Couture L, Naharisoa H, Grebert D, et al. Peptide and immunological mapping of the ectodomain of the porcine LH receptor. J Mol Endocrinol 1996;16:15–25.
8. Baldwin JM. Structure and function of receptors coupled to G proteins. Curr Opinion Cell Biol 1994; 6:180–190.
9. Hoflack J, Hibert MF, Trumpp-Kallmeyer S, Bidart J-M. Three-dimensional models of gonadothyrotropin hormone receptor transmembrane domain. Drug Des Discov 1993;10:157–171.
10. Van Sande J, Parma J, Tonacchera M, Swillens S, Dumont J, Vassart G. Somatic and germline mutations of the TSH receptor gene in thyroid diseases. J Clin Endocrinol Metab 1995;80:2577–2585.
11. Van Sande J, Massart C, Costagliola S, et al. Specific activation of the thyrotropin receptor by trypsin. Mol Cell Endocrinol 1996;119:161–168.
12. Schwartz T.W, Rosenkilde MM. Is there a "lock" for all agonist "keys" in 7TM receptors? Trends Pharmacol Sci 1996;17:213–216.
13. Ji I, Zeng H, Ji TH. Receptor activation of and signal generation by the lutropin/choriogonadotropin receptor. Cooperation of Asp^{397} of the receptor and αLys^{91} of the hormone. J Biol Chem 1993;268: 22,971–22,974.
14. Huang J, Puett D. Identification of two amino acid residues on the extracellular domain of the lutropin/choriogonadotropin receptor important for signaling. J Biol Chem 1995;270:30,023–30,028.
15. Fernandez LM, Puett D. Lys^{583} in the third extracellular loop of the lutropin/choriogonadotropin receptor is critical for signaling. J Biol Chem 1996;271:925–930.
16. Gilchrist RL, Ryu K-S, Ji I, Ji TH. The luteinizing hormone/chorionic gonadotropin receptor has distinct transmembrane conductors for cAMP and inositol phosphate signals. J Biol Chem 1996;271: 19,283–19,287.
17. Shenker A. G protein-coupled receptor structure and function: the impact of disease-causing mutations. Baillieres Clin Endocrinol Metab 1995;9:427–451.
18. van Rhee AM, Jacobson KA. Molecular architecture of G protein-coupled receptors. Drug Dev Res 1996;37:1–38.
19. Hibert MF, Trumpp-Kallmeyer S, Hoflack J, Bruinvels A. This is not a G protein-coupled receptor. Trends Pharmacol Sci 1993;14:7–12.
20. Zhang D, Weinstein H. Signal transduction by a 5-HT$_2$ receptor: a mechanistic hypothesis from molecular dynamics simulations of the three-dimensional model of the receptor complexed to ligands. J Med Chem 1993;36:934–938.
21. Lin Z, Shenker A, Pearlstein R. A model of the lutropin/choriogonadotropin receptor: insights into the structural and functional effects of constitutively activating mutations. Protein Eng, 1997; 10:501–510.
22. Gudermann T, Birnbaumer M, Birnbaumer L. Evidence for dual coupling of the murine luteinizing hormone receptor to adenylyl cyclase and phosphoinositide breakdown and Ca^{2+} mobilization: studies with the cloned murine luteinizing hormone receptor expressed in L cells. J Biol Chem 1992;267:4479–4488.
23. Herrlich A, Kühn B, Grosse R, Schmid A, Schultz G, Gudermann T. Involvement of G$_s$ and G$_i$ proteins in dual coupling of the luteinizing hormone receptor to adenylyl cyclase and phospholipase C. J Biol Chem 1996;271:16,764–16,772.
24. Stone RK. Extraordinary precocity in the development of the male sexual organs and muscular system in a child four years old. Am J Med Sci 1852;24:561–564.

25. Rosenthal SM, Grumbach MM, Kaplan SL. Gonadotropin-independent familial sexual precocity with premature Leydig and germinal cell maturation (familial testotoxicosis): effects of a potent luteinizing hormone-releasing factor agonist and medroxyprogesterone acetate therapy in four cases. J Clin Endocrinol Metab 1983;57:571–578.

26. Holland FJ. Gonadotropin-independent precocious puberty. Endocrinol Metab Clin North Am 1991;20:191–210.

27. Laue L, Jones J, Barnes KM, Cutler GB Jr. Treatment of familial male precocious puberty with spironolactone, testolactone, and deslorelin. J Clin Endocrinol Metab 1993;76:151–155.

28. Manasco PK, Girton ME, Diggs RL, et al. A novel testis-stimulating factor in familial male precocious puberty. N Engl J Med 1991;324:227–231.

29. Kjelsberg MA, Cotecchia S, Ostrowski J, Caron MG, Lefkowitz RJ. Constitutive activation of the α_{1B}-adrenergic receptor by all amino acid substitutions at a single site: evidence for a region which constrains receptor activation. J Biol Chem 1992;267:1430–1433.

30. Robbins LS, Nadeau JH, Johnson KR, et al. Pigmentation phenotypes of variant extension locus alleles result from point mutations that alter MSH receptor function. Cell 1993;72:827–834.

31. Robinson PR, Cohen GB, Zhukovsky EA, Oprian DD. Constitutively active mutants of rhodopsin. Neuron 1992;9:719–725.

32. Shenker A, Laue L, Kosugi S, Merendino JJ Jr, Minegishi T, Cutler GB Jr. A constitutively activating mutation of the luteinizing hormone receptor in familial male precocious puberty. Nature 1993; 365:652–654.

33. Kremer H, Mariman E, Otten BJ, et al. Cosegregation of missense mutations of the luteinizing hormone receptor gene with familial male-limited precocious puberty. Hum Mol Genet 1993;2:1779–1783.

34. Yano K, Hidaka A, Saji M, et al. A sporadic case of male-limited precocious puberty has the same constitutively activating point mutation in luteinizing hormone/choriogonadotropin receptor gene as familial cases. J Clin Endocrinol Metab 1994;79:1818–1823.

35. Kosugi S, Van Dop C, Geffner ME, et al. Characterization of heterozygous mutations causing constitutive activation of the luteinizing hormone receptor in familial male precocious puberty. Hum Mol Genet 1995;4:183–188.

36. Laue L, Chan W-Y, Hsueh AJW, et al. Genetic heterogeneity of constitutively activating mutations of the human luteinizing hormone receptor in familial male-limited precocious puberty. Proc Natl Acad Sci USA 1995;92:1906–1910.

37. Kawate N, Kletter GB, Wilson BE, Netzloff ML, Menon KMJ. Identification of constitutively activating mutation of the luteinising hormone receptor in a family with male limited gonadotropin independent precocious puberty (testotoxicosis). J Med Genet 1995;32:553–554.

38. Rosenthal IM, Refetoff S, Rich B, et al. Response to challenge with gonadotropin releasing hormone agonist in a mother and her two sons with a constitutively activating mutation of the luteinizing hormone receptor. J Clin Endocrinol Metab 1996;81:3802–3806.

39. Kraaij R, Post M, Kremer H, et al. A missense mutation in the second transmembrane segment of the luteinizing hormone receptor causes familial male-limited precocious puberty. J Clin Endocrinol Metab 1995;80:3168–3172.

40. Evans BAJ, Bowen DJ, Smith PJ, Clayton PE, Gregory JW. A new point mutation in the luteinising hormone receptor gene in familial and sporadic male limited precocious puberty: genotype does not always correlate with phenotype. J Med Genet 1996;33:143–147.

41. Yano K, Kohn LD, Saji M, Kataoka N, Okuno A, Cutler GB Jr. A case of male-limited precocious puberty caused by a point mutation in the second transmembrane domain of the luteinizing hormone choriogonadotropin receptor gene. Biochem Biophys Res Commun 1996;220:1036–1042.

42. Latronico AC, Anasti J, Arnhold IJ, et al. A novel mutation of the luteinizing hormone receptor gene causing male gonadotropin-independent precocious puberty. J Clin Endocrinol Metab 1995;80:2490–2494.

43. Yano K, Saji M, Hidaka A, et al. A new constitutively activating point mutation in the luteinizing hormone/choriogonadotropin receptor gene in cases of male-limited precocious puberty. J Clin Endocrinol Metab 1995;80:1162–1168.

44. Laue L, Wu SM, Kudo M, et al. Heterogeneity of activating mutations of the human luteinizing hormone receptor in male-limited precocious puberty. Biochem Mol Med 1996;58:192–198.

45. Müller J, Kosugi S, Shenker A. A severe, non-familial case of testotoxicosis associated with a new mutation (Asp[578] to Tyr) of the lutropin receptor (LHR) gene. Horm Res 1995;41(Suppl):113.

46. Kosugi S, Mori T, Shenker A. The role of Asp[578] in maintaining the inactive conformation of the human lutropin/choriogonadotropin receptor. J Biol Chem 1996;271:31,813–31,817.

47. Nothacker H-P, Grimmelikhuijzen CJP. Molecular cloning of a novel, putative G protein-coupled receptor from sea anemones structurally related to members of the FSH, TSH, LH/CG receptor family from mammals. Biochem Biophys Res Commun 1993;197:1062–1069.

48. Tensen C, van Kesteren ER, Planta RJ, et al. A G protein-coupled receptor with low density lipoprotein-binding motifs suggests a role for lipoproteins in G-linked signal transduction. Proc Natl Acad Sci USA 1994;91:4816–4820.

49. Tonacchera M, Van Sande J, Cetani F, et al. Functional characteristics of three new germline mutations of the thyrotropin receptor gene causing autosomal dominant toxic thyroid hyperplasia. J Clin Endocrinol Metab 1996;81:547–554.

50. Cetani F, Tonacchera M, Vassart G. Differential effects of NaCl concentration on the constitutive activity of the thyrotropin and luteinizing hormone/chorionic gonadotropin receptors. FEBS Lett 1996; 378:27–31.

51. Sklar CA, Conte FA, Kaplan SL, Grumbach MM. Human chorionic gonadotropin-secreting pineal tumor: relation to pathogenesis and sex limitation of sexual precocity. J Clin Endocrinol Metab 1981;53:656–660.

52. Clark PA, Clarke WL. Testotoxicosis: an unusual presentation and novel gene mutation. Clin Pediatr 1995;34:271–274.

53. Berson EL, Rosner B, Sandberg MA, Weigel-DiFranco C, Dryja TP. Ocular findings in patients with autosomal dominant retinitis pigmentosa and rhodopsin, proline-347-leucine. Am J Ophthalmol 1991;111:614–623.

54. Dryja TP, Berson EL, Rao VR, Oprian DD. Heterozygous missense mutation in the rhodopsin gene as a cause of congenital stationary night blindness. Nat Genet 1993;4:280–283.

55. Rao VR, Cohen GB, Oprian DD. Rhodopsin mutation G90D and a molecular mechanism for congenital night blindness. Nature 1994;367:639–642.

56. Samama P, Cotecchia S, Costa T, Lefkowitz RJ. A mutation-induced activated state of the β_2-adrenergic receptor: extending the ternary complex model. J Biol Chem 1993;268:4625–4636.

57. Scheer A, Fanelli F, Costa T, De Benedetti PG, Cotecchia S. Constitutively active mutants of the α_{1B}-adrenergic receptor: role of highly conserved polar amino acids in receptor activation. EMBO J 1996;15:3566–3578.

58. Porter JE, Hwa J, Perez DM. Activation of the α_{1b}-adrenergic receptor is initiated by disruption of an interhelical salt bridge constraint. J Biol Chem 1996;271:28,318–28,323.

59. Neitz M, Neitz J, Jacobs GH. Spectral tuning of pigments underlying red-green color vision. Science 1991;252:971–974.

60. Han M, Lin SW, Minkova M, Smith SO, Sakmar TP. Functional helix–helix interactions in rhodopsin: replacement of phenylalanine 261 by alanine causes reversion of phenotype of a glycine 121 replacement mutant. J Biol Chem 1996;271:32,337–32,342.

61. Lemmon MA, Engelman DM. Specificity and promiscuity in membrane helix interactions. Q Rev Biophys 1994;27:157–218.

62. Lee GF, Dutton DP, Hazelbauer GL. Identification of functionally important helical faces in transmembrane segments by scanning mutagenesis. Proc Natl Acad Sci USA 1995;92:5416–5420.

63. Kudo M, Osuga Y, Kobilka BK, Hsueh AJW. Transmembrane regions V and VI of the human luteinizing hormone receptor are required for constitutive activation by a mutation in the third intracellular loop. J Biol Chem 1996;271:22,470–22,478.

64. Farrens DL, Altenbach C, Yang K, Hubbell WL, Khorana HG. Light activation of rhodopsin requires rigid body motion of transmembrane helices. Science 1996;274:768–770.

65. Blüml K, Mutschler E, Wess J. Functional role in ligand binding and receptor activation of an asparagine residue present in the sixth transmembrane domain of all muscarinic acetylcholine receptors. J Biol Chem 1994;269:18,870–18,876.

66. Högger P, Shockley MS, Lameh J, Sadée W. Activating and inactivating mutations in N- and C-terminal i3 loop junctions of muscarinic acetylcholine Hm1 receptors. J Biol Chem 1995;270:7405–7410.

67. Spalding TA, Burstein ES, Brauner-Osborne H, Hill-Eubanks D, Brann MR. Pharmacology of a constitutively active muscarinic receptor generated by random mutagenesis. J Pharmacol Exp Ther 1995;275:1274–1279.

68. Liu J, Blin N, Conklin BR, Wess J. Molecular mechanisms involved in muscarinic acetylcholine receptor-mediated G protein activation studied by insertion mutagenesis. J Biol Chem 1996;271:6172–6178.

69. Parent J-L, Le Gouill C, de Brum-Fernandes AJ, Rola-Pleszczynski M, Stanková J. Mutations of two adjacent amino acids generate inactive and constitutively active forms of the human platelet-activating factor receptor. J Biol Chem 1996;271:7949–7955.

70. Cho W, Taylor LP, Akil H. Mutagenesis of residues adjacent to the transmembrane prolines alters D_1 dopamine receptor binding and signal transduction. Mol Pharmacol 1996; 50:1338–1345.

71. Schipani E, Langman CB, Parfitt AM, et al. Constitutively activated receptors for parathyroid hormone and parathyroid hormone-related peptide in Jansen's metaphyseal chondrodysplasia. N Engl J Med 1996;335:736–738.

72. Boone C, Davis NG, Sprague GF Jr. Mutations that alter the third cytoplasmic loop of the a-factor receptor lead to a constitutive and hypersensitive phenotype. Proc Natl Acad Sci USA 1993;90: 9921–9925.

73. Konopka JB, Margarit SM, Dube P. Mutation of Pro-258 in transmembrane domain 6 constitutively activates the G-protein-coupled α-factor receptor. Proc Natl Acad Sci USA 1996;93:6764–6769.

74. Subramaniam S, Gerstein M, Oesterhelt D, Henderson R. Electron diffraction analysis of structural changes in the photocycle of bacteriorhodopsin. EMBO J 1993;12:1–8.

75. Brown LS, Váró G, Needleman R, Lanyi JK. Functional significance of a protein conformation change at the cytoplasmic end of helix F during the bacteriorhodopsin photocycle. Biophys J 1995;69: 2103–2111.

76. Sheikh SP, Zvyaga TA, Lichtarge O, Sakmar TP, Bourne HR. Rhodopsin activation blocked by metalion-binding sites linking transmembrane helices C and F. Nature 1996;383:347–350.

77. Grumbach MM, Conte FA. Disorders of sex differentiation. In: Wilson JD, Foster DW eds. Williams Textbook of Endocrinology. W.B. Saunders, Philadelphia, 1992, pp. 853–951.

78. Kremer H, Kraaij R, Toledo SPA, et al. Male pseudohermaphroditism due to a homozygous missense mutation of the luteinizing hormone receptor gene. Nat Genet 1995;9:160–164.

79. Toledo SPA, Brunner HG, Kraaij R, et al. An inactivating mutation of the luteinizing hormone receptor causes amenorrhea in a 46,XX female. J Clin Endocrinol Metab 1996;81:3850–3854.

80. Laue L, Wu S-M, Kudo M, et al. A nonsense mutation of the human luteinizing hormone receptor gene in Leydig cell hypoplasia. Hum Mol Genet 1995;4:1429–1433.

81. Latronico AC, Anasti J, Arnhold IJP, et al. Brief report: testicular and ovarian resistance to luteinizing hormone caused by inactivating mutations of the luteinizing hormone-receptor gene. N Engl J Med 1996;334:507–512.

82. Laue LL, Wu S-M Kudo, M, et al. Compound heterozygous mutations of the luteinizing hormone receptor gene in Leydig cell hypoplasia. Mol Endocrinol 1996;10:987–997

83. Aittomaki K, Lucena JL, Pakarinen P, et al. Mutation in the follicle-stimulating hormone receptor gene causes hereditary hypergonadotropic ovarian failure. Cell 1995;82:959–968.

84. Fernandez LM, Puett D. Identification of amino acid residues in transmembrane helices VI and VII of the lutropin/choriogonadotropin receptor involved in signaling. Biochemistry 1996;35:3986–3993.

85. Hirsch B, Kudo M, Maro F, Conti M, Hsueh AJW. The C-terminal third of the human luteinizing hormone (LH) receptor is important for inositol phosphate release: analysis using chimeric human LH/follicle-stimulating hormone receptors. Mol Endocrinol 1996;10:1127–1137.

9

Inactivating and Activating Mutations of the FSH Receptor Gene

Ilpo T. Huhtaniemi, MD, PhD

INTRODUCTION

It has only recently became apparent that infertility and subfertility may be hereditary conditions. Numerous mutations have been discovered in genes that participate in the regulation of reproductive functions, and those of the gonadotropin receptors (R) have received considerable attention. Since the discovery of the first luteinizing hormone receptor (LHR) mutations in 1993 *(1,2)*, more than 15 mutations have been so far reported in this gene (*see* Chapter 9, and refs. *3,4*). The nature of the mutation determines to what extent the phenotype of the affected individuals is altered. "Loss-of-function" mutations usually require homozygosity or compound heterozygosity for phenotypic alterations, but with "gain-of-function" mutations, heterozygotes display altered hormonal function and phenotype. The first mutations of the follicle-stimulating hormone receptor (FSHR) have just recently been discovered. The purpose of this chapter is to review briefly the structural and functional features of the FSHR, to describe the currently known FSHR mutations, their pathophysiological consequences, and to discuss some future perspectives in the study of the role of FSHR function in reproduction.

From: *Contemporary Endocrinology: G Proteins, Receptors, and Disease*
Edited by: A. M. Spiegel, Humana Press Inc., Totowa, NJ

STRUCTURE AND FUNCTION OF THE FSH RECEPTOR

The cDNA structure of the rat FSHR gene was revealed in 1990 *(5)*, and subsequently, the cDNA sequences of this gene have been published for a number of mammalian species, including humans *(see*, e.g., *6–8)*. This gene, together with those for the receptors of the two other pituitary glycoprotein hormones, luteinizing hormone (LH) and thyroid-stimulating hormone (TSH) *(see*, e.g., *9,10)*, belongs to a new family of the seven times plasma membrane-spanning, G-protein-coupled receptors with an unusually long glycosylated extracellular domain. This domain has an internal repeat structure characteristic of members of the leucine-rich glycoprotein family, and it determines the hormonal selectivity of the receptor *(11)*. In the FSHR gene, the long extracellular part of the receptor is encoded by the first 9 exons, and the transmembrane and intracellular domains, comprising almost half of the 675 amino acid 75-kDa molecule, are encoded by the last long 10th exon *(12)*. There are three N-linked glycosylation sites in the extracellular part of the FSHR *(5,6)*. The genomic structures of the rat FSHR, LHR, and TSH receptor (TSHR) genes are similar *(9,10,12)*, with the exception that the one for LHR has 11 exons. The sequence of the human FSHR cDNA is 89% homologous overall with the cognate rat receptor, and up to 95% homologous in the transmembrane region *(5,6)*. The human FSHR gene is localized in chromosome 2p21 *(13,14)*. Its 5′-flanking region has been characterized *(15)*, but the complete genomic organization of the human FSHR gene has not been published at the time of writing of this chapter.

Some details are known about functions of the putative promoter structures of the rat, mouse, and human FSHR *(15–17)*. The FSHR gene 5′-flanking regions in the three species are homologous in structure (65% within the first 230 nucleotides) and function. The promoters have no TATA or CCAAT consensus sequences. There are no structural similarities between the putative FSHR promoter and that of the LHR, and for instance, the proximal GC-rich 3′-end of the putative LHR promoter, with multiple SP1 binding sites, is missing in the FSHR promoter. Both have features of promoters of constitutively expressed housekeeping genes with multiple transcription initiation sites, located between nucleotides –114 and –79 in the human FSHR promoter *(15)*. Canonical consensus sequences for other known transcription factors have not been characterized in the putative FSHR promoter. Transfection experiments with various reporter genes have revealed that the FSHR promoter function is relatively weak, and its cis- and trans-activators still remain elusive *(15–17)*.

The FSHR mRNA is expressed in multiple splice variants *(18–20)*; at least six of them are present in the human testis, ranging in size from 1.3–6.5 kb, the largest form being the most abundant *(20)*. In contrast, the human ovary contains three splice variants with sizes of 2.5, 4.2, and 7.0 kb, the middle-size message being the most abundant *(21)*. The physiological role of the different splice variants has not yet been explored, but it is a tempting possibility that they reflect differential functional states of the FSHR with respect to tissue specificity, response to various physiological states, and to utilization of various signal transduction mechanisms.

Cyclic AMP (cAMP) is the main second messenger of follicle-stimulating hormone (FSH) action, but there are also data suggesting that other signal transduction mechanisms are involved *(22)*. However, their physiological significance still remains obscure. The stimulatory FSH pathway seems to be under clear negative modulation by high phosphodiesterase activity and adenosine-related G_i protein function *(22)*.

PHYSIOLOGY OF FSH ACTION IN THE FEMALE AND MALE

The granulosa cells express the FSHR gene in the ovary *(23, 24)*. In the ovary, FSH plays a crucial role in the stimulation of follicular growth, which is unable to proceed beyond the early antral stage without proper gonadotropic support *(25)*. Already preantral follicles have FSH receptors in their granulosa cells, and FSH is the primary hormone responsible for the preovulatory follicular growth. As the preovulatory follicle grows, FSH induces in granulosa cells aromatase activity, which is needed for conversion of androgens, produced by the theca cells, into estrogens *(26)*. Estrogen is the major feedback regulator of FSH secretion during the menstrual cycle, but also inhibin plays a role in this action. The most important endocrine effect of FSH is the maintenance of aromatase activity on granulosa cells *(24, 25)*. FSH together with estrogen stimulates granulosa cell mitogenesis, apparently through activation of cyclin D2, a cell-cycle regulator *(27)*, thus enabling follicular maturation. Together with estrogen, FSH also maintains its own receptors in granulosa cells and induces the appearance of LH receptors to granulosa cells of the antral phase *(24)*. Therefore, the two key functions of the ovary, follicular maturation, and estrogen production are intimately related to FSH action, and if this function is disturbed, one would expect a profound disturbance in ovarian function with defective follicular maturation, insufficient estrogen production, and lack of ovulation.

In the male, FSHR are present in Sertoli cells, and FSH is known to stimulate various aspects of Sertoli cell metabolism, indirectly regulating in this way spermatogenesis *(18,22)*. FSH plays an important role in the prepubertal testis, where it stimulates Sertoli cell proliferation *(28,29)*, thereby determining the length of seminiferous tubules and indirectly the final testicular size. FSH has also been considered necessary for the pubertal differentiation of Sertoli cells, stimulation of a variety of specific metabolic events in these cells, and for the initiation of spermatogenesis. In contrast, the connection of FSH and spermatogenesis in the adult testis is less evident *(30, 31)*. It is apparent that FSH and testosterone maintain spermatogenesis in a synergistic fashion in the adult testis. Especially the studies on rodents have shown that spermatogenesis is possible in the presence of high testosterone concentrations, but absence of FSH, but such findings are less convincing in the human and other primates. In contrast, there is evidence from the monkeys and humans *(see below)* that FSH alone, without sufficient androgen support, is able to maintain spermatogenesis in the adult testis. The dogma is thus that although testosterone alone is able to maintain spermatogenesis, FSH is needed for its pubertal initiation and for keeping its rate quantitatively normal. The very recent data on FSHβ knockout mice and inactivating mutation of the FSHR gene in humans will change this concept *(see below)*.

ACTIVATING AND INACTIVATING MUTATIONS OF THE GONADOTROPIN RECEPTOR GENES

It was first observed with TSHR *(32–34)*, and soon thereafter with LHR *(1–4)*, that there are mutations in these two genes leading to either constitutively activated or inactivated forms of the receptors. Such mutations explain certain pathologies in the function of the thyroid gland and gonads. In the thyroid gland, constitutive activation of the TSHR brings about toxic adenomas and hyperplasia, and inactivating mutations cause hypothyroidism *(32–34)*. Concerning gonads, the male-limited familial, gonadotropin-independent form of precocious puberty (testotoxicosis) was found to be owing to a constitutively activating point mutation of the LHR gene *(1,2)*. The first inactivating mutation of the LHR gene, causing male pseudohermaphroditism with Leydig cell hypoplasia, was discovered very recently *(35)*. Subsequently, a variety of activating and inactivating mutations of the LHR gene have been described (*see* Chapter 9). Until the recent studies of Aittomäki et al. *(36)* and Gromoll et al. *(37)*, no mutations in the FSHR gene were known.

An Inactivating Mutation of the FSHR: Hypergonadotropic Ovarian Failure and Variable Impairment of Spermatogenesis

We recently discovered an inactivating mutation of the FSHR gene in connection with hypergonadotropic ovarian failure (HOF) *(36)*. The study was initiated by the population-based investigation *(38)*, where a total of 75 HOF patients were identified in the Finnish population. Segregation analysis confirmed the recessive mode of inheritance of the disease, as well as the existence of several kindreds with two or more affected sisters. Genealogical studies showed a clear-cut founder effect in an isolated subpopulation of the country.

A systematic search for linkage was thereafter carried out in the multiplex affected families, and the HOF locus was mapped to chromosome 2p, with maximum lod score up to 4.71 with chromosome 2p specific markers. Two particularly interesting genes with respect to HOF were localized to chromosome 2p, i.e., those of FSHR *(13,14)* and LHR *(39)*. Inactivating mutation in either gene could potentially cause ovarian dysgenesis. However, the critical role of FSH in the early events of ovarian maturation, including follicular development, as well as the fact that no male pseudohermaphroditism was apparent in the affected families (LHR defect would have caused such a phenotype; ref. *35*), indicated to us that an FSHR mutation was a more likely explanation for the disease.

The majority of the mutations so far detected in the TSHR and LHR genes have been localized to the transmembrane region, in particular, in or near the sixth transmembrane loop (*see above*). We therefore first searched for mutation in the large exon 10 encoding this part of the FSHR molecule. Denaturing gradient gel electrophoresis (DGGE) of several overlapping polymerase chain reaction (PCR) products was used. Only one polymorphism, G2039A, resulting in Asn to Ser conversion, was found in the region of the gene encoding the intracellular tail of the receptor, but it was not related to the disease phenotype. We thereafter went on to screen the first nine exons, encoding the extracellular part of the receptor protein, by amplifying each of them using intron-specific primers and sequencing the PCR products. During the course of the work, we found out that it is also possible to amplify mRNA of the FSHR gene by using reverse transcriptase (RT)-PCR and RNA isolated from white blood cells as template, a phenomenon termed illegitimate transcription *(40)*. This may also be related to the ubiquitous transcription of gonadotropin receptor (especially LHR) genes in various extragonadal tissues (*see*, e.g., *41–43*). Exons 6–9 were amplified in this way, and all affected individuals were found to be homozygous for a C to T transition in position 566 of exon 7 of the FSHR gene, predicting a change of alanine 189 to valine (Fig. 1). When these data were compared with the linkage results, the disease haplotype segregated perfectly with the mutation. All affected individuals displaying the disease haplotype were homozygous for the mutation, and all parents that could be studied (obligatory hetero-zygotes) were heterozygous for the mutation.

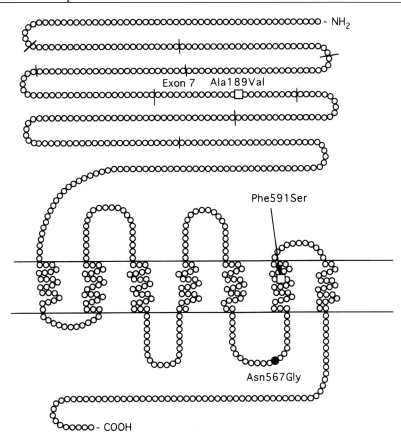

Fig. 1. The inactivating Ala189Val mutation (open square) in exon 7 of the FSHR gene detected in patients with hypergonadotropic ovarian failure *(36)*, the inactivating Phe591Ser mutation (open square) in the sixth transmembrane domain in ovarian stroman tumors *(59)*, and the activating Asn567Gly mutation (filled circle) in the third intracellular loop detected in a hypophysectomized male with sustained spermatogenesis *(37)*. The short lines across the peptide chain depict exon/intron boundaries.

The next step was to study the function of the mutated FSHR gene, in order to prove its role in formation of the disease phenotype. When cDNA encoding the wild-type human FSHR protein was transfected into an immortalized murine Sertoli cell line (MSC-1; ref. *44)*, not expressing the endogenous FSHR gene, a three-to fourfold dose-dependent stimulation of cAMP production was observed with recombinant human (rh) FSH (Fig. 2). In contrast, when the cells were transfected using cDNA of the mutated FSHR, no stimulation of cAMP by rhFSH could be detected. In accordance, when the binding of $[^{125}I]$-labeled rhFSH was measured in the same two transfected cell lines, the binding measured in cells expressing the mutated receptor was only 3% of that measured in cells expressing the wild-type FSHR (Fig. 3). Interestingly, the equilibrium association constant of binding (K_a) in both cases was similar $(4.8–6.7 \times 10^9$ L/mol), which is in good agreement with the affinity of human FSH to receptors in human testicular homogenates *(45)*. It is therefore possible that the conserved alanine to valine mutation mainly affects the trafficking of the receptor protein to the cell membrane or its rate of degradation.

After the mutation of the FSHR gene was discovered, Aittomäki et al. *(46)* carried out a comparison of clinical features of the original HOF patients with ($n = 22$) and without

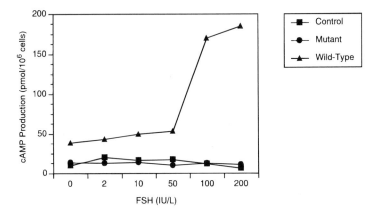

Fig. 2. FSH-stimulated cAMP production of MSC-1 cells transfected with the FSHR expression construct. Triangles denote wild-type, circles mutant, and squares mock-transfected controls. Each batch of cells was cotransfected with a plasmid-expressing bacterial luciferase gene under a powerful viral promoter, and the cAMP production was equalized to a constant amount of luciferase expression and calculated per 10^6 cells after a 3-h incubation. From ref. *36* with permission.

($n = 30$) the mutation. Both groups of patients had similar primary or early secondary amenorrhea, variable development of secondary sex characteristics, and high serum levels of gonadotropins. In contrast, transvaginal sonography or histology of ovarian biopsy revealed in all the receptor-defect patients studied the presence of follicles, whereas only one out of nine of those with unknown etiology had follicles. Therefore, the latter group apparently represents a more profound defect with true ovarian dysgenesis, whereas the receptor defect causes specific arrest of follicular development and maturation owing to absence of FSH action.

Therefore, we have identified a mutation in the FSHR gene, which offers an explanation to the pathogenesis of HOF. Many of the probands were derived from a geographically defined subpopulations in Finland. The minimum frequency of HOF in females for the whole country was calculated as 1 in 8300, which translates into a carrier frequency of 1 in 45. According to our preliminary estimations *(46)*, about 40% of the HOF cases in Finland are owing to the C566T point mutation of the FSHR gene. If similar figures of frequency occur in other populations, HOF resulting from this mutation will turn out to be one of the most common recessively inherited diseases. However, there is a possibility that the mutation discovered belongs to the Finnish heritage of genetic diseases.

Concerning the molecular mechanism of the functional defect of the mutated FSHR, no clear answer is yet available. In this respect, the site-directed mutagenesis study with the rat FSHR gene by Rozell et al. *(47)* is of particular interest. They introduced a single amino acid mutation into position 404 of the first extracellular loop of the FSHR protein. The mutated gene was expressed at protein level, as demonstrated by Western blots. However, the protein was retained intracellularly in the endoplasmic reticulum, and it was unable to bind ligand, possibly because it was in an incompletely folded state. This behavior appeared to be specific for FSHR, since a similar mutation of the LHR gene did not affect ligand binding. Although the C566T mutation is located in a different position of the FSHR peptide chain, it is also possible that this mutation affects the intracellular folding and processing of the mutated receptor protein. It is noteworthy that only a frac-

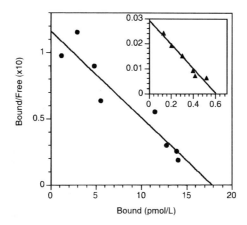

Fig. 3. Scatchard analysis of ^{125}I-labeled FSH binding to transfected MSC-1 cells. Circles denote wild-type and triangles (insert) mutated FSHR expression constructs. In each case, 2×10^6 transfected cells were incubated in triplicate with increasing concentrations of labeled FSH in a total volume of 250 µL. The cells were cotransfected with luciferase. After appropriate corrections, the cell suspension transfected with the wild-type FSHR construct displayed 18.2 pmol/L, and that expressing the mutated construct 0.63 pmol/L of specific FSH binding. The equilibrium association constants (K_a) of FSH binding in the same cell preparations were 6.7 and 4.9×10^9 L/mol, respectively. From ref. *36* with permission.

tion (up to 3%) of the mutated FSHR protein can be detected in the plasma membrane. The rest may be sequestered in incorrectly folded state in the endoplasmic reticulum. Since the C566T mutation was close to one of the three glycosylation sites of the FSHR gene *(5)*, it is also possible that it could interfere with the glycosylation process. Although the carbohydrate structures are not needed for ligand binding of the FSHR, they are necessary for proper intracellular folding of the receptor molecule to a conformation that is capable of binding FSH *(48)*. Studies to explore this matter in more detail are currently in progress in our laboratory.

The families with the disease also have males homozygous for the C566T mutation. The phenotype of these men is of particular interest considering the ongoing uncertainty about the necessity of FSH for male fertility *(31)*. We have recently completed the characterization of five brothers homozygous for the mutation of the affected females *(49)* (Table 1). The affected men were normally masculinized, but had variable reduction of testicular size (4–16 mL). The sperm counts ranged from normal to severe oligozoospermia (0.1–42×10^6/mL), but none was azoospermic. In contrast to their affected sisters, not all men were infertile; two of them had two children each. Serum FSH was moderately elevated (15–40 IU/L), and LH was normal to mildly elevated. The levels of testosterone were normal, and those of inhibin B suppressed in all men. It seems therefore that men with inactivating FSHR mutation have variable degrees of spermatogenic failure, but surprisingly no azoospermia or absolute infertility.

It is of interest to contrast the phenotypic effects of the inactivating mutation of the FSHR gene with the few documented cases of selective FSH deficiency. There is a report on such a male in connection with oligo-azoospermia, normal testosterone production, and normal virilization *(50)*. Another report concerns a young female with primary amenorrhea and postmenopausal LH levels *(51)*. The molecular basis of these two conditions was not technically possible to study at the time of discovery of these

Table 1
Testis Size, Sperm Count, and Some Serum Hormone Levels in Five Men
Homozygous for the Inactivating C566T Mutation of the FSHR Gene *(49)*

Subject	Testis size mL, right/left	Sperm count, 10^6/mL	FSH, IU/L	LH, IU/L	Testosterone, nmol/L	Inhibin B, ng/L
1	4.0/4.0	<0.1	23.5	16.6	14.5	<15
2	15.0/13.8	5.6	12.5	5.6	8.8	33
3	13.5/15.8	<0.1	15.1	4.2	15.8	62
4	8.0/8.0	<1.0	20.6	16.2	26.2	54
5	8.0/6.8	42	39.6	11.1	14.7	53
Reference range		>20	1–10.5	1–8.4	8.2–34.6	76–447

patients. The only known mutation of the FSHβ-subunit gene has been described by Matthews et al. *(52)*. The absence of FSH synthesis was caused by a deletion in the FSHβ gene, resulting in premature termination codon and translation of a truncated FSHβ chain that was not able to couple with the common α-subunit to a biologically active hormone. The phenotype of the affected woman resembled HOF with primary amenorrhea and infertility, but she could be treated by FSH with resulting successful pregnancy. Her mother, an obligate heterozygote for the mutation, had menstrual irregularities and infertility. These types of symptoms are not prevalent in mothers of our HOF patients. The father of the patient was not investigated.

The group of Matzuk has recently achieved targeted disruption (knockout) of the FSHβ gene in the mouse *(53)*. Interestingly, the phenotype of the null mutant mice is practically identical with that of the inactivating FSHR mutation: the females are infertile and display arrest in follicular maturation, whereas the males are fertile, but have reduced testicular size and impaired spermatogenesis. The findings that androgen treatment alone can initiate and maintain spermatogenesis in the hypogonadotropic *hpg* mutant mouse *(54)* also speak against the crucial role of FSH for male fertility. Therefore, the recent data on inactivated FSH secretion or action provide strong evidence that FSH is not essential for the pubertal initiation of spermatogenesis, and that this gonadotropin is more important for female than male fertility.

In addition to HOF, other pathologies of reproductive function have also been suggested to be caused by aberrant FSHR function. Conditions, such as delayed puberty, premature ovarian failure (POF), "resistant ovary syndrome," and idiopathic infertility, have been discussed in this connection. Recently, Whitney et al. *(55)* were unable to detect causative mutations in the FSHR gene in a group of 21 women with POF. Considering the multiple activating and inactivating mutations that have been recently discovered for the LHR gene, it is likely that a number of other FSHR mutations will also be found. The spectrum of reproductive pathologies caused by such mutations is also likely to expand.

An Activating Mutation of the FSHR Gene, Sustaining Autonomous Spermatogenesis in a Hypophysectomized Male

Gromoll et al. *(37)* very recently found a 28-yr-old male who had been hypophysectomized and treated with repeated radiotherapy 8 yr earlier because of a pituitary chromophobe adenoma. The patient had no residual pituitary function, and was treated with glucocorticoids, thyroxine, and testosterone. The circulating gonadotropin levels were nondetectable (<0.5 IU/L), as measured by sensitive immunometric and in vitro bio-assay methods. The concentration of serum testosterone was in the normal male range because of substitution therapy. Despite the history, the testis volume of the patient was in the upper normal range, and spermatogenesis appeared normal, with only slightly subnormal morphology and motility. During the testosterone substitution, the patient impregnated his wife four times, which resulted in births of three normal boys.

The above history led the investigators to the hypothesis that the signal transduction pathway of FSH had to be autonomously activated in the patient. As alluded to earlier, the role of FSH in sustaining male fertility, namely spermatogenesis, has remained a contentious issue (30,31). Although there are studies, in rodents in particular, indicating that testosterone alone is able to sustain and even initiate spermatogenesis (54,56), clinical evidence shows that fertility cannot be achieved in hypogonadal males with testosterone alone (57). Therefore, the hypothesis was feasible that the patient has to have some residual FSH activity, possibly owing to a constitutively activated FSHR. Such a hypothesis was quite natural in light of the numerous activating mutations that have recently been documented for LHR and TSHR (see above).

Exon 10 of the patient's FSHR gene was amplified by PCR from genomic DNA and subjected to single-strand conformation polymorphism analysis and sequencing. A heterozygous A to G mutation was observed in nucleotide 1700 of the gene, which resulted in asparagine to glycine transition in codon 567 of the third intracytoplasmic loop of the transmembrane region (Fig. 1). Interestingly, the same location, and especially the neighboring sixth transmembrane domain, has been shown to be a "hot spot" for activating and inactivating mutations of LHR and TSHR (see Chapters 7 and 8). When the wild-type and mutated receptor cDNAs were transfected into COS 7 cells, the latter consistently resulted in about 50% higher basal cAMP production of the cells. The FSH-stimulated rates of cAMP production were rather similar after both transfections.

These findings are consistent with partial constitutive activation of the mutated FSHR in the absence of ligand, and provide a mechanistic explanation for the sustained spermatogenesis of the patient under testosterone substitution, but without any circulating FSH. It is noteworthy that spermatogenesis of the patient was also sustained when testosterone replacement therapy was interrupted, which provides further evidence for the critical role of the activating FSHR mutation in maintenance of spermatogenesis. The only discordant finding in this interesting case was the persistence of rather high (at least 5 nmol/L) plasma testosterone levels in the absence of testosterone replacement. The control of this testicular activity in a hypophysectomized male remains open, as well as its contribution to the maintenance of spermatogenesis together with the activated FSHR mutation. In accordance with this subject, FSH alone is able to sustain spermatogenesis in monkeys that are rendered pharmacologically hypogonadotrophic by GnRH antagonist therapy (58). In the rat and mouse, spermatogenesis seems to be easier to maintain with testosterone alone (31,54,56,57). Therefore, the information on the physiologic role of FSH in the male obtained from various rodent models has to be extrapolated with caution to humans.

The previous hypophysectomy of the patient enabled the diagnosis of the FSHR mutation. The interrelationship of the two conditions remains elusive. It is questionable whether this type of FSH mutation would cause any phenotypic changes in otherwise healthy men. Chronic FSH hyperstimulation in prepubertal age would potentially lead to increased testis size (which was found in this patient), but Gromoll et al. *(37)* ruled out the association of such a phenotype demonstrating that this mutation was absent in 13 men with megalotestes. It is also possible that the phenotypic change is sex-limited in the same way as the activating LHR mutation that only alters the phenotype in men in the form of precocious puberty (testotoxicosis) (*see* Chapter 8). The constant FSH stimulation could cause in females disturbances of sexual maturation or of the cyclic ovarian function. Constant FSH stimulation could lead to accelerated follicular "consumption" and premature ovarian failure, but no FSHR mutations were recently discovered in this condition *(55)*.

FUTURE PERSPECTIVES

It is apparent that the two mutations so far detected in the FSHR gene will not remain the only ones. As with the LHR (*see above*, and Chapter 8), more activating and inactivating mutations are likely to be found. In the material of Aittomäki et al. *(36,38,46,49)*, there were patients with complete HOF symptoms, but without the described A566T mutation of the FSHR. Other mutations in the same gene are a likely explanation for pathogenesis at least of some of these cases. It also remains to be seen whether other conditions with disturbed reproduction could be owing to other forms of mutation, perhaps activating or with a different degree of affection of the FSH function.

Finally, since the ovaries of the HOF patients with the FSHR mutation appear to maintain follicles, up to the preantral stage, it would be theoretically possible to rescue and stimulate them with appropriate hormonal therapy. Since the FSHR binding is not totally lost (up to 3% maintained), it can be hypothesized that massive FSH doses could be able to stimulate follicular maturation. Also, alternative hormone and growth factor therapies are possible. For this purpose, a suitable animal model would be very useful. One harboring the same mutation through gene targeting is technically feasible.

The role of gonadotropin receptors in gonadal tumorigenesis still remains elusive. In this respect, the recent findings of Kotlar et al. *(59)* are of particular interest. They reported that 9 of 13 ovarian sex cord tumors and 2 of 3 small-cell carcinomas had a heterozygous T to C mutation of the FSHR gene, altering codon 591 in the sixth transmembrane receptor domain from phenylalanine to serine (Fig. 1). These tumors are known to produce endocrine manifestations owing to secretion of estrogens and androgens. Altered signal transduction of the mutated FSHR was found in transfected cells, where the mutation eliminated FSH-stimulated cAMP production. It is of interest that an inactivating heterozygous mutation was found in connection with the tumors, and the causal relationship between these findings remains open. In any case, these findings open up a new avenue for pathogenesis of gonadal tumors.

In conclusion, the recently discovered mutations in the gonadotropin receptor genes represent just the beginning of discoveries likely to be made on molecular pathogenesis of human infertility and subfertility, and possibly even of gonadal tumors. Many conditions affecting reproductive endocrine functions are still idiopathic in nature, including the large proportion of idiopathic infertility. It is likely that future research on genetic basis of such conditions will greatly further our knowledge of their etiology as well as novel strategies for their treatment.

REFERENCES

1. Kremer H, Mariman E, Otten BJ, Moll GW Jr, Stoelinga GB, Wit JM, Jansen M, Drop SL, Faas B, Ropers HH, Brunner HG. Cosegregation of missense mutations of the luteinizing hormone receptor gene with familial male-limited precocious puberty. Hum Mol Genet 1993;2:1779–1783.
2. Shenker A, Laue L, Kosugi S, Merendino JJ Jr, Minegishi T, Cutler GB Jr. A constitutively activating mutation of the luteinizing hormone receptor in familial male precocious puberty. Nature 1993;365:652–654.
3. Huhtaniemi I, Pakarinen P, Haavisto A-M, Nilsson C, Pettersson K, Tapanainen J, Aittomäki K. The polymorphism of gonadotropin action: molecular basis and clinical implications. In: Hansson V, Levy FO, Taskén K, eds. Signal Transduction in Testicular Cells. Springer, Berlin, 1996, pp. 319–341.
4. Themmen APN, Brunner HG. Luteinizing hormone receptor mutations and sex differentiation. Eur J Endocrinol 1996;134:522–540.
5. Sprengel R, Braun T, Nikolics K, Segaloff DL, Seeburg PH. The testicular receptor for follicle-stimulating hormone: structure and functional expression of cloned cDNA. Mol Endocrinol 1990;4:525–530.
6. Minegishi T, Nakamura K, Takakura Y, Ibuki Y, Igarashi M. Cloning and sequencing of human FSH receptor cDNA. Biochem Biophys Res Commun 1991;175:1125–1130.
7. Yarney TA, Sairam MR, Khan H, Ravindranath N, Payne S, Seidah NG. Molecular cloning and expression of the ovine testicular follicle stimulating hormone receptor. Mol Cell Endocrinol 1993;93:219–226.
8. Gromoll H, Dankbar B, Sharma RS, Nieschlag E. Molecular cloning of the testicular follicle stimulating hormone receptor of the nonhuman primate Macaca fascicularis and identification of multiple transcripts in the testis. Biochem Biophys Res Commun 1993;196:1066–1072.
9. Segaloff DL, Ascoli M. The lutropin/choriogonadotropin receptor . . . 4 years later. Endocr Rev 1993;14:324–346.
10. Vassart G, Dumont JE. The thyrotropin receptor and the regulation of thyrocyte function and growth. Endocr Rev 1992;13:596–611.
11. Braun T, Schofield PR, Sprengel R. Amino-terminal leucine rich repeats in gonadotropin receptors determine hormone selectivity. EMBO J 1991;10:1995–1890.
12. Heckert LL, Daly IJ, Griswold MD. Structural organization of the follicle-stimulating hormone receptor gene. Mol Endocrinol 1992;6:70–80.
13. Rousseau-Merck MF, Atger M, Loosfelt H, Milgrom E, Berger R. The chromosomal localization of the human follicle-stimulating hormone receptor gene (FSHR) on 2p21-2p15 is similar to that of the luteinizing hormone receptor gene. Genomics 1993;15:222–224
14. Gromoll J, Ried T, Holtgeve-Grez H, Nieschlag E, Gudermann T. Localization of the human FSH receptor to chromosome 2p21 using a genomic probe comprising exon 10. J Mol Endocrinol 1994;12:265–271
15. Gromoll J, Dankbar B, Gudermann T 1994 Characterization of the 5' flanking regoin of the human follicle-stimulating hormone receptor gene. Mol Cell Endocrinol 102:93–102.
16. Huhtaniemi IT, Eskola V, Pakarinen P, Matikainen T, Sprengel R. The murine luteinizing hormone and follicle-stimulating hormone receptor genes: transcription initiation sites, putative promoter sequences and promoter activity. Mol Cell Endocrinol 1992;88:55–66.
17. Linder CC, Heckert LL, Goetz TL, Griswold MD. Follicle-stimulating hormone receptor gene promoter activity. Endocrine 1994;2:957–966.
18. Heckert LL, Griswold MD. Expression of follicle-stimulating hormone receptor mRNA in rat testis and Sertoli cells. Mol Endocrinol 1991;5:670–677.
19. LaPolt PS, Tilly JL, Aihara T, Nishimori K, Hsueh AJW. Gonadotropin-induced up- and down-regulation of ovarian follicle-stimulating hormone (FSH) receptor gene expression in immature rats: effects of pregnant mare's serum gonadotropin, human chorionic gonadotropin, and recombinant FSH. Endocrinology 1992;130:1289–1295.
20. Gromoll J, Gudermann T, Nieschlag E. Molecular cloning of a truncated isoform of the human follicle stimulating hormone receptor. Biochem Biophys Res Commun 1992;188:1077–1083.
21. Tilly JL, Aihara T, Nishimori K, Jia X-C, Billig H, Kowalski KI, Perlas EA, Hsueh AJW. Expression of recombinant human follicle-stimulating hormone receptor: species-specific ligand binding, signal transduction, and identification of multiple ovarian messenger ribonucleic acid transcripts. Endocrinology 1992;131:799–806.
22. Griswold MD. Actions of FSH on mammalian Sertoli cells. In: Russell LD, Griswold MD, eds. The Sertoli Cell. Cache River, Clearwater, FL, 1993, pp. 493–508.

23. Camp TA, Rahal JO, Mayo KE. Cellular localization and hormonal regulation of follicle-stimulating hormone and luteinizing hormone messenger RNAs in the rat ovary. Mol Endocrinol 1991;5: 1405–1417.

24. Richards JS. Hormonal control of gene expression in the ovary. Endocr Rev 1994;15:725–751.

25. Zeleznik AJ. Dynamics of primate follicular growth. A Physiologic perspective. In: Adashi EY, Leung PCK, eds. The Ovary Raven, New York, 1993, pp. 41–55.

26. Steinkampf MP, Mendelson CR, Simpson ER. Regulation by follicle stimulating hormone of the synthesis of aromatase cytochrome P-450 in human granulosa cells. Mol Endocrinol 1987;1:465–471.

27. Sicinski P, Donaher JL, Geng Y, Parker SB, Gardner H, Park MY, Robker RL, Richards JS, McGinnins LK, Biggers JD, Eppig JJ, Bronson RT, Elledge SJ, Weinberg RA. Cyclin D2 is an FSH-responsive gene involved in gonadal cell proliferation and oncogenesis. Nature 1996;384:470–474.

28. Gondos B, Berndston WE. Postnatal and postpubertal development. In: Russell LD, Griswold MD, eds. The Sertoli Cell. Cache River, Clearwater, FL, 1993, pp. 115–194.

29. Hess RA, Cooke PS, Bunick D, Kirby JD. Adult testicular enlargement induced by neonatal hypothyroidism is accompanied by increased Sertoli and germ cell numbers. Endocrinology 1993;132: 2607–2613.

30. Bremner WJ, Matsumoto AM, Sussman AM, Paulsen CA. Follicle-stimulating hormone and spermatogenesis. J Clin Invest 1981;68:1044–1052.

31. Zirkin B.R., Awoniyi C, Griswold MD, Sharpe RM. Is FSH required for adult spermatogenesis? J Androl 1994;15:273–276.

32. van Sande J, Parma J, Tonacchera M, Swillens S, Dumont J, Vassart G. Somatic and germline mutations of the TSH receptor gene in thyroid diseases. J Clin Endocrinol Metab 1995;80:2577–2585.

33. Utiger RD. Thyrotropin-receptor mutations and thyroid dysfunction. New Engl J Med 1995;332: 183–185.

34. Sunthornthepvarakul T, Gottschalk ME, Hayashi Y, Refetoff S. Brief report: resistance to thyrotropin caused by mutations in the thyrotropin-receptor gene. N Engl J Med 1995;332:155–160.

35. Kremer H, Kraaij R, Toledo SPA, Post M, Friedman JB, Hayashida CY, van Reen M, Milgrom E, Ropers H-H, Mariman E, Themmen APN, Brunner HG. Male pseudohermaphroditism due to a homozygous missense mutation of the luteinizing hormone receptor gene. Nature Gen 1995; 9:160–164.

36. Aittomäki K, Dieguez Lucena JL, Pakarinen P, Sistonen P, Tapanainen J, Gromoll J, Kaskikari R, Sankila E-M, Lehväslaiho H, Reyes Engel A, Nieschlag E, Huhtaniemi I, de la Chapelle A. Mutation in the follicle-stimulating hormone receptor gene causes hereditary hypergonadotropic ovarian failure. Cell 1995;92:959–968.

37. Gromoll J, Simoni M, Nieschlag E. An activating mutation of the follicle-stimulating hormone autonomously sustains spermatogenesis in a hypophysectomized man. J Clin Endocrinol Metab 1996;81:1367–1370.

38. Aittomäki K. The genetics of XX gonadal dysgenesis. Am J Hum Genet 1994;54:844–851.

39. Rousseau-Merck MF, Misrahi M, Atger M, Loosfelt H, Milgrom E, Berger R. Localization of the human LH (luteinizing hormone) receptor gene to chromosome 2p21. Cytogenet Cell Genet 1990; 54:77–79.

40. Chelly J, Concordet J-P, Kaplan J-C, Kahn A. Illegitimate transcription: transcription of any gene in any cell type. Proc Natl Acad Sci USA 1989;86:2617–2621.

41. Lei ZM, Rao ChV, Kornyei JL, Licht P, Hiatt ES. Novel expression of human chorionic gonadotropin/luteinizing hormone receptor gene in brain. Endocrinology 1993;132:2262–2270.

42. Lin J, Lojun S, Lei ZM, Wu WX, Peiper SC, Rao ChV. Lymphocytes from pregnant women express human chorionic gonadotropin/luteinizing hormone receptor gene. Mol Cell Endocrinol 1995;111: R13–R17.

43. Pabon JE, Li X, Lei ZM, Sanfilippo J, Yussman MA, Rao ChV. Novel presence of human luteinizing hormone/chorionic gonadotropin receptors in the human adrenal glands. J Clin Endocrinol Metab 1996;81:2397–2400.

44. Peschon JJ, Behringer RR, Cate RL, Harwood KA, Idzerda RL, Brinster RL, Palmiter RD. Directed expression of an oncogene to Sertoli cells in transgenic mice using Mullerian inhibiting substance regulatory sequences. Mol Endocrinol 1992;6:1403–1411.

45. Wahlström T, Huhtaniemi I, Hovatta O, Seppälä M. Localization of luteinizing hormone, follicle-stimulating hormone, prolactin, and their receptors in human and rat testis using immunohistochemistry and radioreceptor assay. J Clin Endocrinol Metab 1983;57:825–830.

46. Aittomäki K, Herva R, Stenman U-H, Juntunen K, Ylöstalo P, Hovatta O, de la Chapelle A. Clinical features of primary ovarian failure caused by a point mutation in the follicle-stimulating hormone receptor gene. J Clin Endocrinol Metab 1996;81:3722–3726.

47. Rozell TG, Wang H, Liu X, Segaloff DL. Intracellular retention of mutant gonadotropin receptors results in loss of hormone binding activity of the follitropin receptor but not the lutropin/choriogonadotropin receptor. Mol Endocrinol 1995;9:1727–1736.

48. Davis D, Liu L, Segaloff DL. Identification of the sites of N-linked glycosylation on the follicle-stimulating hormone (FSH) receptor and assessment of their role in FSH receptor function. Mol Endocrinol 1995;9:159–170.

49. Tapanainen JS, Aittomäki K, Min J, Vaskivuo T, Huhtaniemi IT. Men homozygous for an inactivating mutation of the follicle-stimulating hormone (FSH) receptor gene present variable suppression of spermatogenesis and infertility. Nature Genet 1997;15:205, 206.

50. Maroulis GB, Parlow AF, Marshall JR. Isolated follicle-stimulating hormone deficiency in man. Fertil Steril 1977;28:818–822.

51. Rabinowitz D, Benveniste R, Lindner J, Lober D, Danniell J. Isolated FSH deficiency revisited. N Engl J Med 1979;300:126–128.

52. Matthews CH, Borgato S, Beck-Peccoz P, Adams M, Tone Y, Gambino G, Casagrande S, Tedeschini G, Benedetti A, Chatterjee VKK. Primary amenorrhoea and infertility due to a mutation in the β-subunit of follicle-stimulating hormone. Nature Genet 1993;5:83–86.

53. Kumar TR, Wang Y, Lu N, Matzuk MM. Follicle stimulating hormone is required for ovarian maturation but not for male fertility. Nature Genet 1997;15:201–204.

54. Singh J, O'Neill C, Handelsman DJ. Induction of spermatogenesis by androgens in gonadotropin-deficient *(hpg)* mice. Endocrinology 1995;136:5311–5321.

55. Whitney EA, Layman LC, Chan PJ, Lee A, Peak DB, McDonough PG. The follicle-stimulating hormone receptor gene is polymorphic in premature ovarian failure and normal controls. Fertil Steril 1995;64:518–524.

56. Awoniyi CA, Zirkin BR, Chandrachekar V, Schlaff WD. Endogenously administered testosterone maintains spermatogenesis quantitatively in adult rats actively immunized against gonadotropin-releasing hormone. Endocrinology 1992;130:3283–3288.

57. Weinbauer GF, Nieschlag E. Hormonal regulation of spermatogenesis. In: de Kretser D, ed. Molecular Biology of the Male Reproductive System. Academic, New York, 1993, pp. 99–142.

58. Weinbauer GF, Behre HM, Fingscheidt U, Nieschlag E. Human follicle-stimulating hormone exerts a stimulatory effect on spermatogenesis, testicular size and serum inhibin levels in the gonadotropin-releasing hormone agonist-treated, non-human primate *(Macaca fascicularis)*. Endocrinology 1991;129:1831–1839.

59. Kotlar TJ, Young RH, Albanese C, Crowley WFJr, Scully RE, Young RH, Jameson JL. A mutation in the follicle-stimulating hormone receptor occurs frequently in human ovarian sex cord tumors. J Clin Endocrinol Metab 1997;82:1020–1028.

10 Nephrogenic Diabetes Insipidus and Vasopressin Receptor Mutations

Daniel G. Bichet, MD

CONTENTS

INTRODUCTION

The conservation of water by the human kidney is the function of the complex architecture of renal tubules within the renal medulla (1). Renal collecting tubules contain selective cells known as principal cells, responsive to the neurohypophyseal antidiuretic hormone arginine-vasopressin (AVP). The major action of AVP is to facilitate urinary concentration by allowing water to be transported passively down an osmotic gradient between the tubular fluid and the surrounding interstitium. The process of this counter multiplication system and the action of AVP on principal collecting duct cells are represented in Fig. 1.

In congenital nephrogenic diabetes insipidus, the renal collecting ducts are resistant to the antidiuretic action of AVP or to its antidiuretic analog dDAVP (2,3). This is a rare, but now well described entity secondary to either mutations in the AVPR2 gene (X-linked nephrogenic diabetes insipidus [Online Mendelian Inheritance in Man, OMIM. Johns Hopkins University, Baltimore, MD. MIM Number: 304800]) that codes for the antidiuretic (V_2) receptor or to mutations in the AQP2 gene (autosomal-recessive nephrogenic diabetes insipidus [Online Mendelian Inheritance in Man, OMIM. Johns Hopkins University, Baltimore, MD. MIM Number: 222000]) that codes for the vasopress-independent water channel (4–6). Of 95 families with congenital nephrogenic diabetes

From: *Contemporary Endocrinology: G Proteins, Receptors, and Disease*
Edited by: A. M. Spiegel, Humana Press Inc., Totowa, NJ

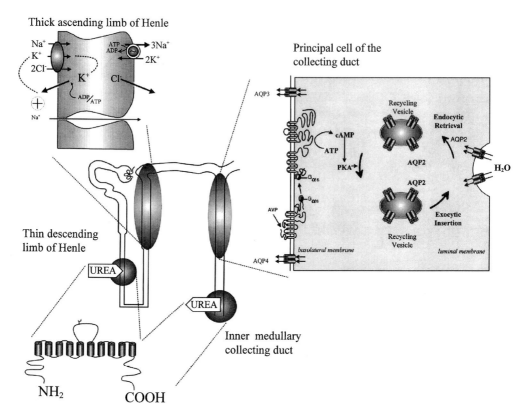

Fig. 1. Schematic representation of the nephron with selected areas involved in the urinary concentrating mechanism. *(1)* The reabsorption of NaCl, but not water from the ascending limbs of Henle initiate countercurrent multiplication within the renal medulla. The Na-K-2Cl cotransporter (inhibited by bumetanide) in the medullary thick ascending limb is shown. *(2)* Plasma AVP increases water permeability in collecting ducts: the hormone is bound to the vasopressin V_2 receptor (a G-protein-linked receptor) on the basolateral membrane. AVP activates adenylyl cyclase increasing the intracellular concentration of cAMP. The topology of adenylyl cyclase is characterized by two tandem repeats of six hydrophobic putative transmembrane domains separated by a large cytoplasmic loop and terminating in a large intracellular tail. Generation of cAMP follows receptor-linked activation of the heterometric G protein (G_s) and interaction of the free $G\alpha_s$ chain with the adenylyl cyclase catalyst. A cAMP-dependent protein kinase (PKA) is the target of the generated cAMP. Cytoplasmic vesicles carrying the water channel proteins (represented as homotetrameric complexes) are fused to the luminal membrane in response to vasopressin, thereby increasing the water permeability of this membrane. When vasopressin is not available, water channels are retrieved by an endocytic process, and water permeability returns to its original low rate. AQP3 and AQP4 *(see text)* are expressed on the basolateral membrane. ATP, adenosine triphosphate. *(3)* Vasopressin also increases the permeability of the terminal part of the collecting duct to urea, resulting in movement of urea into the medullary interstitium. This process is provided by urea transporters (represented here with 10 transmembrane domains). Both the inner medullary collecting duct and thin descending limbs of short loops of Henle express a urea transporter.

insipidus referred to our laboratory in Montreal, 87 families have *AVPR2* mutations and 8 have *AQP2* mutations.

CELLULAR ACTIONS OF VASOPRESSIN AND MOLECULAR BIOLOGY OF NEPHROGENIC DIABETES INSIPIDUS

Vasopressin Isoreceptors and Postreceptor Events

Vasopressin binds at least three distinct subtypes of receptors, V_{1a}, V_{1b}, and V_2, now cloned and sequenced *(7–14)* all belonging to the G-protein-coupled receptor super-family characterized by seven putative transmembrane helices *(15)*. The vasopressin isoreceptors are strikingly similar in both size and amino acid sequence, but differ in their coupling: V_{1a} and V_{1b} receptors through their $Gq/_{11}$ coupling mediate the activation of distinct isoforms of phospholipase C_β resulting in the breakdown of phosphoinositide lipids *(16)*. The V_2 receptor preferentially activates the G protein G_s resulting in activation of adenylyl cyclase. The classical vascular smooth muscle contraction, platelet aggregation, and hepatic glycogenolysis actions of AVP are mediated by a V_{1a} vasopressin receptor that increases cytosolic calcium. *In situ* hybridization histochemistry using ^{35}S-labeled cRNA probes specific for the V_{1a} receptor mRNA showed high levels of V_{1a} receptor transcripts in the liver among hepatocytes surrounding central veins and in the renal medulla among the vascular bundles, the arcuate, and interlobular arteries *(17)*. Vasopressin V_{1a} receptor mRNA was found to be extensively distributed throughout the brain where vasopressin may act as a neurotransmitter or a neuromodulator in addition to its classical role on vascular tone *(18)*. Specifically, brain vasopressin receptors have been proposed to mediate the effect of vasopressin on memory and learning, antipyresis, brain development, selective aggression and partner preference in rodents, cardiovascular responsivity, blood flow to the choroid plexus and cerebrospinal fluid production, regulation of smooth muscle tone in superficial brain vasculature, and analgesia. It is, however, not known whether V_{1a} brain receptors respond to AVP released within the brain proper or whether the receptors also respond to vasopressin from the peripheral circulation *(18)*.

V_{1b} (or V_3) receptors are not only expressed in the anterior pituitary *(11)* and kidney *(12)* as originally reported, but Lolait et al. recently cloned and sequenced the rat pituitary V_{1b} vasopressin receptor, and demonstrated by RNA blot analysis, reverse transcription PCR, and *in situ* hybridization experiments that numerous tissues, such as brain, uterus, thymus, heart, breast, and lung, also expressed the V_{1b} vasopressin receptor gene *(13)*. The physiological role of these extrapituitary V_{1b} receptors remains unknown, but some functions of AVP attributed in the past to V_{1a} receptors or oxytocin receptors may be a result of the activation of V_{1b} receptors *(13)*. In the rat adrenal medulla, vasopressin may regulate the adrenal functions by paracrine/autocrine mechanisms involving distinct vasopressin receptor subtypes: V_{1a} in the adrenal cortex and V_{1b} in the adrenal medulla *(19)*.

V_2 transcripts are heavily expressed in cells of the renal collecting ducts (in humans and rodents) and in cells of the thick ascending limbs of the loops of Henle (in rodents only) *(17)*.

Receptor Functional Domains Underlying Binding of Vasopressin to Its Receptors

A 3-D model of the V_{1a} vasopressin receptor was constructed by Mouillac et al. *(20)* to dock its endogenous ligand AVP. AVP was found to be completely embedded into a

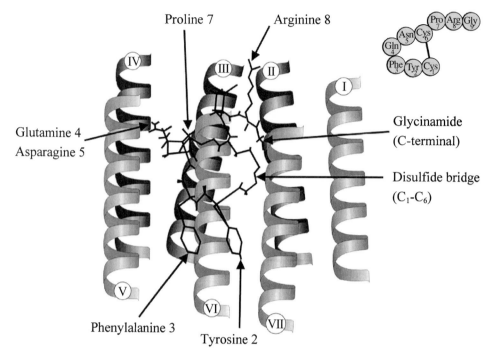

Fig. 2. Hypothetical model of interaction between AVP and its V_{1a} receptor. A schematic lateral view of the seven-transmembrane α-helices (I–VII) of the receptor and of the vasopressin docked in the rat V_{1a} receptor is represented. Each individual amino acid of the vasopressin molecule is represented. Redrawn from data published by Mouillac et al. *(20).*

15–20 Å deep cleft defined by the transmembrane helices 2–7 of the receptor (Fig. 2). Mouillac et al. (20) proposed that residues highly conserved in vasopressin and oxytocin transmembrane domains formed the same agonist binding site shared by all members of this receptor family. The conserved residues were mutated to alanine, which decreased the affinity of the receptor for agonists, but not for antagonists. These results indicate a different binding mode for agonists and antagonists in the vasopressin receptor.

Receptor Functional Domains Underlying G-Protein Coupling

The vasopressin receptor family is unique among all classes of peptide receptors, since its individual members couple to different subsets of G proteins *(16)*. Hybrid receptors with different intracellular domains exchanged between V_{1a} and V_2 receptors were expressed in COS-7 cells by Liu and Wess *(16)*. All mutant receptors containing V_{1a} receptor sequence in the second intracellular loop were able to stimulate the phosphatidylinositol pathway. On the other hand, only those hybrid receptors containing V_2 receptor sequences in the third intracellular loop were capable of stimulating cAMP production. These studies will lead to 3-D models of vasopressin receptor G-protein binding/activation interactions.

Molecular Biology of Nephrogenic Diabetes Insipidus

The first step in the action of AVP on water excretion is its binding to AVP type 2 receptors (V_2 receptors) on the basolateral membrane of the collecting duct cells

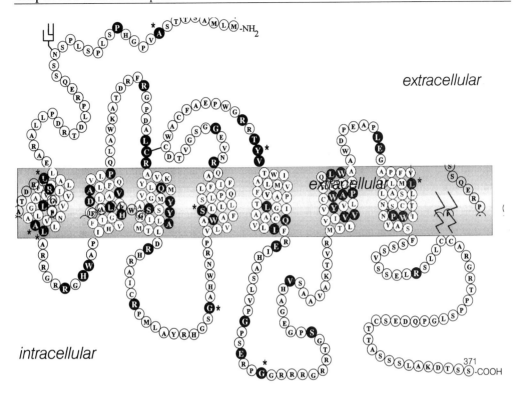

Fig. 3. Schematic representation of the V_2 receptor and identification of 72 *AVPR2* mutations, consisting of 36 missense, 10 nonsense, 18 frameshift, 2 inframe deletions, 1 splice-site, and 5 large deletion mutations. The four large deletions are characterized incompletely and are not included in the figure. Predicted amino acids are given as the one-letter code. Solid symbols indicate the predicted location of the mutations; an asterisk indicates two different mutations in the same codon. The names of the mutations were assigned according to the conventional nomenclature. The extracellular (E_I–E_{IV}), cytoplasmic (C_I–C_{IV}), and transmembrane domains (TM_I–TM_{VII}) are labeled from the N-terminus to the C-terminus according to Sharif and Hanley *(42)*. E_I 98del28, 98ins28, 113delCT. TM_I: L44F, L44P, L53R, L62P. TM_I and C_I: 253del35, 255del9. C_I: 274insG, W71X. TM_{II}: H80R, L83P, D85N, V88M, 337delCT, P95L. E_{II}: R106C, 402delCT, C112R, R113W. TM_{III}: Q119X, Y124X, S126F, Y128S, A132D. C_{II}: R137H, R143P, 528del7, 528delG. TM_{IV}: W164S, S167L, S167T. E_{III}: R181C, G185C, R202C, T204N, 684delTA, Y205C, V206D. TM_V: L219R, Q225X, 753insC. C_{III}: E231X, 763delA, 786delG, E242X, 804insG, 804delG, 834delA, 855delG. TM_{VI}: V277A, ΔV278, Y280C, W284X, A285P, P286L, P286R, L292P, W293X. E_{IV}: 977delG, 982–2A→G. TM_{VII}: L312X, P322H, P322S, W323R. C_{IV}: R337X.

(Fig. 1). The human V_2 receptor gene, *AVPR2,* is located in chromosome region Xq28, and has three exons and two small introns *(8,21)*. The sequence of the cDNA predicts a polypeptide of 371 amino acids with a structure typical of guanine-nucleotide (G) protein-coupled receptors with seven transmembrane, four extracellular, and four cytoplasmic domains *(15; see also* Fig. 3). The activation of the V_2 receptor on renal collecting tubules stimulates adenylyl cyclase via the stimulatory G protein (G_s) and promotes the cyclic adenosine monophosphate (cAMP)-mediated incorporation of water channels (aquaporins) into the luminal surface of these cells. This process is the molecular basis of the vasopressin-induced increase in the osmotic water permeability of the apical membrane of the collecting tubule.

Aquaporin-1 (AQP1, also known as CHIP, channel-forming integral membrane protein of 28 kDa) was the first protein shown to function as a molecular water channel *(6)*, and is constitutively expressed in mammalian red cells, renal proximal tubules, thin descending limbs, and other water-permeable epithelia *(22)*. At the subcellular level, AQP1 is localized in both apical and basolateral plasma membranes, which may represent entrance and exit routes for transepithelial water transport. In contrast to AQP2, limited amounts of AQP1 are localized in membranes of vesicles or vacuoles. In the basolateral membranes, AQP1 is localized to both basal and lateral infoldings. AQP2 is the vasopressin-regulated water channel in renal collecting ducts. It is exclusively present in principal cells of inner medullary collecting duct cells and is diffusely distributed in the cytoplasm in the euhydrated condition, whereas apical staining of AQP2 is intensified in the dehydrated condition or after vasopressin administration. These observations are thought to represent the exocytic insertion of preformed water channels from intracellular vesicles into the apical plasma membrane (the shuttle hypothesis) (Fig. 1). AQP3 is the water channel in basolateral membranes of renal medullary collecting ducts.

CLINICAL CHARACTERISTICS OF NEPHROGENIC DIABETES INSIPIDUS, INCIDENCE, POPULATION GENETICS, ANCESTRAL MUTATIONS, AND *DE NOVO* MUTATIONS, MECHANISMS OF *AVPR2* MUTATIONS

Males who have an *AVPR2* mutation have a phenotype characterized by early dehydration episodes, hypernatremia, and hyperthermia as early as the first week of life *(2)*. The dehydration episodes can be so severe that they lower arterial blood perfusion pressure to a degree that is not sufficient to sustain adequate oxygenation to the brain, kidneys, and other organs. Mental and physical retardations and renal failure are the classical "historical" consequences of a late diagnosis and lack of treatment. Heterozygous females exhibit variable degrees of polyuria and polydipsia because of skewed X chromosome inactivation. The onset and severity of the clinical manifestations of autosomal-recessive nephrogenic diabetes insipidus are similar to those of X-linked nephrogenic diabetes insipidus.

In Quebec, the incidence of this disease among males was estimated to be approx 4 in 1,000,000 *(23)*. A founder effect for a particular *AVPR2* mutation in Ulster Scot immigrants resulted in an elevated prevalence of X-linked nephrogenic diabetes insipidus in their descendants and was estimated to afflict approx 24 in 1000 males in certain communities in Nova Scotia. The W71X mutation was identified as the cause of nephrogenic diabetes insipidus in the extended "Hopewell" kindred and in families in the Canadian Maritime provinces *(24–26)*. The W71X mutations of these patients are likely identical by descent, although a common ancestor has not been identified in all cases. Among X-linked nephrogenic diabetes insipidus patients in North America, the W71X mutation is more common than any other *AVPR2* mutation.

Seventy-two different putative disease-causing mutations in the *AVPR2* gene have now been reported in 102 unrelated families with X-linked nephrogenic diabetes insipidus (Fig. 3). The diversity of *AVPR2* mutations (described in Fig. 3) found in many ethnic groups (Caucasians, Japanese, African-Americans, Africans) and the rareness of the disease are consistent with an X-linked recessive disease that was lethal in the past for

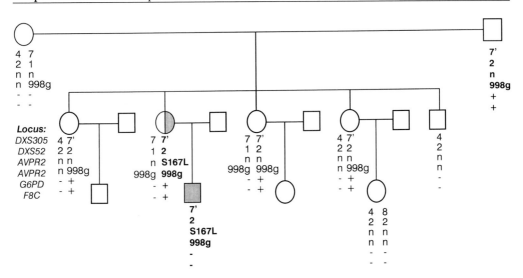

Fig. 4. Parental origin of a *de novo* mutation. The mother of the affected male (solid symbol) is a carrier of the S167L mutation. None of her three sisters carry this mutation, although all the daughters received the same haplotype from their father. These data are consistent with a new mutation arising during spermatogenesis in the maternal grandfather of the patient. The distance spanned by the markers is sufficiently large that recombination between the markers has been observed *(28)*. In this pedigree, the affected male inherited a recombinant chromosome; recombination occurred between *AVPR2* and *G6PD*. Reprinted from ref. *3* with permission.

male patients and was balanced by recurrent mutations. In X-linked nephrogenic diabetes insipidus, loss of mutant alleles from the population occurs because of the higher mortality of affected males compared to normal males, whereas gain of mutant alleles occurs by mutation. If affected males with a rare X-linked recessive disease do not reproduce and if mutation rates are equal in mothers and fathers, then at genetic equilibrium, one-third of new cases of affected males will be owing to new mutations *(27)*. The gametic origins of new mutations could be identified or inferred in 18 families, and consist of 5 maternal, 9 grandpaternal, 2 grandmaternal gametes, 1 great-grandmaternal gamete, and 1 gamete that was either of grandpaternal or grandmaternal origin *(28–31)*. Figure 4 illustrates the identification of a new mutation.

Eleven different *AVPR2* mutations were observed in more than one independent nephrogenic diabetes insipidus family, suggesting that there are hot spots for mutations. For example, mutations at serine 167 have been described in at least eight unrelated families *(28–30,32)*.

Seven of nine mutations at CpG nucleotide in the *AVPR2* gene (V88M, R113W, R137H, S167L, R181C, R202C, and R337X) are recurrent mutations, that is, they have arisen *de novo* in unrelated families. The hypermutability of methylated CpG dinucleotides (scholarly reviewed in ref. *33*) is a frequent cause of single basepair substitution. Thirteen of 18 small deletion or insertion mutations (1–35 bp) involved direct or complementary repeats (2–9 bp) or strings of 4–6 guanines. This finding suggests that these deletions, like many others that have been described in other genes, resulted from DNA strand slippage and mispairing during replication *(33)*. Examples of mutations generated by the slipped mispairing model are represented in Fig. 5.

B

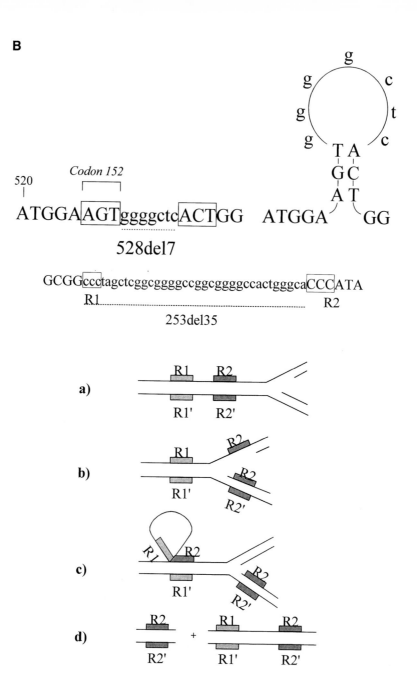

Fig. 5. Proposed mechanisms of mutagenesis. Boxes enclose repeat units considered to be involved in the generation of a deletion. The codons are numbered according to ref. *28* Dashes (–) indicate nucleotide deletions. (**A**) The mechanism generating the 253del35 mutation *(28)* is consistent with the slipped-mispairing model *(33)*. This mechanism involves the misalignment, during DNA replication, of short direct repeats of 2–11 bp. If the direct repeat in box R2 forms base pairs with the complementary box R1 repeat (R1′), a single-stranded loop containing the R1 repeat, and the intervening sequence between box R1 and box R2 is generated. Excision of the loop and rejoining of the sequence would generate the 35-bp deletion. (a) Duplex DNA containing direct repeat sequence; (b) duplex becomes single-stranded at replication fork; (c) backward slip of the template strand and formation of a single-stranded loop; (d) daughter duplexes: one of which contains only one of the two repeats and lacks the intervening sequence. (**B**) Slipped-mispairing stabilized by a hairpin could generate the 528del7 mutation. Transient complementary base pairing between *box 1* and *box 2* could form a hairpin stem; the 7 bp in the loop are excised; the sequence is linearized and ligated. Modified from ref. *3*.

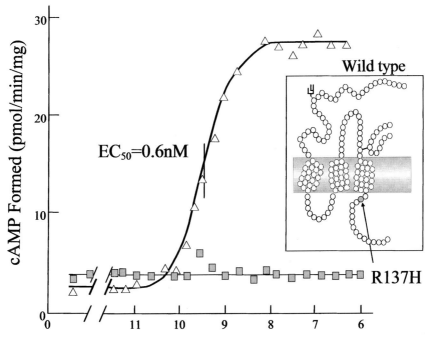

Fig. 6. Expression of the R137H *AVPR2* mutant in "L" cells. The R137H mutant had unaltered affinity for triated tritiated AVP, but failed to stimulate the G_s/adenylyl cyclase system. The insert shows the localization of the missense amino acid in the AVPR2 protein. Only the first three transmembrane domains are represented (data from ref. *35*).

EXPRESSION OF *AVPR2* MUTANTS

The cause of loss of function or dysregulation of 28 different mutant V_2 receptors has been studied using in vitro expression systems *(34–38)*. Cells have been transiently or stably transfected with plasmids encoding the mutant receptors. Major disturbances on the transcriptional level have not been observed. In addition to characterizing the defect, it has been possible to differentiate between mutations that are disease-causing and those that are benign sequence variants. A classification system similar to the classification of LDL receptor mutations *(39)* based on the phenotypic effects of the protein has been proposed by Tsukaguchi et al. *(34)* to help understand the molecular pathophysiology of X-linked nephrogenic diabetes insipidus. Type 1 receptors reach the cell surface, but have impaired binding; type 2 receptors have defective intracellular transport; and type 3 receptors are ineffectively translated and/or rapidly degraded.

Truncated polypeptides, which are expected to be nonfunctional, or absent protein are expected in the case of nonsense mutations (W71X, Q119X, Y124X, Q225X, E231X, E242X, W284X, W293X, L312X, and R337X). A missense mutation could result in misfolding of the protein and trapping in the endoplasmic reticulum, or alteration of the binding pocket or the contact surface that activates the stimulatory G protein. The R137H mutant protein expressed in cultured kidney cells from African green monkey (COS cells) from transfected mutant cDNA exhibited a normal binding affinity for AVP, but failed to stimulate the G_s/adenylyl cyclase system *(35)* (Fig. 6). The R113W

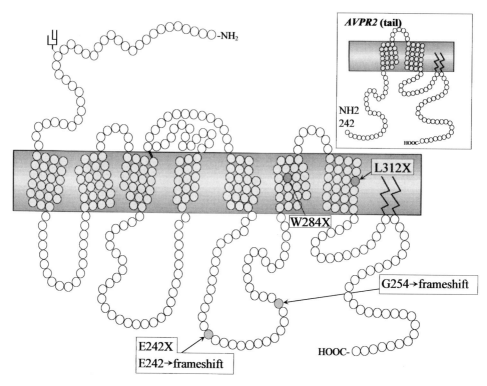

Fig. 7. Functional rescue of mutant V_2 vasopressin receptors proposed by Schöneberg and coworkers *(40)*. The human vasopressin V_2 receptor amino acid sequence is represented, and naturally occurring mutations responsible for nephrogenic diabetes insipidus are indicated (E242X, E242 frameshift, G254 frameshift, W284X, L312X). The insert in the upper part of the figure is representing the V_2 (tail) polypeptide (Glu 242 to Ser 371) used by Schöneberg and coworkers to complement the various truncated receptor mutants and restore, in vitro, cAMP stimulation. Redrawn from the data of Schöneberg et al. *(40)*.

mutant cDNA was also transfected into COS cells and the mutant protein exhibited a combination of functional defects: lowered affinity for vasopressin, diminished ability to stimulate adenylyl cyclase, and diminished ability to reach the cell surface *(36)*. A similar result has been obtained for the Y205C mutant *(37)*. No adenylyl cyclase activity was detected in COS cells transfected with cDNA of a nonsense mutation (Q119X), frameshift mutation (763delA or 855delG), or missense mutations *(37)*. In addition, functional analysis of *AVPR2* mutations provided evidence that the 810del12 mutation is not the cause of NDI in a patient who had this mutation as well as the R181C mutation *(37)*. The R181C mutant receptor had less than half of the normal adenylyl cyclase activity, and although it was expressed at the same level as the normal V_2 receptor, the EC_{50} for adenylyl cyclase stimulation was increased presumably owing to its altered structure.

Schöneberg and coworkers *(40)* pharmacologically rescued truncated V_2 receptors by coexpression of a polypeptide consisting of the last 130 amino acids of the V_2 receptor (Fig. 7). Four of the six truncated receptors (E242X, 804delG, 834delA, and W284X) regained considerable functional activity as demonstrated by an increase in the number of binding sites and stimulation of adenylate cyclase activity.

CARRIER DETECTION AND POSTNATAL DIAGNOSIS

How is this new molecular knowledge transferred to the care of patients with X-linked nephrogenic diabetes insipidus? When the disease-causing mutation has been identified, carrier and perinatal testing can be done by mutation analysis. If a large deletion is observed *(41)* or if a mutation has not yet been identified (family C), reliable testing can be performed using Southern blot analysis (for large deletions) or haplotype analysis using an informative sequence variant in the *AVPR2* gene or closely linked markers *(25,28)*. We encourage physicians who follow families with X-linked nephrogenic diabetes insipidus to recommend molecular genetic analysis, because early diagnosis and treatment of male infants can avert the physical and mental retardation associated with episodes of dehydration. Diagnosis of X-linked nephrogenic diabetes insipidus was accomplished by mutation testing of a sample of cord blood in three of our patients. These patients were immediately treated with abundant water intake, a low-sodium diet, and hydrochlorothiazide. They never experienced episodes of dehydration, and their physical and mental development is normal. They can wait safely for further developments in pharmacotherapeutics and possibly somatic gene therapy.

REFERENCES

1. Knepper MA, Rector FC Jr. Urine concentration and dilution. In: Brenner BM, ed. Brenner & Rector's The Kidney, 5th ed., vol. 1. Saunders, Philadelphia, 1996, pp., 532–570.
2. Bichet DG. Nephrogenic diabetes insipidus. In: Cameron JS, Davison AM, Grünfeld JP, Kerr DNS, Ritz E, eds. Oxford Textbook of Clinical Nephrology. 2nd ed. Oxford University Press, New York, 1997, in press.
3. Fujiwara TM, Morgan K, Bichet DG. Molecular biology of diabetes insipidus. In: Coggins CH, ed. Annual Review of Medicine, vol. 46. Annual Reviews Inc., Palo Alto, CA, 1995, pp. 331–343.
4. Deen PMT, Verdijk MAJ, Knoers NVAM, Wieringa B, Monnens LAH, van Os CH, van Oost BA. Requirement of human renal water channel aquaporin-2 for vasopressin-dependent concentration of urine. Science 1994;264:92–95.
5. van Lieburg AF, Verdijk MAJ, Knoers NVAM, van Essen AJ, Proesmans W, Mallmann R, Monnens LAH, van Oost BA, van Os CH, Deen PMT. Patients with autosomal nephrogenic diabetes insipidus homozygous for mutations in the aquaporin 2 water-channel gene. Am J Hum Genet 1994;55:648–652.
6. Agre P, Brown D, Nielsen S. Aquaporin water channels: unanswered questions and unresolved controversies. Curr Opinion Cell Biol 1995;7:472–483.
7. Morel A, O'Carroll A-M, Brownstein MJ, Lolait SJ. Molecular cloning and expression of a rat V1a arginine vasopressin receptor. Nature 1992;356:523–526.
8. Birnbaumer M, Seibold A, Gilbert S, Ishido M, Barberis B, Antaramian A, Brabet P, Rosenthal W. Molecular cloning of the receptor for human antidiuretic hormone. Nature 1992;357:333–335.
9. Lolait SJ, O'Carroll A-M, McBride OW, Konig M, Morel A, Brownstein MJ. Cloning and characterization of a vasopressin V2 receptor and possible link to nephrogenic diabetes insipidus. Nature 1992;357:336–339.
10. Thibonnier M, Auzan C, Madhun Z, Wilkins P, Berti-Mattera L, Clauser E. Molecular cloning, sequencing, and functional expression of a cDNA encoding the human V1a vasopressin receptor. J Biol Chem 1994;269:3304–3310.
11. Sugimoto T, Saito M, Mochizuki S, Watanabe Y, Hashimoto S, Kawashima H. Molecular cloning and functional expression of a cDNA endocing the human V1b vasopressin receptor. J Biol Chem 1994;269:27,088–27,092.
12. de Keyzer Y, Auzan C, Lenne F, Beldjord C, Thibonnier M, Bertagna X, Clauser E. Cloning and characterization of the human V3 pituitary vasopressin receptor. FEBS Lett. 1994;356:215–220.
13. Lolait SJ, O'Carroll A-M, Mahan LC, Felder CC, Button DC, Young WS III, Mezey E, Brownstein MJ. Extrapituitary expression of the rat V1b vasopressin receptor gene. Proc Natl Acad Sci USA 1995;92:6783–6787.
14. Rozen F, Russo C, Banville D, Zingg HH. Structure, characterization, and expression of the rat oxytocin receptor gene. Proc Natl Acad Sci USA 1995;92:200–204.

15. Watson S, Arkinstall S. The G Protein Linked Receptor FactsBook. FactsBook Series: Academic, London, 1994.

16. Liu J, Wess J. Different single receptor domains determine the distinct G protein coupling profiles of members of the vasopressin receptor family. J Biol Chem 1996;271:8772–8778.

17. Ostrowski NL, Young II WS, Knepper MA, Lolait ST. Expression of vasopressin V1a and V2 receptor messenger ribonucleic acid in the liver and kidney of embryonic, developing, and adult rats. Endocrinology 1993;133:1849–1859.

18. Ostrowski NL, Lolait SJ, Young III WS. Cellular localization of vasopressin V1a receptor messenger ribonucleic acid in adult male rat brain, pineal, and brain vasculature. Endocrinology 1994;135:1511–1528.

19. Grazzini E, Lodboerer AM, Perez-Martin A, Joubert D, Guillon G. Molecular and functional characterization of V1b vasopressin receptor in rat adrenal medulla. Endocrinology 1996;137:3906–3914.

20. Mouillac B, Chini B, Balestre M-N, Elands J, Trumpp-Kallmeyer S, Hoflack J, Hibert M, Jard S, Barberis C. The binding site of neuropeptide vasopressin V1a receptor. J Biol Chem 1995;270: 25,771–25,777.

21. Seibold A, Brabet P, Rosenthal W, Birnbaumer B. Structure and chromosomal localization of the human antidiuretic hormone receptor gene. Am J Hum Genet 1992;51:1078–1083.

22. Nielsen S, Marples D, Frøkiær J, Knepper M, Agre P. The aquaporin family of water channels in kidney: an update on physiology and pathophysiology of aquaporin-2. Kidney Int 1996;49:1718–1723.

23. Bichet DG, Hendy GN, Lonergan M, Arthus MF, Ligier S, Pausova Z, Kluge R, Zingg H, Saenger P, Oppenheimer E, Hirsch DJ, Gilgenkrantz S, Salles JP, Oberlé I, Mandel JL, Gregory MC, Fujiwara TM, Morgan K, Scriver CR. X-linked nephrogenic diabetes insipidus: From the ship Hopewell to restriction fragment length polymorphism studies. Am J Hum Genet 1992;51:1089–1102.

24. Bode HH, Crawford JD. Nephrogenic diabetes insipidus in North America—the Hopewell hypothesis. N Engl J Med 1969;280:750–754.

25. Bichet DG, Arthus MF, Lonergan M, Hendy GN, Paradis AJ, Fujiwara TM, Morgan K, Gregory MC, Rosenthal W, Didwania A, Antaramian A, Birnbaumer M. X-linked nephrogenic diabetes insipidus mutations in North America and the Hopewell hypothesis. J Clin Invest 1993;92:1262–1268.

26. Holtzman EJ, Kolakowski LF Jr, O'Brien D, Crawford JD, Ausiello DA. A null mutation in the vasopressin V2 receptor gene (AVPR2) associated with nephrogenic diabetes insipidus in the Hopewell kindred. Hum Mol Genet 1993;2:1201–1204.

27. Vogel F, Motulsky AG. Human Genetics: Problems and Approaches, 2nd ed. Springer, Berlin, 1986;347–349.

28. Bichet DG, Birnbaumer M, Lonergan M, Arthus MF, Rosenthal W, Goodyer P, Nivet H, Benoit S, Giampietro P, Simonetti S, Fish A, Whitley CB, Jaeger P, Gertner J, New M, DiBona FJ, Kaplan BS, Robertson GL, Hendy GN, Fujiwara TM, Morgan K. Nature and recurrence of AVPR2 mutations in X-linked nephrogenic diabetes insipidus. Am J Hum Genet 1994;55:278–286.

29. Knoers NVAM, van den Ouweland AMW, Verdijk M, Monnens LAH, van Oost BA. Inheritance of mutations in the V_2 receptor gene in thirteen families with nephrogenic diabetes insipidus. Kidney Int 1994;46:170–176.

30. Wildin RS, Antush MJ, Bennett RL, Schoof JM, Scott CR. Heterogeneous AVPR2 gene mutations in congenital nephrogenic diabetes insipidus. Am J Hum Genet 1994;55:266–277.

31. Pan Y, Metzenberg A, Das S, Jing B, Gitschier J. Mutations in the V2 vasopressin receptor gene are associated with X-linked nephrogenic diabetes insipidus. Nature Genet 1992;2:103–106.

32. Oksche A, Dickson J, Schülein R, Seyberth HW, Müller M, Rascher W, Birnbaumer M, Rosenthal W. Two novel mutations in the vasopressin V2 receptor gene in patients with congenital nephrogenic diabetes insipidus. Biochem Biophys Res Comm 1994;205:552–557.

33. Cooper DN, Krawczak M, Antaonarakis SE. The nature and mechanisms of human gene mutation. In: Scriver CR, Beaudet AL, Sly WS, Valle D, eds. The Metabolic and Molecular Bases of Inherited Disease, 7th ed. vol. 1. McGraw-Hill, New York, 1995, pp. 259–291.

34. Tsukaguchi H, Matsubara H, Taketani S, Mori Y, Seido T, Inada M. Binding-, intracellular transport-, and biosynthesis-defective mutants of vasopressin type 2 receptor in patients with X-linked nephrogenic diabetes insipidus. J Clin Invest 1995;96:2043–2050.

35. Rosenthal W, Antaramian A, Gilbert S, Birnbaumer M. Nephrogenic diabetes insipidus: a V_2 vasopressin receptor unable to stimulate adenylyl cyclase. J Biol Chem 1993;268:13,030–13,033.

36. Birnbaumer M, Gilbert S, Rosenthal W. An extracellular congenital nephrogenic diabetes insipidus mutation of the vasopressin receptor reduces cell surface expression, affinity for ligand, and coupling to the G_s/adenylyl cyclase system. Mol Endocrinol 1994;8:886–894.

37. Pan Y, Wilson P, Gitschier J. The effect of eight V2 vasopressin receptor mutations on stimulation of adenylyl cyclase and binding to vasopressin. J Biol Chem 1994;269:31,933–31,937.

38. Oksche A, Schülein R, Rutz C, Liebenhoff U, Dickson J, Müller H, Birnbaumer M, Rosenthal W. Vasopressin V2 receptor mutants causing X-linked nephrogenic diabetes insipidus: analysis of expression, processing and function. Mol Pharmacol 1996;50:820–828.

39. Hobbs HH, Russell DW, Brown MS, Goldstein JL. The LDL receptor locus in familial hypercholesterolemia: mutations analysis of a membrane protein. Annu Rev Genet 1990;24:133–170.

40. Schöneberg T, Yun J., Wenkert D, Wess J. Functional rescue of mutant V2 vasopressin receptors causing nephrogenic diabetes insipidus by a coexpressed receptor polypeptide. EMBO J 1996;15:1283–1291.

41. Arthus M-F, Lonergan M, Platzer M, Rosenthal A, Robertson G, Fujiwara M, Morgan K, Bichet DG. Large deletions/rearrangements of the *AVPR2* gene causing X-linked nephrogenic diabetes insipidus. J Am Soc Nephrol 1996;7:1610 (Abstract no. A1806).

42. Sharif M, Hanley MF. Stepping up the pressure. Nature 1992;357:279,280.

11

Disorders with Increased or Decreased Responsiveness to Extracellular Ca^{2+} Owing to Mutations in the Ca$_\text{o}^{2+}$-Sensing Receptor

Edward M. Brown, MD, Martin Pollak, MD, Mei Bai, PHD, and Steven C. Hebert, MD

CONTENTS

INTRODUCTION

Calcium (Ca^{2+}) ions are of vital importance for numerous intra- and extracellular functions *(1,2)*. Cytosolic free calcium (Ca$_\text{i}^{2+}$) is a key second messenger and enzymatic cofactor that coordinates and controls cellular processes as diverse as muscular contraction, secretion, and glycogen metabolism as well as cellular proliferation, differentiation, and motility *(2)*. The basal level of Ca$_\text{i}^{2+}$, generally ~100 nM, is much lower than the extracellular ionized calcium concentration (Ca$_\text{o}^{2+}$) (~1 mM) and undergoes large, rapid fluctuations owing to release of Ca^{2+} from intracellular stores and/or uptake of Ca^{2+} through the plasma membrane. Ca$_\text{o}^{2+}$, in contrast, remains nearly constant, varying by only a few percent under normal circumstances *(1,3–5)*. Ca$_\text{o}^{2+}$ also has numerous critical funtions, including promoting blood clotting, regulating neuromuscular excitability, and maintaining skeletal integrity.

Ca$_\text{o}^{2+}$ is maintained nearly invariant through a homeostatic system comprising two central elements (Fig. 1) *(1,3–5)*. The first consists of Ca$_\text{o}^{2+}$-sensing cells secreting cal-

From: *Contemporary Endocrinology: G Proteins, Receptors, and Disease*
Edited by: A. M. Spiegel, Humana Press Inc., Totowa, NJ

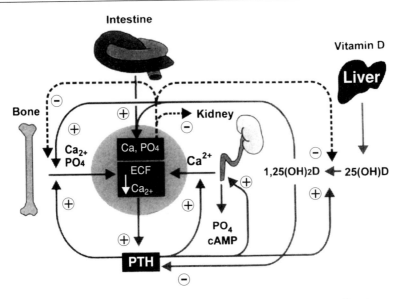

Fig. 1. Schematic diagram illustrating the regulatory system maintaining $[Ca^{2+}]_o$ homeostasis. The solid arrows and lines show the effects of PTH and $1,25(OH)_2D_3$; the dotted arrows and lines demonstrate examples of how Ca^{2+} or phosphate ions exert direct actions on target tissues. Abbreviations are the following: Ca^{2+}, calcium; PO_4, phosphate; ECF, extracellular fluid; PTH, parathyroid hormone; $1,25(OH)_2D$, 1,25-dihydroxyvitamin D; 25(OH)D, 25-hydroxyvitamin D; minus signs indicate inhibitory actions, and plus signs show positive effects. Reproduced with permission from ref. 5a.

ciotropic hormones (i.e., parathyroid cells, thyroidal C-cells, and renal proximal tubular cells). With changes in Ca_o^{2+}, these cells modulate their secretion of these hormones (parathyroid hormone [PTH], calcitonin [CT], and 1,25-dihydroxyvitamin D [1,25 $(OH)_2D$], respectively) in order to normalize the extracellular calcium concentration. Calciotropic hormones then act on the second element of the system, effector tissues (e.g., bone, kidney, and intestine—see Fig. 1) that modify their transport of calcium and/or phosphate ions so as to normalize Ca_o^{2+}. The cloning and characterization of a G-protein-coupled, Ca_o^{2+}-sensing receptor (CaR) (6) has shed considerable light on how Ca_o^{2+}-sensing cells detect the Ca_o^{2+} signal and on the mechanisms underlying normal calcium metabolism. In addition, it enabled documentation that inherited human hyper- or hypocalcemic disorders result from inactivating or activating mutations, respectively, in the CaR (7,8). This chapter will outline the clinical and molecular features of these disorders after a brief description of how the CaR governs the level of Ca_o^{2+} "set" by the calcium homeostatic system.

ROLE OF THE CaR IN NORMAL MINERAL ION HOMEOSTASIS

Cloning and Characterization of a G-Protein-Coupled CaR

Expression cloning in *Xenopus laevis* has been a useful approach for cloning phosphoinositide (PI)-coupled receptors for which no molecular probes are available. Previous studies had shown that parathyroid cells respond to elevated levels of Ca_o^{2+} with activation of phospholipase C (PLC) (9,10), transient followed by sustained increases in Ca_i^{2+} *(11)*, and a pertussis-toxin-sensitive inhibition of adenylyl cyclase *(12)*, suggesting that the CaR was a G-protein-coupled receptor linked positively and negatively, respectively, to PLC and adenylyl cyclase *(1)*. Racke et al. *(13)* and Chen T. et al. *(14)* subsequently showed that injection of *X. laevis* oocytes with parathyroid mRNA renders them responsive to Ca_o^{2+}. Brown et al. *(6)* then utilized a similar assay system to screen a bovine parathyroid cDNA library and isolate a full-length clone of a CaR. The use of hybridization-based screening techniques permitted the later cloning of additional, highly homologous CaRs from human parathyroid (Figure 2) *(15)* and kidney *(16)*, rat kidney *(17)* and brain *(18)*, and a rat C-cell-derived cell line (rMTC44-2 cells) *(19)*.

The various CaRs share three principal structural domains. The first is a predominantly hydrophilic, amino terminal extracellular domain (ECD) containing over 600 amino acids. A second, generally hydrophobic region follows, with 250 amino acids and 7 predicted, membrane-spanning segments characteristic of the superfamily of G-protein-coupled receptors (GPCRs). The third is a cytoplasmic, carboxyl-terminal tail of some 200 amino acids. The recognition of polycationic CaR agonists has been shown to take place within the ECD through the use of receptors that are chimeras of the CaR and the structurally related, metabotropic glutamate receptors (mGluRs). For example, a receptor construct in which the ECD of the CaR is fused to the transmembrane domains and carboxyl-terminal tail of the mGluR recognizes CaR and not mGluR agonists *(20)*. The CaR presumably couples through its intracellular loops and carboxyl-terminal tail to its respective G proteins (most likely $G_{q/11}$ for activation of PLC *(21)* and G_i for inhibition of adenylyl cyclase *(12,21,22)*, although the cloned receptor has not yet been definitively shown to couple directly to adenylyl cyclase). There are multiple isoforms of mGluRs, each of which couples to one predominant effector system (e.g., mGluRs 1 and 5 couple to PLC, for instance) *(23)*. Thus, although it is possible that there is only a single isoform of the CaR linking to multiple second messenger pathways, the existence of additional CaR isoforms has by no means been excluded.

Tissue Distribution and Physiological Roles of the CaR

Transcripts for the CaR are present in diverse tissues, not all of which play obvious roles in mineral ion homeostasis *(6,15,17,18)*. These include the parathyroid glands, C-cells, kidney, intestine, lung, and various regions of brain. *In situ* hybridization and immunohistochemistry with specific, anti-CaR antibodies has enabled more detailed localization of the CaR in these tissues as described below *(17,18)*. Moreover, this information, combined with physiological and biochemical data described later, have elucidated significantly the roles of the CaR in the tissues expressing it.

In the parathyroid, the CaR activates PLC, phospholipase A_2 (PLA_2), and phospholipase D (PLD) *(23a)*, and may also inhibit adenylyl cyclase, as noted above *(1,12)*. Which, if any, of these intracellular messenger pathways is the principal one through which the CaR inhibits rather than stimulates PTH secretion, however, remains an important unsolved problem. Nevertheless, the marked impairment of high Ca_o^{2+}-mediated inhibition of PTH secretion in patients with homozygous inactivating mutations in the CaR *(24,25)* or in mice homozygous for targeted disruption of the CaR gene *(26)* (see Neonatal Severe Hyperparathyroidism [NSHPT] and Mouse Models of FHH and NSHPT) provides strong support for the central role of the CaR in Ca_o^{2+}-regulated PTH

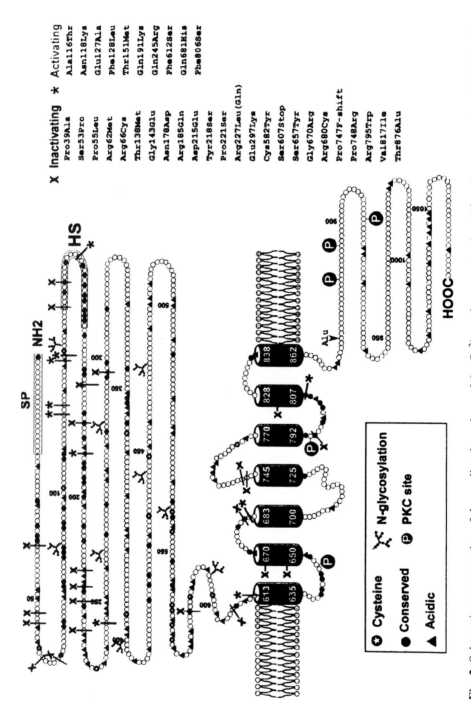

Fig. 2. Schematic representation of the predicted topology of the Ca_o^{2+}-sensing receptor cloned from human parathyroid gland with activating and inactivating mutations. Abbreviations: SP, signal peptide; HS, hydrophobic segment. Also shown are missense and nonsense mutations that cause either FBHH or ADH, which are indicated with the three-letter amino acid code. The normal amino acid is indicated before and the mutant amino acid after the number of the relevant codon. Reproduced with permission from ref. *15a*.

release. Moreover, the use of "calcimimetic" CaR agonists has shown that the CaR likely also mediates the high Ca$_o^{2+}$-induced decrease in preproPTH mRNA levels *(27)*. Finally, the conspicuous chief cell hyperplasia in both NSHPT *(28,29)* and in mice homozygous for targeted disruption of the CaR gene *(26)* provides indirect evidence that the receptor directly or indirectly suppresses parathyroid cellular proliferation. In contrast to its effects on PTH secretion, the CaR probably mediates Ca$_o^{2+}$-evoked calcitonin secretion *(19)*.

The CaR is expressed within nearly all segments of the nephron, including the glomerulus, proximal convoluted and straight tubules, medullary thick ascending limb (MTAL) and cortical thick ascending limb (CTAL), distal convoluted tubule (DCT) and cortical (CCD), outer medullary (OMCD) and inner medullary collecting ducts (IMCD) *(17,30)*. In the CTAL, where CaR transcripts and protein are expressed at the highest levels, the CaR is located prominently on the basolateral surface of the cells, where it likely senses systemic (e.g., blood) levels of Ca$_o^{2+}$. The CaR in CTAL and probably also in DCT appears to regulate tubular Ca^{2+} and Mg^{2+} handling, increasing their reabsorption when Ca$_o^{2+}$ is low and reducing it when Ca$_o^{2+}$ is high *(31)*. There is coexpression of the CaR and PTH receptors in CTAL and DCT, permitting mutually antagonistic interactions between the effects of the two receptors on Ca$_o^{2+}$ reabsorption in the distal nephron *(32,33)*. In the IMCD, the CaR is principally on the apical (e.g., luminal) cell surface, enabling monitoring of urinary levels of Ca$_o^{2+}$ *(33)*. Recent studies suggest that it inhibits vasopressin-stimulated transepithelial water flow in a manner that could diminish the risk of renal stone formation when renal Ca^{2+} excretion is increased *(33)*. In addition, by inhibiting NaCl transport in the MTAL, the CaR may further decrease maximal urinary concentrating capacity by reducing the medullary hypertonicity that drives vasopressin-mediated, transepithelial water flow in the collecting duct *(34)*. In contrast to our rapidly increasing understanding of the role of the CaR in tissues involved in maintaining mineral ion homeostasis, much remains to be learned about the function(s) of the CaR in those that are not, such as the brain and lung *(18,35)*.

SYNDROMES OF EXTRACELLULAR CALCIUM RESISTANCE

Familial Benign Hypocalciuric Hypercalcemia (FBHH)

CLINICAL FEATURES OF FBHH

In 1972, Foley, et al. *(36)* pointed out the unusually benign clinical features of a hypercalcemic syndrome that they called familial benign hypercalcemia (FBH). Several forms of familial hypercalcemia had been described previously, but this report first outlined clearly the distinctive clinical features of individuals with this syndrome. Subsequently, a large number of families with this condition were investigated by several groups in the late 1970s and 1980s, particularly those of Marx et al. *(37)* and Heath and coworkers *(38)*. These studies confirmed and extended the initial description of FBH. Marx et al. called this syndrome familial hypocalciuric hypercalcemia (FHH) because of the characteristic alteration in renal Ca^{2+} handling in affected family members *(39)*. Although there has never been an overall consensus concerning the name that should be employed for this inherited abnormality in calcium homeostasis, we employ the hybrid term FBHH in this chapter.

FBHH is a rare genetic syndrome that is inherited in an autosomal-dominant fashion and is characterized by lifelong, generally asymptomatic hypercalcemia of mild to moderate severity (usually <12 mg/dL) *(37–39)*. Despite being hypercalcemic, affected patients generally have few, if any, of the characteristic symptoms and complications of other hypercalcemic disorders. The latter include most commonly gastrointestinal abnormalities, particularly anorexia, nausea and constipation, mental disturbances, and renal complications (i.e., impaired renal function, a defective urinary concentration, and nephrolithiasis or nephrocalcinosis) *(3,40)*. Occasionally in families, affected individuals exhibit higher serum calcium concentrations than in most kindreds with FBHH with this condition (e.g., 12–13 mg/dL or rarely even higher *(37)*). Even these individuals, however, are generally remarkably free of symptoms. Nonspecific manifestations encountered in other forms of hypercalcemia, such as fatigue, were reported in some early studies of FBHH *(37)*, but were not confirmed in later reports *(38,41)*. Ascertainment bias perhaps attributed symptoms in FBHH probands to the disease that were not present more commonly, in fact, in affected than in unaffected family members in more systematic analyses of entire kindreds.

Affected members of some FBHH kindreds have presented with pancreatitis or chondrocalcinosis (calcification of the cartilage covering the joint surfaces) *(37)*, suggesting that these might represent true complications of this syndrome. Pancreatitis, however, does not appear to be more prevalent in affected than in unaffected family members of FBHH kindreds or in the general population, and most patients with FBHH who developed pancreatitis had other predisposing factors (e.g., alcoholism or gallstones) *(41)*. Subsequent studies likewise have not confirmed that chondrocalcinosis is more common in FBHH than in the general population *(38,41)*. Law and Heath *(38)* described an apparent increase in the incidence of gallstones in FBHH, but most large series of FBHH kindreds have not described this as a complication of the disorder.

BIOCHEMICAL FEATURES OF FBHH

The degree of hypercalcemia in FBHH is comparable to that in patients with primary hyperparathyroidism (PHPT) of mild to moderate severity, with equivalent increases in both the serum total and ionized calcium concentrations *(37,38)*. Individuals with FBHH often have some mild reduction in serum phosphate concentration, although to a lesser extent than those with PHPT *(37,38)*, and the serum phosphate concentration in FBHH is usually within the lower half of the normal range. Serum magnesium concentrations are in the upper part of the normal range or mildly elevated. Hypermagnesemia may be more common in kindreds in which the serum calcium concentration is more elevated, since there is a positive relationship between the serum calcium and magnesium concentrations in FBHH, in contrast to PHPT in which there is an inverse relationship between these parameters *(37)*.

A very characteristic biochemical feature of patients with FBHH is an inappropriately normal circulating (PTH) level in spite of their hypercalcemia *(41)*, particularly when measured using assays for intact parathyroid hormone (PTH) *(42,43)*. Less commonly PTH levels are in the lower part of the normal range or frankly elevated *(44)*. In the latter situation, it is difficult to distinguish patients with FBHH from those with mild primary hyperparathyroidism on the basis of the PTH level alone, particularly in the 5–10% of cases of PHPT where the level of intact PTH is in the upper part of the normal range. Patients with FBHH also exhibit dysregulation of PTH secretion during the administration of agents raising or lowering the serum ionized calcium concentration, showing an elevated "set point" (the Ca_o^{2+} that half-maximally suppresses PTH levels)

(45,46). That is, to reduce PTH to a given extent, individuals with FBHH require a serum calcium concentration that is 10–15% higher than that lowering PTH to a comparable degree in normals. Thus, there is mild to moderate resistance to the inhibitory effects of Ca_o^{2+} on PTH secretion in FBHH. A similar, but somewhat more severe defect in set point is present in most patients with PHPT (47); pathological parathyroid glands in this condition also have additional defects in secretory control, such as increases in maximal and minimal secretory rates at low and high Ca_o^{2+}, respectively (46,47). Given their generally normal circulating levels of intact PTH, it is not surprising that the parathyroid glands in FBHH generally exhibit normal histology or very mild parathyroid hyperplasia (48,49).

A number of patients with FBHH have undergone total or partial parathyroidectomy because they were thought to have primary hyperparathyroidism. The distinctly atypical course following surgical intervention in FBHH provided additional clues that this disorder differed in some fundamental way from typical PHPT. In 27 patients with FBHH who underwent from 1–4 neck explorations each, hypercalcemia recurred within a few days or weeks in 21; only two remained permanently normocalcemic without further treatment (41). More commonly, long-term normocalcemia was only achieved after patients with FBHH were rendered totally aparathyroid and then treated with vitamin D (5 of the 27 patients described above). Recurrence of hypercalcemia following removal of a parathyroid adenoma, in contrast, is unusual, whereas in the various forms of primary parathyroid hyperplasia, if recurrence of hypercalcemia takes place at all, it only occurs after several years (3,40).

Serum levels of 25(OH)D and 1,25(OH)$_2$D are usually within the normal range in FBHH (50–52), with intestinal absorption of calcium that is normal or slightly reduced. Some individuals with FBHH have a blunted homeostatic response to reduced dietary calcium intake, exhibiting smaller than expected increments in gastrointestinal Ca^{2+} absorption and 1,25(OH)$_2$D levels (52). In contrast, patients with PHPT frequently have elevated levels of these latter two parameters (40). Although indices of bone turnover, such as urinary hydroxyproline excretion, can be slightly elevated (53,54), bone mineral density is normal in FBHH (38,53,55), and there is no increased risk of fractures. Several family members in a recently reported FBHH kindred from Oklahoma had evidence of osteomalacia, but this form of bone disease is very uncommon in other FBHH kindreds (56). Moreover, the kindred from Oklahoma has a form of FBHH genetically distinct from that responsible for most cases of the syndrome (see below).

Another characteristic biochemical feature in FBHH is excessively avid renal tubular reabsorption of Ca^{2+} and Mg^{2+} in spite of the concomitant hypercalcemia (39,44). The parameter of renal Ca^{2+} handling employed most commonly to document this abnormality is the renal calcium to creatinine clearance ratio, which is <0.01 in some 80% of persons with FBHH. In contrast, this clearance ratio is higher than 0.01 in the great majority of patients with PHPT and markedly so in other hypercalcemic disorders, in which the accompanying suppression of PTH secretion further reduces renal tubular reabsorption of calcium. Therefore, a low calcium to creatinine clearance ratio combined with a normal PTH level and the autosomal-dominant inheritance of mild, asymptomatic hypercalcemia generally make the diagnosis of FBHH straightforward.

Occasional FBHH kindreds have been reported in which hypercalciuria and even overt renal stone disease are present in some family members (57). It is not currently known whether the disorder present in such families represents a variant of FBHH, or coexistence of a derangement in renal Ca^{2+} handling that promotes increased calcium excretion and outweighs the hypocalciuric effect of the FBHH gene(s). Interestingly, the enhanced renal tubular reabsorption of calcium remains even following total parathyroidectomy *(50,58)*. Therefore, the abnormal renal handling of calcium is not dependent on PTH, but is an entirely separate alteration in renal sensing/handling of Ca_o^{2+}. One study found that the abnormal renal Ca^{2+} handling was present in the thick ascending limb (TAL) *(58)*, but another suggested that it resided within the proximal tubule *(59)*.

Several additional aspects of renal function in FBHH have suggested altered renal responsiveness to Ca_o^{2+}. Renal blood flow and glomerular filtration rate are both normal, despite being reduced in a sizable fraction of patients with other forms of hypercalcemia *(37)*. In addition, persons with FBHH concentrate their urine normally *(60)*, even though hypercalcemia of other causes frequently impairs urinary concentrating ability and can sometimes produce overt nephrogenic diabetes insipidus *(34)*.

Thus, both the clinical and biochemical features of FBHH provided compelling evidence that it represented an inherited abnormality in the sensing and/or handling of Ca_o^{2+} by kidney, parathyroid, and perhaps other tissues (i.e., there is an apparent lack of the other gastrointestinal or mental symptoms found in other forms of hypercalcemia). Both because of its benign clinical course and because it is so difficult to obtain a biochemical "cure" (an accomplishment of dubious value in an otherwise asymptomatic patient), a consensus has emerged that surgical intervention should not be undertaken in FBHH *(41)*. The clinical differentiation of PHPT from FBHH, therefore, is of importance in order to avoid unnecessary and futile exploration of the neck in the latter.

GENETICS OF FBHH

FBHH is inherited as an autosomal-dominant trait with a penetrance of >90% *(37,38,41)*, and the biochemical abnormalities have been detected in the immediate postnatal period in affected infants. The disease gene was first mapped to chromosome 3 (band q21–24) using linkage analysis by Chou al. in four large FBHH families *(43)*. Moreover, formal genetic analysis proved that individuals with FBHH have one copy of the abnormal gene and are, therefore, heterozygous for the FBHH gene *(43,61)*. Subsequent studies showed that 90% or more of families large enough for genetic analysis exhibit linkage of the disease gene to the chromosome 3 locus *(62,63)*. One family, however, showed linkage of a phenotypically indistinguishable disorder to the short arm of chromosome 19, band 19p13.3 *(62)*, confirming the genetic heterogeneity of the disorder. In addition, the Oklahoma kindred noted above with atypical features (osteomalacia in a few affected family members and a tendency to show progressive increases in serum PTH with age) was linked to neither chromosome 3 nor 19 *(56,64)*. A severe form of hyperparathyroidism in infants (NSHPT) can be encountered occasionally in FBHH kindreds and, in some cases, represents the homozygous form of the disease that is linked to chromosome 3 *(61,65)*. NSHPT will be discussed in detail later (*see* Neonatal Severe Primary Hyperparathyroidism).

DISCOVERY AND FUNCTIONAL EXPRESSION OF CaR MUTATIONS IN FBHH3Q

Because of the abnormal Ca_o^{2+}-sensing by parathyroid, kidney, and probably other tissues in FBHH, the newly cloned CaR was an obvious candidate for the disease gene in FBHH. Pollak et al. *(8)* initially showed that the CaR gene was located on the long arm of chromosome 3 and then used a ribonuclease A (RNase A) protection assay to screen for mutations in this gene in three unrelated families with FBHH previously shown to be linked to chromosome 3. They identified a unique missense mutation in each family (i.e., a change in a single nucleotide base that substitutes a new amino acid for the one that is normally coded for—in these three cases, arg185gln,* glu297lys, and arg795trp). Moreover, these mutations were not found in genomic DNA of 50 normocalcemic individuals (Fig. 2). Subsequent studies have identified additional CaR mutations in families with FBHH linked to chromosome 3 *(63,66–69)*. In most cases, each family has its own unique mutation. Most are missense mutations clustered within several distinct regions of the CaR (Fig. 2):

1. The first half of the extracellular domain;
2. A region in the ECD immediately preceding TM1 (the first membrane-spanning helix); and
3. The transmembrane domains, intra- and/or extracellular loops.

Several apparently benign polymorphisms have also been described in the C-terminal tail of the CaR that are present in a substantial proportion of the population (~10–30%) *(67)*.

Several additional types of mutations have been described recently in FBHH. One family harbors a nonsense mutation just proximal to TM1 (e.g., ser607stop, which substitutes a stop codon for the normally encoded serine) *(63)* that would result in a presumptively inactive, truncated receptor lacking all of its membrane-spanning domains. Another mutation with both a one-nucleotide deletion and a transversion of an adjacent nucleotide (change from one nucleotide to another) within codon 747 would modify the downstream reading frame and result in premature termination of the protein following residue 776 within the transmembrane domains *(63)*. A Nova Scotian family harbors the insertion of a 383-bp Alu repetitive sequence at codon 876 *(66)*. This alu element is in the opposite orientation to the CaR gene and contains an unusually long poly A tract. Stop signals present within all three reading frames of the Alu sequence would predict a truncated CaR protein containing a long stretch of repeated phenylalanines within its carboxyl-terminus (encoded by the repeating AAA codons resulting from translation of the poly A tract). Of interest, the size of the alu repetitive element has undergone an approximate doubling in size in a later generation of this family *(70)*. Only about two-thirds of families with FBHH linked to chromosome 3, however, have identifiable mutations within the CaR coding sequence. In the rest, there are presumably mutations within introns or within the gene's upstream or downstream regulatory domains that interfere with normal expression of the gene.

Recent studies have expressed mutant CaRs engineered to include several of the mutations defined to this point in mammalian expression systems *(71)*. Figure 3 illustrates the effects of several such point mutations on high Ca²⁺ₒ-elicited elevations in the Ca²⁺ᵢ in transiently transfected human embryonic kidney (HEK293) cells. Some mutations, including arg185gln and arg795trp, markedly decrease the apparent affinity and/or maximal biological activity of the mutated receptors. In other cases (e.g., thr138met or arg62met), the mutations only modestly diminish apparent affinity, without altering the maximal response *(71)*. Many of the mutant CaRs that show the

---

* Note that this mutation was inadvertently reported as arg186glu in the original publication and that the numbering for the amino acid residues within the bovine CaR *(8)* is numerically one higher than that for the human CaR *(63)* because of the presence of an extra amino acid in the ECD of the former.

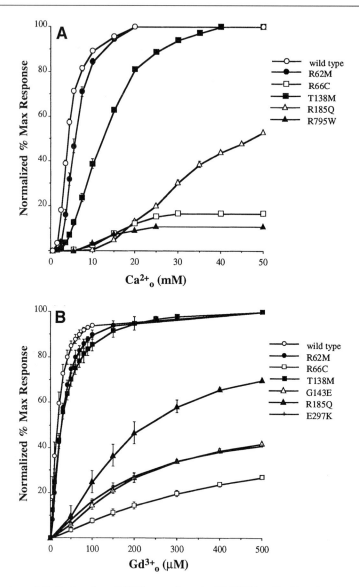

Fig. 3. Expression of CaRs bearing FBHH mutations in HEK293 cells. Results show the effects of varying levels of Ca_o^{2+} or Gd_o^{3+} on the cytosolic calcium concentration (Ca_i^{2+}) in HEK293 cells transiently transfected with the wild-type CaR or the indicated mutant CaRs. Results are normalized to percent of the maximal response of the wild-type human CaR. Reproduced from ref. *71* with permission.

most dramatic reductions in biological activity show reduced quantities of the putatively mature, glycosylated form of the receptor as assessed by Western analysis of crude plasma membrane preparations. Interestingly, the elevations in serum calcium concentration in these families are, in general, mild. Indeed, the family with the nonsense mutation at codon 607 exhibits serum calcium concentrations at or slightly above the upper limit of normal *(63)*. Moreover, as described in greater detail below, mice with targeted disruption of one allele of the CaR also have very mild hypercalcemia *(26)*. In contrast, mutations that markedly impair the biological function of the receptor despite showing an apparently normal pattern on western analysis can, in some cases, produce a greater degree of hypercalcemia. The arg795trp or arg185gln mutations *(71)*, for example, are associated with serum calcium concentrations in affected family members that average over 2 mg/dL and about 3 mg/dL higher, respectively, than those in unaffected family members of the same families. Indeed, although coexpression of normal and mutant receptors (to mimic the heterozygous state of FBHH patients in vivo) has no detectable effect on the function of the normal receptor when the mature form of the latter is expressed in reduced amounts, both arg795trp and arg185gln shift the EC_{50} (the effective concentration of agonist evoking half of the maximal response) of the wild-type receptor rightward. These latter two mutant receptors most likely interfere in some fashion with the function of the normal CaR. This could occur through several possible mechanisms:

1. A decrease in the amount of the normal CaR reaching the cell surface;
2. A reduction in the effective concentration of G protein(s) available to the normal CaR owing to the formation of an inactive complex of G protein(s) with the inactive receptor; and/or
3. The presence of inactive complexes of normal and mutant receptors on the cell surface.

Available data do not permit differentiation among these possibilities at present.

Transient transfection has also been carried out with cDNAs encoding two mutant receptors that contain the deletion and transversion in codon 747 *(71a)* or the inserted alu repetitive element at codon 876 *(71b)*. In both cases, the transfected receptors exhibited no biological activity, and truncated proteins were produced on Western analysis that were of the sizes predicted from the premature stop codons introduced by these two mutations.

Several tentative conclusions can be drawn about the structure–function relationships for the CaR from the work just outlined. Some missense mutations in the ECD produce a spectrum of alterations in the apparent affinity of the CaR for Ca_o^{2+} (as well as for Gd_o^{3+}) without clear-cut changes in the level of expression of the mature CaR protein, at least as assessed by Western analysis *(71)*. Therefore, the altered amino acid might directly or indirectly modify the affinity of the CaR for its polycationic ligands. Eventual elucidation of the 3-D structure of the ECD will be required to understand the precise interactions of the protein with its polycationic ligands. The Hill coefficient for stimulation of the transiently expressed CaR by Ca_o^{2+} is approximately three, suggesting that there are at least three interacting binding sites for Ca_o^{2+} *(71)*. The Hill coefficient for activation of the receptor by Gd_o^{3+}, on the other hand, is around one; therefore, trivalent cations may interact with the receptor differently from Ca_o^{2+}. Interestingly, Hammerland et al. *(20)* showed that a mutant CaR lacking virtually the entire ECD was no longer activated by Ca_o^{2+}, but still exhibited relatively robust responses to Gd_o^{3+}. This result raises the possibility that there is a binding site for Gd_o^{3+}, but perhaps not for Ca_o^{2+}, within the extracellular loops or even within the TMDs of the receptor, or that binding of Ca_o^{2+} to this site is by itself insufficient to initiate signal transduction. These results obtained with the CaR deletion mutant may also explain why mutant CaRs identified in some FBHH families exhibit no responses to Ca_o^{2+} but are activated reasonably well by Gd_o^{3+} *(71)*.

The mutations within the transmembrane segments of the CaR probably interfere with receptor activation by reducing its cell-surface expression and/or disrupting conformational changes of the transmembrane domains (TMDs) and or intracellular loops (ICLs) needed for interactions with and activation of G protein(s). As noted before, the single FBHH mutation described to date having a mutation within an ICL (arg795trp, within the third ICL) severely impairs activation of PLC despite normal amounts of the mature receptor protein (71). The third intracellular loop is thought to play a critical role in determining the specificity of the coupling of many GPCRs to their respective G proteins (72,73), although in the mGluRs, the second loop may be most important in this regard (74).

From these results, we draw the following conclusions:

1. FBHH is genetically heterogeneous, but at least 90% of families probably have the form of the disorder linked to chromosome 3.
2. About two-thirds of all persons with FBHH that is linked to chromosome 3_q harbor inactivating mutations in the coding region of the CaR. Most commonly, each family has its own unique mutation. The majority of mutations reside within the extracellular domain, and likely reduce the affinity of the receptor for Ca_o^{2+} or interfere with its biosynthesis or cell-surface expression. Some mutations within transmembrane or cytoplasmic domains may disrupt the processes required for productive signal transduction. All mutations probably interfere with the responsiveness of the CaR to Ca_o^{2+}, rendering patients with FBHH mildly to moderately "resistant" to extracellular Ca_o^{2+}.
3. The remaining one-third of persons with FBHH that is linked to the chromosome 3 locus, but who do not have detectable mutations in the coding region may have mutations in promoter or enhancer sequences of the CaR gene.
4. The alterations in parathyroid dynamics in persons with FBHH confirm that the CaR plays a key role in Ca_o^{2+} regulated PTH secretion. In addition, the PTH-independent changes in the regulation of renal Ca^{2+}, Mg^{2+}, and water handling by Ca_o^{2+} (i.e., excessively avid renal tubular reabsorption of these two divalent cations despite hypercalcemia and the absence of the normal inhibitory action of high Ca_o^{2+} on urinary concentration) provide in vivo evidence supporting a key role for the CaR in controlling several aspects of renal function.
5. In an occasional family, the gene defect maps to additional, as yet undefined genes on chromosome 19p or elsewhere. The identification of these genes may lead to isolation of additional Ca_o^{2+}-sensing receptors or other components needed for normal function of the CaR.
6. Because the disorder is genetically heterogeneous and a substantial minority of patients with $FBHH_{3q}$ do not have detectable mutations within the CaR coding region, the diagnosis of FBHH will likely continue to include the documentation of mild, PTH-dependent hypercalcemia with relative hypocalciuria (calcium to creatinine clearance ratio <0.01) with an autosomal-dominant pattern of inheritance. Direct mutational analysis could be useful in specific clinical settings, such as in the differentiation of FBHH from PHPT in individuals without available relatives for genetic screening or in patients with apparently de novo CaR mutations.
7. Finally, since patients with FBHH generally have a benign clinical course, parathyroidectomy should not be performed, except in very unusual clinical circumstances where patients are suffering adverse consequences of their hypercalcemia.

Neonatal Severe Primary Hyperparathyroidism (NSHPT)

CLINICAL AND BIOCHEMICAL FEATURES OF NSHPT

Neonatal primary hyperparathyroidism often has a dramatic presentation as severe, symptomatic hypercalcemia in association with hyperparathyroid bone disease before the age of 6 mo; in such cases, it is appropriately called NSHPT *(41)*. This latter syndrome was described well before FBHH *(75)*. A recent review of 49 cases of NSHPT found that the majority presented at birth or shortly afterward, usually during the first week of life *(41)*. Affected infants often exhibited anorexia, constipation, failure to thrive, hypotonia, and respiratory distress. Additional clinical findings have included chest wall deformity, and less frequently, dysmorphic facies, craniotabes, and recto-vaginal or anovaginal fistulas *(29,76–79)*. Respiratory complications may arise owing to thoracic deformity, sometimes with a flail chest syndrome resulting from multiple rib fractures that can cause substantial morbidity *(41,76)*.

The hypercalcemia in NSHPT is most commonly severe, in the range of 14–20 mg/dL; levels as high as 30.8 mg/dL have been described *(79)*. Despite the marked hypercalcemia, relative hypocalciuria has been noted in some cases, even without a family history of FBHH *(80)*. When available, serum magnesium concentrations have sometimes been elevated well above normal *(69)*. Serum PTH levels have been high in most cases, usually being 5- to 10-fold elevated, although the degree of the increase can sometimes be modest *(24,81)*. Skeletal X-rays often show profound undermineralization, with fractures of the long bones and ribs, subperiosteal erosions, widening of the metaphyses, and occasionally rickets *(76,82)*. Bone histology reveals typical osteitis fibrosa cystica *(78)*. At parathyroidectomy, all four parathyroid glands are generally enlarged, commonly being many times the normal mass of the parathyroid glands at this age, and exhibit chief cell or water-clear-cell hyperplasia. Sometimes, when glandular enlargement is less marked, the normally low content of fat in the parathyroid glands of children complicates interpretation of the parathyroid histology *(41,78,83)*. No cases have been reported in which a parathyroid adenoma caused NSHPT.

Sometimes, the hypercalcemia in neonatal hyperparathyroidism is less severe, on the order of 11–12 mg/dL, and occasional cases have been described in which the disorder ran a self-limited course, reverting to milder hypercalcemia at 6–7 mo following conservative therapy *(76)*. The recent discovery that mutations in the CaR cause NSHPT will likely widen the spectrum of the disease further as milder cases are uncovered. A particularly interesting case was recently identified of a homozygous female who was the product of a consanguineous union of two individuals with FBHH. The parents' serum calcium concentrations were in the upper part of the normal range *(69)*. This homozygous child did not present as NSHPT, but was only diagnosed at age 32, when her homozygous state was identified by mutational analysis. Despite serum calcium concentrations of 15–17 mg/dL, she was essentially asymptomatic, although mildly retarded. Her serum magnesium concentration was elevated to a similar extent (~50% above the upper limit of the normal range), and her serum intact PTH level was at the upper limit of normal. Despite the marked hypercalcemia, her renal function was normal, including urinary concentrating ability.

Prior to 1982 *(41)*, NSHPT often had a fatal outcome in severe cases without prompt, aggressive medical and surgical management. This has not been invariably true in more recent clinical experience, however, and wider recognition of the broadening clinical spectrum of the disease combined with improvements in the medical treatment of severe hypercalcemia have resulted in successful medical management in a number of cases during the past 15 yr. In symptomatic cases, initial management includes vigorous hydration, the use of inhibitors of bone resorption, and respiratory support. If the infant's condition is very severe or deteriorates during medical therapy, total parathyroidectomy with autotransplantation of part of one of the glands is generally recommended within the first month of life (25,41,81). Some authors recommend total parathyroidectomy followed by lifelong management of the resultant hypoparathyroidism with oral calcium and vitamin D therapy (generally with 1,25[OH]$_2$ D) as needed to prevent symptomatic hypocalcemia (24,78). There is generally rapid and dramatic clinical improvement after parathyroidectomy, with rapid healing of the skeletal lesions, even though the hypercalcemia generally recurs rapidly with less than a total parathyroidectomy or following autotransplantation (41,78). Similar clinical improvement has been observed more recently in infants with NSHPT managed medically (41), indicating that biochemical improvement in the degree of hyperparathyroidism can be part of the natural history of NSHPT, a point that will be returned to later.

GENETICS OF NSHPT

Early descriptions of FBHH described the presence in these kindreds of children with NSHPT (37,65,78,84). In 15 kindreds with FBHH, three patients from two families had NSHPT (37), suggesting that in some cases, NSHPT can be the homozygous form of FBHH. In another family with two children affected by NSHPT, the parents, who were related, had mild increases in serum ionized calcium concentration (despite total calcium levels being normal) and hypocalciuria (65), again suggesting that NSHPT could be the homozygous form of FBHH. Pollak and coworkers (61) later showed in an additional study of 11 families in whom the abnormal gene mapped to chromosome 3q that consanguineous marriages of affected individuals in four families resulted in children with NSHPT. The pattern of inheritance of genetic markers closely linked to the FBHH gene in these families provided very strong evidence that NSHPT can be the homozygous form of the same disorder. Subsequent studies of FBHH arising from mutations in the CaR gene confirmed that inheriting two abnormal copies of the gene can cause NSHPT (8,66,68). As a result of having no normal CaR genes, these patients exhibit much more severe clinical and biochemical findings than in the heterozygous state (FBHH) as a result of having severe parathyroid resistance to Ca$_o^{2+}$.

HETEROZYGOUS CaR MUTATIONS ALSO CAUSE NSHPT

Not all cases of NSHPT, however, represent homozygous FBHH. Most cases occur sporadically or in FBHH families with only one affected parent (29,85,86). What are the possible explanations for these cases? Such children with NSHPT could conceivably be compound heterozygotes, harboring two CaR alleles, each with a distinct mutation—one producing manifest hypercalcemia in one parent, but the other being so mild as to be biochemically undetectable in the other parent. Alternatively, there might be a mutation in one allele of the CaR gene as well as in one allele of another gene causing an FBHH-like clinical picture, such as the one on chromosome 19p (62) or that linked to neither chromosome 3 nor 19 (64). No clear documentation of any such scenarios, however, has been achieved to date.

Another possible factor that has been suggested to contribute to the development of NSHPT in a child with a single abnormal CaR allele arising from a father with FBHH, but a normal mother might be the impact of normal maternal calcium homeostasis on the abnormal Ca$_o^{2+}$-sensing of the affected fetus in utero (65). Calcium is actively transported across the placenta from mother to fetus, generating a higher fetal than maternal calcium concentration *(65)*. Thus a normal mother would expose fetal parathyroid glands with even modestly abnormal Ca_o^{2+}-sensing owing to FBHH to a Ca_o^{2+} level that would be recognized as relatively hypocalcemic. The latter would, in turn, "over-stimulate" the fetal parathyroids, resulting in additional "secondary" fetal/neonatal hyperparathyroidism superimposed on the abnormal Ca_o^{2+}-sensing already present because of the FBHH mutation by itself. This possibility is supported by the occurrence of cases of NSHPT with autosomal-dominant inheritance in situations where the father had familial benign hypocalciuric hypercalcemia and the mother was apparently normal *(41,78,87)*. Postnatally, the "secondary" hyperparathyroidism would eventually subside, leading to the clinical and biochemical features of FBHH. In most cases, however, children with FBHH who are born to a normal mother do not have more severe hypercalcemia than those born to an affected mother, and there are no apparent differences between mice heterozygous for knockout of the CaR born to normal mothers and those heterozygous for CaR knockout *(26)*.

Recent studies have demonstrated that clinically severe, neonatal hyperparathyroidism can result from heterozygous *de novo* CaR mutations *(63)* (i.e., caused by a single *de novo* CaR mutation in the child of normal parents). Two such infants had hyperparathyroid bone disease, but less severe hypercalcemia than seen in NSHPT owing to homozygous FBHH *(63)*. We recently documented another case of *de novo* heterozygous NSHPT in a child with the same arg185gln mutation described previously that is associated with a greater elevation in serum calcium than in most FBHH cases *(8,78,87a)*. In this case, the relatively large disparity between the set points of the maternal and fetal parathyroid glands may have promoted more prenatal hyperparathyroidism with resultant hyperparathyroid bone disease in the newborn infant.

Thus, the clinical and biochemical findings in NSHPT, which in homozygous cases represents a "knockout" of the human CaR gene, suggest the following additional conclusions about the receptor's function in humans: (1) they highlight its importance in fetal and neonatal calcium homeostasis, and (2) they indicate that, in addition to its role in Ca_o^{2+}-regulated PTH release, which is markedly abnormal in NSHPT, particularly that owing to homozygous FBHH, the CaR has a potential function in inhibiting parathyroid cellular proliferation, since there is substantial parathyroid hyperplasia in NSHPT.

Mouse Models of FHH and NSHPT

Recently, Ho et al. *(26)* utilized targeted disruption of the CaR gene to generate mice that are heterozygous or homozygous for inactivation of the CaR gene and provide animal models of FBHH and NSHPT, respectively. Introduction of DNA encoding the neomycin resistance gene into the third exon of the CaR gene resulted in essentially complete absence of detectable CaR protein in parathyroid and kidney of homozygous mice, and approx 50% reductions in the levels of the protein in heterozygotes. Phenotypically, the heterozygous mice were normal in appearance, fertile, and had a normal life-span. Their serum calcium concentration averaged 10.4 mg/dL, which is about 10% higher than that of their normal littermates. The heterozygotes also had modest, but significant elevations in their serum magnesium concentrations. Serum PTH levels were approx 50% higher in heterozygotes than in normals, and the calcium concentration in bladder urine was slightly reduced compared to the normal mice. Skeletal X-rays were normal. Thus, mice heterozygous for targeted disruption of the CaR gene share many of the phenotypic and biochemical features of persons with FBHH.

It is of interest that in the heterozygous mice there appears to be little, if any, up-regulation of the production of the CaR protein from the remaining normal gene despite the complete lack of CaR production from the inactivated allele, since the levels of expression of the CaR protein in kidney and parathyroid are about half those in wild-type animals (26). This ~50% reduction in the expression of the CaR protein in the parathyroid glands produces a mild (~10%) increase in the apparent set point of Ca_o^{2+}-regulated PTH release, similar to that seen in FBHH families with mutations expected to produce a totally inactive CaR from the mutant allele (e.g., ser607stop). Thus, the results obtained in the heterozygous mice support further the concept that the abnormal CaR allele in FBHH often acts as a null mutation (i.e., it produces no gene product or a totally inactive one), and the abnormality in parathyroid function results simply from a reduction in the number of normally functioning CaRs on the cell surface (37,38,41). This pathophysiology is similar to that which we recently postulated to occur in parathyroid adenomas, which have not been found to harbor mutations in the CaR gene (88), but show an average 60% reduction in CaR immunoreactivity on immunohistochemistry (89). Parathyroid adenomas usually exhibit a somewhat greater increase in set point in vitro and in vivo than is observed in FBHH (89), perhaps related to the greater reduction in the level of the CaR protein on the cell surface.

Mice homozygous for inactivation of the CaR, in contrast, although nearly normal in size at birth, grew much more slowly than their normal or heterozygous littermates (26). This poor growth may have occurred, in part, because they competed poorly with their more vigorous normal and heterozygous littermates for maternal milk. The homozygotes had severe hypercalcemia, with serum calcium concentrations that averaged 14.8 mg/dL. Their magnesium levels, in contrast, were slightly, but not significantly greater than those of heterozygous mice. Serum levels of PTH were nearly 10-fold higher than those of the normal mice, an increase comparable to that in infants with NSHPT. Despite the severe hypercalcemia, the calcium concentration in bladder urine was significantly lower than in the normal mice (26). Skeletal X-rays showed numerous abnormalities, with substantial reductions in apparent mineral density, bowing of the long bones, and kyphoscoliosis. Most of the homozygous mice died during the first 2 wk postnatally, and only occasionally some survived for up to 3–4 wk of age. Thus, the biochemical and clinical features of mice homozygous for targeted disruption of the CaR gene exhibited many similarities to the human disorder, NSHPT. Much work remains to be carried out employing this animal model to investigate abnormalities in Ca_o^{2+}-sensing in tissues that normally express the CaR, including those not thought to be involved in calcium homeostasis, such as the brain.

SYNDROME OF EXTRACELLULAR Ca_o^{2+} OVERRESPONSIVENESS

Clinical and Biochemical Features of ADH

Familial isolated hypoparathyroidism is a rare disease that occurs in several forms—autosomal-recessive, autosomal-dominant, or X-linked (90). The molecular basis for the autosomal-recessive and X-linked forms has not been uncovered to date. A study of eight families with autosomal-dominant hypoparathyroidism found linkage of the disorder to the PTH gene in two *(91)*, one of whom was later shown to harbor a mutation in the signal peptide-encoding region of the preproPTH gene *(92)*. Another family has subsequently been identified with a mutation within a splice junction of the same gene *(93)*. The identification of inactivating mutations in the CaR gene in FBHH, coupled with the identification of activating mutations in other GPCRs *(94,95)*, raised the possibility that autosomal-dominant hypocalcemia (ADH) could result from activating mutations of the CaR. The recent studies described below showed that this is, in fact, the case.

ADH has only been recognized as a distinct clinical entity for 2 yr. Nevertheless, the disorder has certain characteristic clinical findings that are generally predictable from the presence of activating CaR mutations that "reset" downward the set points of both parathyroid and kidney for Ca_0^{2+} *(7,96–98)*. Thus, this disorder is the clinical expression of mild to moderate increases in responsiveness of target tissues to Ca_0^{2+} (vs the resistance to Ca_0^{2+} present in FBHH [*31*]). The identification of additional families will doubtless provide a more detailed picture of the presentation and clinical course of this syndrome.

Individuals with ADH have mild to moderate hypocalcemia (~6–8 mg/dL) *(7,96–99)*, although one patient with an apparently *de novo* CaR mutation had more severe hypocalcemia (4.8 mg/dL) *(96)*. Some individuals with ADH have relatively few symptoms despite their hypocalcemia *(99)*, although others exhibit the signs and symptoms found in other hypocalcemic disorders, such as paresthesias, muscle cramps, and laryngospasm *(96,97)*. Seizures are common, especially in younger patients, although the seizures in several cases occurred during febrile episodes and were not difficult to control *(97)*. Individuals with ADH, like those with classical primary hypoparathyroidism, tend to have hyperphosphatemia. In some kindreds, however, the serum phosphate concentrations of affected individuals may be normal *(7)*, perhaps in those individuals who have normal PTH levels *(see below)*. Serum magnesium levels are often low-normal or are even frankly subnormal in the untreated state *(97)*. Intact PTH levels are usually in the lower half of the normal range *(7,96,97)*. In one case, induced lowering of serum calcium concentration in a patient with ADH caused a brisk rise in serum PTH, consistent with a leftward shift in the set point for Ca_0^{2+}-regulated PTH release *(100)*, the converse of what is observed in FBHH. The levels of 1,25(OH)₂ D have been measured in relatively few cases and were generally normal *(97)*. Urinary calcium excretion has been found to be higher in untreated patients with ADH than in patients with classical hypoparathyroidism, in spite of the fact that PTH levels are often lower in the latter than in ADH *(96,97,99)*. The latter observation presumably reflects direct inhibition of renal tubular reabsorption of Ca^{2+} (and Mg^{2+}) by mutant CaRs activated at inappropriately low levels of Ca_0^{2+}, again the opposite of the effects of inactivating FBHH mutations on renal calcium handling.

From the available data, patients with ADH appear to respond to therapy with vitamin D in a characteristic manner that differs from patients with true hypoparathyroidism. Patients with ADH seem unusually susceptible to marked hypercalciuria and the renal complications of overtreatment with vitamin D, even in the absence of overt hypercalcemia *(97)*. These deleterious consequences of vitamin D therapy have included nephrocalcinosis, renal stones, reversible (and, in some cases, irreversible) decreases in renal function, as well as polydipsia and polyuria, probably as a result of poor urinary concentrating ability *(97)*. In other words, patients with ADH suffer from "hypercalcemic"

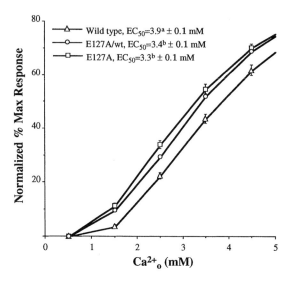

Fig. 4. Expression of a mutant CaR bearing an ADH mutation (glu127ala) in HEK293 cells. Results show the effects of the indicated levels of Ca_o^{2+} on the cytosolic calcium level in HEK293 cells transiently transfected with the wild-type CaR, a mutant CaR bearing the ADH mutation, glu127ala, or cotransfected with both the wild-type and mutant receptors. Reproduced from ref. *71* with permission.

complications during vitamin D treatment even when normocalcemic, presumably as a consequence of "resetting" of their mineral ion homeostatic mechanism owing to increased responsiveness of target tissues to Ca_o^{2+}.

Description of Linkage of ADH to Chromosome 3 and Identification of CaR Mutations

Finegold and coworkers showed that ADH was linked to a locus on chromosome 3 in the vicinity of the CaR locus *(101)*. Shortly thereafter, Pollak et al. *(7)* identified a heterozygous missense mutation in codon 127 of the CaR (glu127ala). Subsequent studies have identified additional missense mutations in approx 10 ADH families *(7,96,97,102)* and in a case of sporadic hypocalcemia *(96)* (Fig. 2). Some are present within the CaR ECD, providing further support for the importance of this part of the receptor in the mechanisms of the CaR's activation by Ca_o^{2+}, where several families also harbor mutations within the transmembrane domains of the receptor *(96)*. To date, no cases of homozygous ADH have been described.

Expression of several of the known ADH mutations in HEK293 cells showed a clear leftward shift in Ca_o^{2+}-evoked increases in Ca_i^{2+} (Fig. 4) *(71,97)*. Activating mutations in other GPCRs, like the TSH and LH receptors, are present in transmembrane domains, and presumably facilitate the process of signal transduction or mimic the active state of the receptor if the activation of the receptor is truly ligand-independent *(103,104)*. Those mutations in the transmembrane domains of the CaR may act in a similar fashion. Mutations within the CaR ECD, in contrast, may increase the affinity of the CaR for Ca_o^{2+}, thereby favoring the active conformation of the receptor and initiating subsequent events in signal transduction at inappropriately low levels of Ca_o^{2+}.

Diagnostic and Therapeutic Implications of Activating CaR Mutations

Thus, ADH is an entity distinct from typical hypoparathyroidism, and further studies will likely uncover a larger number of cases of ADH or *de novo* activating mutations in the CaR that previously would have been classified as familial isolated or sporadic hypoparathyroidism. This distinction is of clinical importance, because individuals with ADH may suffer irreversible renal damage during overly aggressive therapy with calcitriol to normalize their serum calcium concentration *(97)*. Identifying this disorder requires careful clinical and genetic evaluation. The diagnosis of ADH should be entertained in cases with a presumptive diagnosis of familial hypoparathyroidism, especially in those individuals who develop severe hypercalciuria and/or renal impairment during therapy with vitamin D.

SUMMARY

The cloning of the CaR directly documents that several cell types recognize and respond to even minute perturbations in Ca_o^{2+} through a receptor-mediated mechanism similar to that through which numerous cells respond to a wide variety of hormones, neurotransmitters, and other extracellular messengers. Therefore, Ca_o^{2+} can function as an extracellular, first messenger in addition to serving its better-recognized role as a key intracellular second messenger. Of the tissues expressing the CaR, several are important elements within the mineral ion homeostatic system that have been known to sense Ca_o^{2+} for many years. The presence of the CaR on a variety of renal cells, however, strongly suggests that several of the direct, but poorly understood actions of Ca_o^{2+} on kidney function could also be mediated by the CaR. The latter include the increased urinary excretion of calcium and magnesium owing to the effects of hypercalcemia *per se* on CaRs in the distal tubule, which acts in concert with the reduction in renal calcium reabsorption resulting from the concomitant, high Ca_o^{2+}-induced suppression of PTH release. The decrease in urinary concentration noted in some hypercalcemic individuals probably is a manifestation of a functionally relevant coordination of the homeostatic mechanisms governing calcium and water handling by the kidney. The purpose of integrating and coordinating these systems is presumably to minimize the risk of renal calcium deposition and resultant damage during disposal of calcium loads. Human syndromes of Ca_o^{2+} "resistance" or "over-responsiveness" owing to loss-of-function or gain-of-function mutations in the CaR, respectively, provide additional support for the role of the CaR in regulating renal function. Much remains to be learned, however, about the role of the CaR in parts of the body, such as the brain, where it probably responds to local rather than systemic changes in Ca_o^{2+}. The development of drugs that activate or inhibit the CaR has great potential utility for the treatment of conditions where the receptor is either under- or overactive. Clinical trials are currently under way assessing the efficacy of calcimimetic CaR agonists for the treatment of primary and secondary hyperparathyroidism *(105)*. Finally, there may well be further receptors for Ca_o^{2+} *(106–109)*, perhaps encoded by the additional genetic loci producing the syndrome of FBHH, or for other ions (indeed, the CaR probably acts as a physiologically relevant Mg_o^{2+}-receptor).

ACKNOWLEDGMENTS

The authors gratefully acknowledge the generous grant support provided by the USPHS (DK41415, 44588, 46422, [to E. M. B.], 48330 [to E. M. B. and S. C. H.]) and

DK09436 (to M. B.), the St. Giles Foundation, and NPS Pharmaceuticals, Inc., Salt Lake City, UT.

REFERENCES

1. Brown E. Extracellular Ca^{2+} sensing, regulation of parathyroid cell function, and role of Ca^{2+} and other ions as extracellular (first) messengers. Physiol Rev 1997;71:371–411.
2. Pietrobon D, Di Virgilio F, Pozzan T. Structural and functional aspects of calcium homeostasis in eukaryotic cells. Eur J Biochem 1990;120:599–622.
3. Aurbach G, Marx S, Spiegel A. Parathyroid Hormone, Calcitonin, and the Calciferols. In: Wilson JD, Foster D, eds, 7th ed. Saunders, Philadelphia, PA. Textbook of Endocrinology 1985, pp. 1137–1217.
4. Kurokawa K. The kidney and calcium homeostasis. Kidney Int 1994;45(Suppl 44):S97–S105.
5. Parfitt A. Bone and plasma calcium homeostasis. Bone 8 1987;(Suppl. 1):1–8.
5a Brown EM, Pollak M, Hebert SC. Cloning and characterization of extracellular Ca^{2+}-sensing receptors from parathyroid and kidney: Molecular physiology and pathophysiology of Ca^{2+}-sensing. The Endocrinologist 1994;4:419–426.
6. Brown E, Gamba G, Riccardi D, Lombardi D, Butters R, Kifor O, Sun A, Hediger M, Lytton J, Hebert S. Cloning and characterization of an extracellular Ca^{2+}-sensing receptor from bovine parathyroid. Nature 1993;366:575–580.
7. Pollak M, Brown E, Estep H, McLaine P, Kifor O, Park J, Hebert S, Seidman C, Seidman J. An autosomal dominant form of hypocalcemia caused by a mutation in the human Ca^{2+}-sensing receptor gene. Nature Genet 1994;8:303–308.
8. Pollak M, Brown E, Chou Y-H, Hebert S, Marx S, Steinmann B, Levi T, Seidman C, Seidman J. Mutations in the human Ca^{2+}-sensing receptor gene cause familial hypocalciuric hypercalcemia and neonatal severe hyperparathyroidism. Cell 1993;75:1297–1303.
9. Kifor O, Kifor I, Brown EM. Effects of high extracellular calcium concentrations on phosphoinositide turnover and inositol phosphate metabolism in dispersed bovine parathyroid cells. J Bone Miner Res 1992;7:1327–1335.
10. Shoback D, Membreno L, McGhee J. High calcium and other divalent cations in increase inositol trisphosphate in bovine parathyroid cells. Endocrinology 1988;123:382–389.
11. Nemeth EF, Wallace J, Scarpa A. Stimulus-secretion coupling in bovine parathyroid cells. Dissociation between secretion and net changes in cytosolic Ca^{++}. J Biol Chem 1986;261: 2668–2674.
12. Chen C, Barnett J, Congo D, Brown E. Divalent cations suppress $3',5'$-adenosine monophosphate accumulation by stimulating a pertussis toxin-sensitive guanine nucleotide-binding protein in cultured bovine parathyroid cells. Endocrinology 1989;124:233–239.
13. Racke F, Hammerland L, Dubyak G, Nemeth E. Functional expression of the parathyroid calcium receptor in *Xenopus oocytes*. FEBS Lett 1993;333:132–136.
14. Chen T, Pratt S, Shoback D. Injection of parathyroid poly(A)+ RNA into *Xenopus oocytes* confers sensitivity to high extracellular calcium. J Bone Miner Res 1994;9:293–300.
15. Garrett J, Capuano I, Hammerland L, Hung B, Brown E, Hebert S, Nemeth E, Fuller F. Molecular cloning and characterization of the human parathyroid calcium receptor. J Biol Chem 1995;270: 12,919–12,925.
15a. Brown EM, Bai, M, and Pollak M. Familial benign hypocalciuric hypercalcemia and other syndromes of altered responsiveness to extracellular calcium. In: Krane SM, and Avioli LV, eds. Metabolic Bone Diseases, 3rd ed. Academic, San Diego, in press.
16. Aida K, Koishi S, Tawata M, Onaya T. Molecular cloning of a putative Ca^{2+}-sensing receptor cDNA from human kidney. Biochem Biophys Res Commun 1995;214:524–529.
17. Riccardi D, Park J, Lee W-S, Gamba G, Brown E, Hebert S. Cloning and functional expression of a rat kidney extracellular calcium-sensing receptor. Proc Natl Acad Sci USA 1995;92:131–135.
18. Ruat M, Molliver M, Snowman A, Snyder S. Calcium sensing receptor: Molecular cloning in rat and localization to nerve terminals. Proc Natl Acad Sci USA 1995;92:3161–3165.
19. Garrett JE, Tamir H, Kifor O, Simin RT, Rogers KV, Mithal A, Gagel RF, Brown EM. Calcitonin-secreting cells of the thyroid gland express an extracellular calcium-sensing receptor gene. Endocrinology 1995;136:5202–5211.
20. Hammerland LG, Krapcho KJ, Alasti N, Garrett JE, Capuano IV, Hung BCP, Fuller F. Cation binding determinants of the calcium receptor revealed by functional analysis of chimeric receptors and a deletion mutant. J Bone Miner Res 1995;10:S156 (Abstract).

21. Varrault A, Rodriguez-Pena M, Goldsmith P, Mithal A, Brown E, Spiegel A. Expression of G-protein alpha-subunits in bovine parathyroid. Endocrinology 1995;136:4390–4396.

22. Rogers K, Dunn C, Hebert S, Brown E, Nemeth E. Pharmacological comparison of bovine parathyroid, human parathyroid, and rat kidney calcium receptors expressed in HEK 293 cells. J Bone Miner Res 1995;10:S483 (Abstract T516).

23. Nakanishi S. Metabotropic glutamate receptors: synaptic transmission, modulation and plasticity. Neuron 1994;13:1031–1037.

23a. Kifor O, Diaz R, Butters R, Brown EM. The Ca^{2+}-sensing receptor (CaR) activates phospholipase C, A$_2$, and D in bovine parathyroid and CaR-transfected, human embryonic kidney (HEK293) cells. L Bone Mineral Res 1997;12:715–725.

24. Marx S, Lasker R, Brown E, Fitzpatrick L, Sweezey N, Goldbloom R, Gillis D, Cole D. Secretory dysfunction in parathyroid cells from a neonate with severe primary hyperparathyroidism. J Clin Endocrinol Metab 1986;62:445–449.

25. Cooper L, Wertheimer J, Levey R, Brown E, LeBoff M, Wilkinson R, Anast C. Severe primary hyperparathyroidism in a neonate with two hypercalcemic parents: management with parathyroidectomy and heterotopic autotransplantation. Pediatrics 1986;78:263–268.

26. Ho C, Conner DA, Pollak M, Ladd DJ, Kifor O, Warren H, Brown EM, Seidman CE, Seidman JG. A mouse model for familial hypocalciuric hypercalcemia and neonatal severe hyperparathyroidism. Nature Genet 1995;11:389–394.

27. Garrett JE, Steffey ME, Nemeth EF. The calcium receptor agonist R-568 suppresses PTH mRNA levels in cultured bovine parathyroid cells. J Bone Miner Res 1995;10:S387 (Abstract).

28. Randall C, and Lauchlan S. Parathyroid hyperplasia in an infant. Am J Dis Child 1963;105:364–367.

29. Spiegel A, Harrison H, Marx S, Brown E, Aurbach G. Neonatal primary hyperparathyroidism with autosomal dominant inheritance. J Pediatr 1977;90:269–272.

30. Riccardi D, Plotkin M, Lee W-S, Lee K, Segre G, Brown E, Hebert S. Colocalization of the Ca^{2+}-sensing receptor and PTH/PTHrP receptor in rat kidney. J Am Soc Nephrol. 1995;6:954 (Abstract).

31. Brown E, Hebert S. A cloned Ca^{2+}-sensing receptor: A mediator of direct effects of extracellular Ca^{2+} on renal function? J Am Soc Nephrol 1995;6:1530–1540.

32. Chabardes D, Imbert M, Clique A, Montegut M, Morel F. PTH-sensitive adenyl cyclase activity in different segments of the rabbit nephron. Pflugers Arch 1975;354:229–239.

33. Baum M, Chattopadhyay M, Brown E, Ruddy M, Hosselet C, Riccardi D, Hebert S, Harris H. Perinatal expression of aquaporins-2 and 3 and the calcium receptor in developing rat kidney collecting ducts. J Am Soc Nephrol 1995;6:319 (Abstract).

34. Suki W, Eknoyan G, Rector F. The renal diluting and concentrating mechanism in hypercalcemia. Nephron 1969;6:50–61.

35. Brown E, Vassilev P, Hebert S. Calcium as an extracellular messenger. Cell 1995;83:679–682.

36. Foley T, Harrison H, Arnaud C, Harrison H. Familial benign hypercalcemia. J Pediatr 1972;81: 1060–1067.

37. Marx SJ, Attie MF, Levine MA, Spiegel AM, Downs RWJ, Lasker RD. The hypocalciuric or benign variant of familial hypercalcemia: Clinical and biochemical features in fifteen kindreds. Medicine (Baltimore) 1981;60:397–412.

38. Law WJ, Heath H III. Familial benign hypercalcemia (hypocalciuric hypercalcemia). Clinical and pathogenetic studies in 21 families. Ann Int Med 1985;105:511–519.

39. Marx S, Speigel A, Brown E, Koehler J, Gardner D, Brennan M, Aurbach G. Divalent action metabolism. Familial hypocalciuric hypercalcemia versus typical primary hyperparathyroidism. Am J Med 1978;65:235–242.

40. Stewart A, Broadus A. Mineral Metabolism. In: Felig P, Baxter JD, Broadus AE, Frohman LA, eds. Endocrinology and Metabolism, 2nd ed. McGraw-Hill, New York, 1987, p. 1317–1453.

41. Heath D. Familial Hypocalciuric Hypercalcemia. In: Bilezikian JP, Marcus RM, Levine MA, eds. The Parathyroids, Raven New York, 1994, pp. 699–710.

42. Gunn I, Wallace J. Urine calcium and serum ionised calcium, total calcium and parathyroid hormone concentrations in the diagnosis of primary hyperparathyroidism and familial benign hypercalcemia. Ann Clin Biochem 1992;29:52–58.

43. Chou Y-H, Brown E, Levi T, Crowe G, Atkinson A, Arnquist H, Toss G, Fuleihan G-H, Seidman J, Seidman C. The gene responsible for familial hypocalciuric hypercalcemia maps to chromosome 3 in four unrelated families. Nature Genet 1992;1:295–300.

44. Heath H III. Familial benign (hypocalciuric) hypercalcemia, a troublesome mimic of primary hyper-parathyroidism. Endocrinol Metab Clin North Am 1989;18:723–740.

45. Auwerx J, Demedts M, Bouillon R. Altered parathyroid set point to calcium in familial hypocalciuric hypercalcemia. Acta Endocrinologica 1984;106:215–218.

46. Khosla S, Ebeling PR, Firek AF, Burritt MM, Kao PC, Heath H III. Calcium infusion suggests a "set-point" abnormality of parathyroid gland function in familial benign hypercalcemia and more complex disturbances in primary hyperparathyroidism. J Clin Endocrinol Metab 1993;76:715–720.

47. Brown E. Four parameter model of the sigmoidal relationship between PTH release and extracellular calcium concentration in normal and abnormal parathyroid tissue. J Clin Endocrinol Metab 1983;56:572–581.

48. Law WJ, Carney J, Heath H III. Parathyroid glands in familial benign hypercalcemia (familial hypocalciuric hypercalcemia). Am J Med 1984;76:1021–1026.

49. Thogeirsson U, Costa J, Marx S. The parathyroid glands in familial benign hypocalciuric hyper-calcemia. Hum Pathol 1981;12:229–237.

50. Davies M, Adams P, Lumb G. Familial hypocalciuric hypercalcemia: Evidence for continued enhanced renal tubular reabsorption of calcium following total parathyroidectomy. Acta Endocrinol 1984;106:499–504.

51. Kristiansen J, Rodbro P, Christiansen C, Brochner Mortensen J, Carl J. Familial hypocalciuric hypercal-cemia II: intestinal calcium absorption and vitamin D metabolism. Clin Endocrinol 1985;23: 511–515.

52. Law WJ, Bollman S, Kumar R, Heath H III. Vitamin D metabolism in familial benign hypercalcemia (hypocalciuric hypercalcemia) differs from that in primary hyperparathyroidism. J Clin Endocrinol Metab 1984;58:744–747.

53. Kristiansen J, Rodbro P, Christiansen C, Johansen J, Jensen J. Familial hypocalciuric hypercalcemia III: bone mineral metabolism. Clin Endocrinol 1987;26:713–716.

54. Menko F, Bijouvet O, Fronen J, et al. Familial benign hypercalcemia: study of a large family. Q J Med 1983;206:120–140.

55. Abugassa S, Nordenstrom J, Jarhult J. Bone mineral density in patients with familial hypocalciuric hypercalcemia. Eur J Surg 1992;158:397–402.

56. McMurtry C, Schranck F, Walkenhorst D, Murphy W, Kocher D, Teitelbaum S, Rupich R, Whyte M. Significant developmental elevation in serum parathyroid hormone levels in a large kindred with familial benign (hypocalciuric) hypercalcemia. Am J Med 1992;93:247–258.

57. Pasieka J, Anderson M, Hanley D. Familial benign hypercalcemia: hypercalciuria and hypocalciuria in affected members of a small kindred. Clin Endocrinol 1990;33:429–433.

58. Attie M, Gill JJ, Stock J, Spiegel A, Downs RJ, Levine M, Marx S. Urinary calcium excretion in familial hypocalciuric hypercalcemia. J Clin Invest 1983;72:667–676.

59. Kristiansen J, Brochner-Mortensen J, Pederson K. Renal tubular reabsorption of calcium in familial hypocalciuric hypercalcemia. Acta Endocrinol 1986;112:541–546.

60. Marx SJ, Attie MF, Stock JL, Spiegel AM, Levine MA. Maximal urine-concentrating ability: Familial hypocalciuric hypercalcemia versus typical primary hyperparathyroidism. J Clin Endocrinol Metab 1981;52:736–740.

61. Pollak M, Chou Y-H, Marx S, Steinmann B, Cole D, Brandi M, Papapoulos S, Menko F, Hendy G, Brown E, Seidman C, Seidman J. Familial hypocalciuric hypercalcemia and neonatal severe hyper-calcemia: The effects of mutant gene dosage on phenotype. J Clin Invest 1994;93:1108–1112.

62. Heath H, Jackson C, Otterud B, Leppert M. Genetic linkage analysis of familial benign (hypocalci-uric) hypercalcemia: evidence for locus heterogeneity. Am J Hum Genet 1993;53:193–200.

63. Pearce S, Trump D, Wooding C, Besser G, Chew S, Heath D, Hughes I, Thakker R. Calcium-sensing receptor mutations in familial benign hypercalcaemia and neonatal hyperparathyroidism. J Clin Invest 1995;96:2683–2692.

64. Trump D, Whyte M, Wooding C, Pang J, Pearce S, Kocher D, Thakker R. Linkage studies in a kin-dred from Oklahoma with familial benign (hypocalciuric) hypercalcemia and developmental eleva-tions in serum parathyroid hormone levels, indicate a third locus for FHH. Hum Genet 1995;96:183–187.

65. Marx S, Fraser D, Rapoport A. Familial hypocalciuric hypercalcemia. Mild expression of the disease in heterozygotes and severe expression in homozygotes. Am J Med 1985;78:15–22.

66. Janicic N, Pausova Z, Cole DEC, Hendy GN. Insertion of an alu sequence in the Ca^{2+}-sensing recep-tor gene in familial hypocalciuric hypercalcemia and neonatal severe hyperparathyroidism. Am J Hum Genet 1995;56:880–886.

67. Heath H III, Odelberg S, Jackson C, Teh B, Hayward N, Larsson C, Buist N, Krapcho K, Hung B, Capuano I, Garrett J, Leppert M. Clustered inactivating mutations and benign polymorphisms of the calcium receptor gene in familial benign hypocalciuric hypercalcemia suggest receptor functional domains. J Clin Endocrinol Metab 1996;81:1312–1317.

68. Chou Y-H, Pollak M, Brandi M, Toss G, Arnqvist H, Atkinson A, Papapoulos S, Marx S, Brown E, Seidman J, Seidman C. Mutations in the human calcium-sensing receptor gene. Am J Hum Genet 1995;56:1075–1079.

69. Aida K, Koishi S, Inoue M, Nakazato M, Tawata M, Onaya T. Familial hypocalciuric hypercalcemia associated with mutation in the human Ca^{2+}-sensing receptor gene. J Clin Endocrinol Metab 1995;80:2594–2598.

70. Janicic N, Pausova Z, Cole D, Hendy G. De novo expansion of an alu insertion mutation of the Ca^{2+}-sensing receptor gene in familial hypocalciuric hypercalcemia and neonatal severe hyperparathyroidism. J Bone Miner Res 1995;10 (Suppl 1):S191.

71. Bai M, Quinn S, Trivedi S, Kifor O, Pearce S, Pollak M, Krapcho KK, Hebert S, Brown E. Expression and characterization of inactivating and activating mutations of the human Ca$_o^{2+}$-sensing receptor. J Biol Chem 1996;271:19,537–19,545.

71a. Pearce SHS, Bai M, Quinn SJ, Brown EM, Thakker RV. Functional characterization of calcium-sensing receptor mutations expressed in human embryonic kidney cells. J Clin Invest 1996;98:1860–1866.

71b. Bai M, Janicic N, Trivedi S, Quinn SJ, Cole DEC, Brown EM, Hendy GN. Markedly reduced activity of mutant calcium-sensing receptor with an inserted Alu element from a kindred with familial hypocalciuric hypercalcemia and neonatal severe hyperparathyroidism. J Clin Invest 1997;99:1917–1925.

72. Bockaert J. G proteins, G-protein-coupled receptors: structure, function and interactions. Curr Opinion Neurobiol 1991;1:1132–1142.

73. Jackson T. Structure and function of G protein coupled receptors. Pharm Ther 1991;50:425–442.

74. Pin J-P, Gomeza T, Joly C, Bockaert J. The metabotropic glutamate receptors: their second intracellular loop plays a critical role in the G-protein coupling specificity. Biochem Soc Trans 1994;23:910–96.

75. Landon J. Parathyroidectomy in generalized osteitis fibrosa cystica. J Pediatr 1932;1:544–560.

76. Eftekhari F, Yousufzadeh D. Primary infantile hyperparathyroidism: clinical, laboratory and radiographic features in 21 cases. Skeletal Radiol 1982;8:201–208.

77. Steinmann B, Gnehm H, Rao V, Kind H, Prader A. Neonatal severe primary hyperparathyroidism and alkaptonuria in a boy born to related parents with familial hypocalciuric hypercalcemia. Helv Paediatr Acta 1984;39:171–186.

78. Marx S, Attie M, Spiegel A, Levine M, Lasker R, Fox M. An association between neonatal severe primary hyperparathyroidism and familial hypocalciuric hypercalcemia in three kindreds. N Engl J Med 1982;306:257–284.

79. Gaudelus J, Dandine M, Nathanson M, Perelman R, Hassan M. Rib cage deformity in neonatal hyperparathyroidism. Am J Dis Child 1983;137:408–409.

80. Mallette L. The Functional and Pathologic Spectrum of Parathyroid Abnormalities in Hyperparathyroidism. In: Bilezikian JP, Marcus RM, Levine MA, eds. The Parathyroids. Raven New York, 1994, pp. 423–455.

81. Fujimoto Y, Hazama H, Oku K. Severe primary hyperparathyroidism in a neonate having a parent with hypercalcemia: treatment by total parathyroidectomy and simultaneous heterotopic autotransplantation. Surgery 1990;108:933–938.

82. Grantmyre E. Roentgenographic features of "primary" hyperparathyroidism in infancy. J Can Assoc Radiol 1974;24:257–260.

83. Fujita T, Watanabe N, Fukase M, Tsutsumi M, Fukami T, Imai Y, Sakaguchi K, Okada S, Matsuo M, Takemine H. Familial hypocalciuric hypocalcemia involving four members of a kindred including a girl with severe neonatal primary hyperparathyroidism. Miner Electrolyte Metab 1983;9:51–54.

84. Matsuo M, Okita K, Takemine H, Fujita T. Neonatal primary hyperparathyroidism in familial hypocalciuric hypercalcemia. Am J Dis Child 1982;136:728–731.

85. Harris S, D'Ercole A. Neonatal hyperparathyroidism: the natural course in the absence of surgical intervention. Pediatrics 1989;83:53–56.

86. Page L, Haddow J. Self limited neonatal hyperparathyroidism in familial hypocalciuric hypercalcemia. J Pediatr 1987;111:261–264.

87. Heath D. Familial benign hypercalcemia. Trends Endocrinol Metab 1989;1:6–9.

87a. Bai M, Pearce SHS, Kifor O, Trivedi S, Stauffer UG, Thakker RV, Brown EM, Steinmann B. In vivo and in vitro characterization of neonatal hyperparathyroidism resulting from a de novo, heterozygous mutation in the Ca^{2+} -sensing receptor gene: Normal maternal calcium homeotasis as a causeof secondary hyperparathyroidism in familial benign hypocalciuric hypercalcemia. J Clin Invest 1997;99:88–96.

88. Hosokawa Y, Pollak M, Brown E, Arnold A. Mutational analysis of the extracellular Ca^{2+}-sensing receptor gene in human parathyroid tumors. J Clin Endocrinol Metab 1995;80:3107–3110.

89. Kifor O, Moore FJ, Wang P, Goldstein M, Vassilev P, Kifor I, Hebert S, Brown E. Reduced immuno-staining for the extracellular Ca^{2+}-sensing receptor in primary and uremic secondary hyperpara-thyroidism. J Clin Endocrinol Metab 1996;81:1598–1606.

90. Eastell R, Heath H III. The Hypocalcemic States: Their Differential Diagnosis and Management. In: Coe F, Favus M, eds. Disorders of Bone Metabolism. Raven, New York; 1992, pp. 571–585.

91. Ahn T, Antonarakis S, Kronenberg H, Igarishi T, Levine M. Familial isolated hypoparathyroidism: a molecular genetic analysis of 8 families with 23 affected persons. Medicine 1986;65:73–81.

92. Arnold A, Horst S, Gardella T, Baba H, Levine M, Kronenberg H. Mutation of the signal peptide-encoding region of the preproparathyroid hormone gene in familial isolated hypoparathyroidism. J Clin Invest 1990;86:1084–1087.

93. Parkinson D, Thakker R. A donor splice mutation in the parathyroid hormone gene in association with autosomal recessive hypoparathyroidism. Nature Genet 1992;1:149–153.

94. Lefkowitz R, Premont R. Diseased G-protein-coupled receptors. J Clin Invest 1993;92:2089.

95. Coughlin S. Expanding horizons for receptors coupled to G-proteins-diversity and disease. Curr Opinion Cell Biol 1994;6:191–197.

96. Baron J, Winer K, Yanovski J, Cunningham A, Laue L, Zimmerman D, Cutler G Jr. Mutations in the Ca^{2+}-sensing receptor gene cause autosomal dominant and sporadic hypoparathyroidism. Hum Mol Genet 1996;5:601–606.

97. Pearce S, Coulthard M, Kendall-Taylor P, Thakker R. Autosomal dominant hypocalcaemia associated with a mutation in the calcium-sensing receptor. J Bone Miner Res 1995;10:S176 (Abstract 149).

98. Perry Y, Finegold D, Armitage M, Ferell R. A missense mutation in the Ca-sensing receptor causes familial autosomal dominant hypoparathyroidism. Am J Hum Genet 1994;55 (Suppl):A17(Abstract).

99. Davies M, Mughal Z, Selby P, Tymms D, Mawer E. Familial benign hypocalcemia. J Bone Miner Res 1995;10 (Suppl 1):S507.

100. Estep H, Mistry Z, Burke P. In Proceedings and Abstracts of the 63rd Annual Meeting of the Endocrine Society. Endocrine Society, Cincinnati, 1981, abstract 750, p. 270.

101. Finegold D, Armitage M, Galiani M, Matise, TC, Pandian MR, Perry YM, Deka R, Ferrell RE. Preliminary localisation of a gene for autosomal dominant hypoparathyroidism to chromosome 3q13. Pediatr Res 1994;36:414–417.

102. Lovlie R, Eiken H, Sorheim J, Boman H. The Ca^{2+}-sensing receptor gene PCAR1) mutation T151M in isolated autosomal dominant hypoparathyroidism. Hum Genet 1996;98:129–133.

103. Parma J, Sande JV, Swillens S, Tonacchera M, Dumont J, G GV. Somatic mutations causing consti-tutive activity of the thyrotropin receptor are a major cause of hyperfunctioning thyroid adenomas: Identification of additional mutations activating both the cyclic adenosine $3',5'$-monophosphate and inositol phosphate-Ca^{2+} cascades. Mol Endocrinol 1995;9:725–733.

104. Shenker A, Laue L, Kosugi S, Merendino JJ, Mineyshi T, Cutler GJ. A constitutively acti-vating mutation of the luteinizing hormone receptor in familial male precocious puberty. Nature 1993;65:652–654.

105. Nemeth E. Ca^{2+} receptor-dependent regulation of cellular function. News in Physiol Sci 1995;10:1–5.

106. Malgaroli A, Meldolesi J, Zambone-Zallone A, Teti A. Control of cytosolic free calcium in rat and chicken osteoclasts. The role of extracellular calcium and calcitonin. J Biol Chem 1989;264: 14,342–14,349.

107. Lundgren S, Hjalm G, Hellman P, Ek B, Juhlin C, Rastad J, Klareskog L, Akerstrom G, Rask L. A protein involved in calcium sensing of the human parathyroid and placental cytotrophoblast cells belongs to the LDL-receptor protein superfamily. Exp Cell Res 1994;212:344–350.

108. Saito A, Pietromonaco S, Loo AK-C, Farquhar M. Complete cloning and sequencing of rat gp330/"megalin," a distinctive member of the low density lipoprotein receptor gene family. Proc Natl Acad Sci USA 1994;91:9725–9729.

109. Zaidi M, Datta H, Patchell A, Moonga B, MacIntyre I. "Calcium-activated" intracellular calcium ele-vation: a novel mechanism of osteoclast regulation. Biochem Biophys Res Commun 1989;183: 1461–1465.

12

Constitutively Active PTH/PTHrP Receptors Cause Jansen's Metaphyseal Chondrodysplasia

Harald Jüppner, MD

CONTENTS

INTRODUCTION

Endocrine disorders are typically caused by excessive or insufficient production of an otherwise normal hormone. However, in recent years, several endocrine disorders were shown to be caused by other defects, i.e., mutations in peptide hormones, their cognate receptors, G proteins, or downstream effectors *(1)*. Although such defects are extremely uncommon and thus provide only a rare diagnostic challenge, their definition at the molecular level often provided important novel insights into the biological significance of the affected protein and/or its functional properties. This is illustrated by the discovery that Jansen's metaphyseal chondrodysplasia, a rare genetic disorder characterized by short-limbed dwarfism and severe hormone-independent hypercalcemia, is caused by activating mutations in the parathyroid hormone (PTH) PTH-related peptide (PTHrP) receptor. These findings are likely to have significant implications for understanding the biological importance of the PTH/PTHrP receptor in addition to its role in regulating mineral ion homeostasis.

From: *Contemporary Endocrinology: G Proteins, Receptors, and Disease*
Edited by: A. M. Spiegel Humana Press Inc., Totowa, NJ

BIOLOGICAL IMPORTANCE OF PTH AND PTHRP

PTH, through its actions on bone and kidney, has long been known to be the most important peptide hormone for maintaining the circulating concentrations of calcium and phosphorus within narrow limits (2). The more recently isolated PTHrP was first discovered as the factor responsible for the humoral hypercalcemia of malignancy syndrome (3–6). In patients with certain malignancies, e.g., squamous cell carcinoma and renal cell carcinoma, its excessive release into the blood circulation causes changes in mineral ion homeostasis that are similar to those in patients with primary hyper-parathyroidism (3,6–8). With regard to mineral ion homeostasis, PTHrP thus has bio-logical properties that are similar to or indistinguishable from those of PTH (9–13). However, in contrast to PTH, which is produced by the parathyroid glands (2) and prob-ably in small amounts by the hypothalamus (14), PTHrP is not only found in tumors, but also in a large variety of normal fetal and adult tissues (6). This finding and its expression during early embryonic development (15,16) suggested that PTHrP serves other, yet incompletely understood roles in mammalian biology that are unrelated to the regulation of calcium and phosphorus homeostasis.

A SINGLE G-PROTEIN-COUPLED RECEPTOR MEDIATES THE ACTIONS OF TWO HORMONES

The amino-terminal portion of PTH binds to and activates two closely related G-protein-coupled receptors, the PTH/PTHrP receptor (17–19) and the recently isolated PTH2-receptor, which serves yet unknown biological functions (20). In contrast to PTH, the amino-terminal portion of native PTHrP acts only through the PTH/PTHrP receptor (20,21). This common receptor thus mediates the functions of two distinct ligands, PTH and PTHrP, which presumably have different biological roles.

The PTH/PTHrP receptor belongs to a distinct family of receptors, which unlike most other G-protein-coupled receptors, typically activate at least two effector systems, adenylyl cyclase and phospholipase C (17–19). Members of this presumably ancient receptor family were isolated from multiple mammalian species, as well as from birds, insects, and nema-todes (22–24). All these receptors share, in addition to their common structure with seven membrane-spanning helices, about 50 strictly conserved amino acid residues, including eight extracellular cysteines that appear to be functionally important (Fig. 1) (25). PTH/PTHrP receptor homologs that were recently isolated from frogs and fishes, share more than 70% amino acid sequence identity with the mammalian receptor homologs (26,27). Owing to this evolutionary conservation and its expression in early embryonic development (28), it appeared likely that the PTH/PTHrP receptor serves additional functions, which are distinct from its role in mineral ion homeostasis.

PTH/PTHRP RECEPTORS ARE ABUNDANTLY EXPRESSED IN BONE, KIDNEY, AND GROWTH PLATE CHONDROCYTES

Similar to the wide expression of PTHrP (6), mRNA transcripts encoding the PTH/PTHrP receptor are not only found in kidney and bone, but also in a large variety of fetal and adult tissues (29–31), including the growth plates (32,33). In kidney and bone, PTH/PTHrP receptors mediate the endocrine actions of PTH, and thus increase the urinary excretion of phosphorus and cAMP, maintain the circulating blood calcium

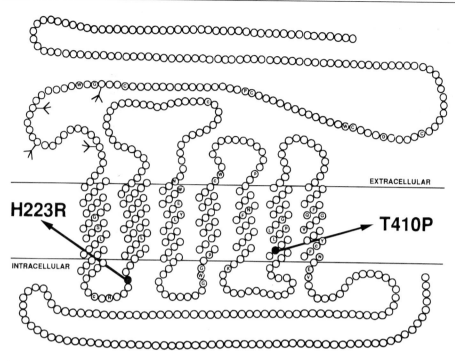

Fig. 1. Schematic presentation of the human PTH/PTHrP receptor. Residues that are strictly conserved in all mammalian members of this family of G-protein-coupled receptors are shown; two amino acid substitutions that were identified in patients with Jansen's metaphyseal chondrodysplasia are indicated *(40–42)*.

levels, and enhance bone turnover *(2)*. In addition to their expression in these tissues, which are important for mineral ion homeostasis, abundant concentrations of the PTH/PTHrP receptors are also found in growth plate chondrocytes where they are thought to mediate the autocrine/paracrine actions of PTHrP, which is now known to have an important role in bone elongation *(22)*.

Evidence for this previously unrecognized function of PTHrP, which is mediated by the PTH/PTHrP receptor, first became apparent when PTHrP-ablated mice showed a perinatally lethal phenotype with severely impaired bone formation *(34)*. In these animals, bones that are formed through an endochondral process undergo premature ossification, and thus remain short, indicating that PTHrP has a major role in bone elongation by inhibiting the differentiation of proliferating chondrocytes into hypertrophic chondrocytes *(33,35)*. Recent findings show that this chondrocyte differentiation process involves several autocrine/paracrine factors, including PTHrP and Indian hedgehog (Ihh) *(22)*. Ihh belongs to the hedgehog family of secreted proteins that are known to provide in several species key signals for embryonic patterning. Its mRNA is expressed in prehypertrophic and hypertrophic chondrocytes, and it is thought to interact, directly or indirectly, with receptors that are likely to share some homology of two recently isolated *Drosophila* proteins. These proteins are patched, a large glycoprotein that is predicted to contain 12 membrane-spanning domains, and smoothened, most likely a G- (G$_i$) protein-coupled receptor with 7 membrane-spanning helices *(36,37)*. Ihh increases the expression of PTHrP in the periarticular perichondrium, which subsequently activates

PTH/PTHrP receptors in prehypertrophic chondrocytes and thus inhibits their differentiation into hypertrophic chondrocytes (22). Consistent with this signaling pathway, bone explants from PTH/PTHrP receptor-ablated mice, but not those from normal littermates, show no suppression of hypertrophic differentiation when cultured in the presence of either PTHrP or sonic hedgehog (Shh) (which has in vitro properties that are indistinguishable from those of Ihh) (38). Consequently, animals that lack both alleles encoding the PTH/PTHrP receptor have a similar skeletal phenotype as PTHrP-ablated animals (38), which furthermore confirms that the PTH/PTHrP receptor mediates the effects of PTHrP on endochondral bone formation.

ACTIVATING PTH/PTHRP RECEPTOR MUTATIONS IN JANSEN'S METAPHYSEAL CHONDRODYSPLASIA

These advances in understanding the biological importance of the PTH/PTHrP receptor for the bone formation process were essential for determining the molecular defect in Jansen's metaphyseal chondrodysplasia. This rare genetic disorder, which is characterized by short-limbed dwarfism secondary to abnormal growth plate development and by severe PTH- and PTHrP-independent hypercalcemia, was first described in 1934 (39). However, because of the involvement of multiple organ systems, this interesting metabolic disorder of growth and mineral ion homeostasis had remained enigmatic.

PTH/PTHrP receptors are abundantly expressed in bone, kidney, and growth plates (29–33), i.e., in those tissues that contribute most significantly to the metabolic and phenotypic abnormalities in Jansen's disease. Genomic DNA from several affected patients was therefore screened for activating PTH/PTHrP receptor mutations, since a PTH- and PTHrP-independent stimulation of effectors downstream of the common PTH/PTHrP receptor would have provided a plausible genetic explanation for the abnormalities in mineral ion homeostasis and growth plate development.

Thus far, two different heterozygous PTH/PTHrP receptor mutations were identified in the genomic DNA of six unrelated patients with Jansen's disease (40–42) (Fig. 1). Both mutations are located close to or at the cytoplasmic surface of the PTH/PTHrP receptor, and are thought to affect, directly or indirectly, the interaction with stimulatory G proteins. The H223R mutation, which changes a conserved histidine residue at the junction between the first intracellular loop and the second membrane-spanning domain to arginine, was identified in the genomic DNA of five patients with Jansen's disease, but not in the DNA of their healthy parents and siblings, and its presence was furthermore excluded in the genomic DNA of healthy controls (40–42). In one family, an affected child and her affected mother both had the same receptor mutation (41), confirming that the disease is inherited in an autosomal-dominant fashion, as proposed previously (43–45). The H223R mutation, which is caused by an adenine-to-guanine transition, is so far the most frequent cause of the disease, and it appears to occur irrespective of the ethnic background (42).

The second PTH/PTHrP receptor mutation (T410P), caused by an adenine-to-cytosine transversion, which changes a conserved threonine to proline, was identified in only one patient with the disease (41). The mutated amino acid residue is predicted to be located in the sixth membrane-spanning helix close to the third intracellular loop, and is thus at a location similar to that of activating mutations in other G-protein-coupled receptors (46–51).

FUNCTIONAL PROPERTIES OF CONSTITUTIVELY ACTIVE PTH/PTHRP RECEPTORS

When expressed in COS-7 cells, PTH/PTHrP receptors with either the H223R or the T410P mutation showed constitutive, agonist-independent accumulation of cAMP (Fig. 2), yet no measurable increase in basal inositol trisphosphate. In comparison to cells expressing the wild-type PTH/PTHrP receptor, intracellular cAMP levels in cells transfected with mutant receptors were four- to eight-fold higher, despite considerably lower levels of cell-surface expression *(40,41,52)*. Consistent with findings in other G-protein-coupled receptors *(46,47,53,54)*, both constitutively active PTH/PTHrP receptor mutants displayed an increased binding affinity for agonists, i.e. [Nle^{8,18}, Tyr^{34}]bPTH(1-34)amide and [Tyr^{36}]PTHrP(1-34)amide bound two- to five-fold more tightly to receptors with either the H223R or the T410P mutation than to the wild-type PTH/PTHrP receptor *(40,41,52)*.

Interestingly, truncated PTH and PTHrP analogs, previously developed as potent antagonists of PTH action *(55–58)*, are inverse agonists when tested with either of the two constitutively active PTH/PTHrP receptor mutants *(52)*. Increasing concentrations of [D-Trp^{12}, Tyr^{34}]bPTH(7-34)amide or [Leu^{11}, D-Trp^{12}]PTHrP(7-34)amide dose-dependently inhibited the constitutive formation of cAMP by up to approx 50% (Fig. 3). This effect appears to be dependent on D-Trp^{12}, since similarly truncated PTH and PTHrP analogs with the native glycine at position 12 lacked inverse agonist activity. However, it remains uncertain whether D-Trp^{12} *per se* is an important determinant of inverse agonism, or whether the D-amino acid simply enhances the potency of analogs with otherwise weaker receptor binding affinity. The identification of peptide analogs with inverse agonist activity could lead to the development of nonpeptide compounds with inverse agonist properties, which may provide pharmacological approaches for the treatment of Jansen's disease and possibly other disorders caused by activating mutations in other G-protein-coupled receptors *(49,51,59,60)*.

IN VIVO PROPERTIES OF CONSTITUTIVELY ACTIVE PTH/PTHRP RECEPTORS

The constitutive accumulation of cAMP by PTH/PTHrP receptors with the H223R or the T410P mutation reached approximately one-forth of the second messenger concentrations typically obtained with wild-type receptors that are challenged with maximal stimulatory concentrations of either PTH or PTHrP (Fig. 2). The ligand-independent accumulation of cAMP by the mutant, constitutively active PTH/PTHrP receptors was therefore similar to that obtained with wild-type receptors stimulated with approx 0.1 nM PTH or PTHrP. Similar or higher ligand concentrations are typically detected in the circulation of patients with primary hyperparathyroidism or with the humoral hypercalcemia of malignancy syndrome, respectively *(7,8)*. The degree of constitutive PTH/PTHrP receptor activation that is induced by the H223R or the T410P mutation, therefore, appears to be sufficient to explain in Jansen's disease the changes in mineral ion homeostasis and bone turnover. In fact, patients with either nonprogressive primary hyperparathyroidism or Jansen's disease have comparable levels of tubular calcium reabsorption, phosphate excretion, and cAMP excretion, and biochemical and histological evidence shows an equivalent increase in bone turnover for both disorders

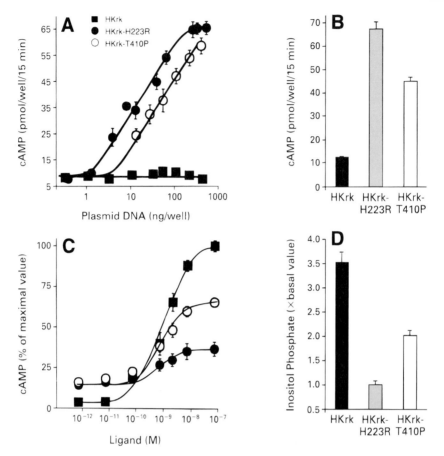

Fig. 2. Functional properties of wild-type (HKrk) and mutant PTH/PTHrP receptors (HKrk-H223R and HKrk-T410P) that are transiently expressed in COS-7 cells. Basal cAMP accumulation of COS-7 cells that express increasing concentrations of wild-type or mutant PTH/PTHrP receptors (**A**), basal (**B**) and PTH-stimulated (**C**) cAMP accumulation, and PTH-stimulated inositol phosphate accumulation (**D**) using COS-7 cells expressing maximal concentrations of wild-type or mutant PTH/PTHrP receptors. (■), Wild-type human PTH/PTHrP receptor, HKrk (●), HKrk-H223R (○), HKrk-T410P. Reprinted from ref. *41* with permission.

(61). The changes in bone- and kidney-specific functions are thus indistinguishable from those in primary hyperparathyroidism, and therefore explain the well-established changes in serum calcium and phosphate homeostasis in Jansen's disease *(62–67)* (Fig. 4).

The expression of constitutively active PTH/PTHrP receptors in prehypertrophic chondrocytes would also provide a plausible explanation for the skeletal changes in Jansen's disease *(68)*. At birth, patients with Jansen's disease usually present with one or several dysmorphic features, and radiological studies at this age usually show metaphyseal changes in long bones that are reminiscent of vitamin D-deficient rickets, i.e., widening, fraying, and cupping. However, distinct from the findings in rickets, metatarsals and metacarpals are also involved, whereas the calvaria and the base of the skull show increased density. Enlarged joints, prominent supraorbital ridges, and fronto-nasal hyperplasia become obvious in childhood. Radiological studies during this period typically show metaphyseal changes with patches of partially calcified cartilage

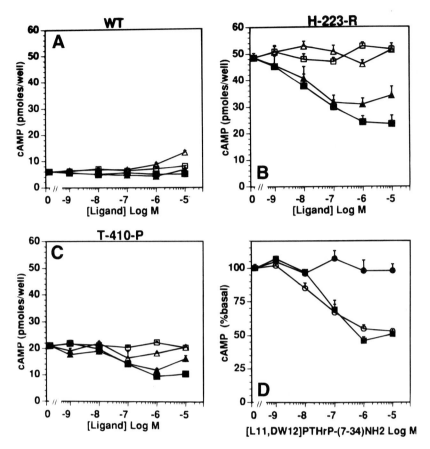

Fig. 3. Constitutive cAMP accumulation of COS-7 cells expressing wild-type (HKrk) or mutant (HKrk-H223R and HKrk-T410P) PTH/PTHrP receptors is partially reversed by PTH or PTHrP analogs. Effect of [D-Trp^{12}, Tyr^{34}]bPTH(7-34)amide (▲), [Leu^{11}, D-Trp^{12}]PTHrP(7-34)amide (■), [Nle^{8,18}, Tyr^{34}]bPTH(7-34)amide (△), or PTHrP(7-34)amide (□) is shown with COS-7 cells expressing the wild-type PTH/PTHrP receptor (**A**), HKrk-H223R (**B**), or HKrk-T410P (**C**). In panel **D** the data generated with [Leu^{11}, D-Trp^{12}]PTHrP(7-34)amide were replotted as percent of basal cAMP accumulation; (●), wild-type PTH/PTHrP receptor; (■), HKrk-H223R; or (○) HKrk-T410P. Reprinted from ref. *51* with permission.

that protrude into the diaphyses; these changes gradually resolve after pubertal development. Histological data show wide, irregular masses of abnormal, protruding cartilage, a lack of the regular columnar architecture of the maturing cartilage cells, and a severe delay in endochondral ossification of the metaphysis *(45,62–67,69–71)*.

Like the changes in mineral ion homeostasis, these abnormalities in endochondral bone formation are most likely caused by constitutively active PTH/PTHrP receptors, which are abundantly expressed in prehypertrophic growth plate chondrocytes *(32,33,38)*. During the normal bone formation process, PTHrP (which is synthesized in the perichondrium and the subarticular cartilage) activates PTH/PTHrP receptors that are expressed in prehypertrophic chondrocytes. This delays the differentiation of these cells into hypertrophic chondrocytes and their subsequent replacement by bone-forming osteoblasts *(22,38)*. The inhibitory activity of PTHrP thus allows the bone elongation

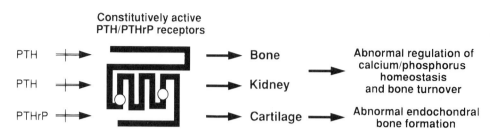

Fig. 4. Endocrine/metabolic consequences that are owing to the expression of constitutively active PTH/PTHrP receptors in kidney, bone, and growth plate cartilage.

process to proceed until full growth potential is reached at the end of puberty, and growth plates undergo mineralization.

In mice, this tightly regulated chondrocyte differentiation process can be disrupted through different genetic manipulations, and results in the abnormal elongation of all those bones that are formed through an endochondral process. For example, the growth plates of mice, in which the genes encoding PTHrP or the PTH/PTHrP receptor are ablated, show an accelerated differentiation into hypertrophic chondrocytes, which results in premature ossification of all growth plates and therefore short bones *(34,38)*. Dwarfed animals are also generated when overexpressing PTHrP in proliferating growth plate chondrocytes *(72,73)*. These animals, in which PTHrP expression is under the control of the type II collagen promotor, show histological growth plate changes that resemble those seen in patients with Jansen's disease *(69)*, in particular, a severe delay in the metaphyseal mineralization process. The overexpression of PTHrP in proliferating chondrocytes thus appears to have similar consequences as the expression of constitutively active PTH/PTHrP receptors in prehypertrophic chondrocytes, the normal target cells of PTHrP action in the growth plate (Fig. 4). In mice, both the ablation of the PTHrP gene and the targeted overexpression of PTHrP result in shortened bones and, thus, dwarfism. Skeletal changes similar to those in mice that overexpress PTHrP in the growth plate are also found in patients with Jansen's disease. The apparent paradox that lack of PTH/PTHrP receptor activation and expression of constitutively active PTH/PTHrP receptors result in short bones requires additional studies to clarify further the role of PTHrP and its receptor in chondrocyte proliferation, differentiation, and apoptosis.

IMPLICATIONS FOR THE PATHOPHYSIOLOGICAL ROLE OF PTH/PTHRP RECEPTORS IN OTHER DISORDERS

The presented findings may have considerable implications for the understanding of other endocrine disorders of mineral ion homeostasis, i.e., pseudohypoparathyroidism type Ib (PHP-Ib) and other forms of end-organ resistance toward PTH (and presumably PTHrP) that lack $G\alpha_s$ mutations and are consequently not associated with other endocrine deficiencies. In Jansen's disease, constitutively activate PTH/PTHrP receptors affect calcium/phosphorus homeostasis and chondrocyte differentiation, and subsequently bone elongation. Inactivating PTH/PTHrP receptor mutations should, therefore, result at least when both receptor alleles are affected *(38)*, in hypocalcemia owing to resistance toward PTH in kidney and bone, and in skeletal changes owing to resistance toward PTHrP in the growth plates such skeletal changes may be similar to those observed in Albright hereditary osteodystrophy *(74)*. Consistent with these considerations, inactivating mutations in the PTH/PTHrP receptor were excluded for patients with PHP-Ib *(75–77)* who present with hypocalcemia owing to resistance toward PTH, but lack skeletal abnormalities and are therefore unlikely to have resistance toward PTHrP.

REFERENCES

1. Spiegel AM. Mutations in G proteins and G protein-coupled receptors in endocrine disease. J Clin Endocrinol Metab 1996;81:2434–2442.
2. Kronenberg HM, Bringhurst FR, Nussbaum S, Jüppner H, Abou-Samra AB, Segre GV, Potts JT Jr. Parathyroid hormone: Biosynthesis, secretion, chemistry, and action. In: Mundy GR, Martin TJ, eds. Handbook of Experimental Pharmacology: Physiology and Pharmacology of Bone. Springer-Verlag, Heidelberg, Germany, 1993, pp. 185–201.
3. Stewart AF, Horst R, Deftos LJ, Cadman EC, Lang R, Broadus AE: Biochemical evaluation of patients with cancer-associated hypercalcemia. Evidence for humoral and non-humoral groups. N Engl J Med 1980;303:1377–1381.
4. Strewler GJ, Stern PH, Jacobs JW, Eveloff J, Klein RF, Leung SC, Rosenblatt M, Nissenson RA. Parathyroid hormone-like protein from human renal carcinoma cells. Structural and functional homology with parathyroid hormone. J Clin Invest 1987;80:1803–1807.
5. Martin JT, Moseley JM, Gillespie MT. Parathyroid hormone-related protein: biochemistry and molecular biology. Crit Rev Biochem Mol Biol 1991;26:377–395.
6. Broadus AE, Stewart AF. Parathyroid hormone-related protein: Structure, processing, and physiological actions. In: Bilzikian JP, Levine MA, Marcus R. eds. The Parathyroids, Basic and Clinical Concepts. Raven, New York, 1994, pp. 259–294.
7. Burtis WJ, Brady TG, Orloff JJ, Ersbak JB, Warrell RP, Olsen BR, Mitnick ME, Broadus AE, Stewart AF. Immunochemical characterization of circulating parathyroid hormone related protein in patients with humoral hypercalcemia of cancer. N Engl J Med 1990;322:1106–1112.
8. Segre GV, Potts JT Jr. Differential diagnosis of hypercalcemia. In: DeGroot LJ, ed. Endocrinology. Saunders, Philadelphia, 1995, pp. 1075–1093.
9. Jüppner H, Abou-Samra AB, Uneno S, Gu WX, Potts JT Jr, Segre GV. The parathyroid hormone-like peptide associated with humoral hypercalcemia of malignancy and parathyroid hormone bind to the same receptor on the plasma membrane of ROS 17/2.8 cells. J Biol Chem 1988;263:8557–8560.
10. Shigeno C, Yamamoto I, Kitamura N, Noda T, Lee K, Sone T, Shiomi K, Ohtaka A, Fujii N, Yajima H, Konish J. Interaction of human parathyroid hormone-related peptide with parathyroid hormone receptors in clonal rat osteosarcoma cells. J Biol Chem 1988;34:18,369–18,377.
11. Orloff JJ, Wu TL, Stewart AF. Parathyroid hormone-like proteins: biochemical responses and receptor interactions. Endocr Rev 1989;10:476–495.
12. Fraher LJ, Hodsman AB, Jonas K, Saunders D, Rose CI, Henderson JE, Hendy GN, Goltzman D. A comparison of the in vivo biochemical responses to exogenous parathyroid hormone-(1-34) [PTH-(1-34)] and PTH-related peptide-(1-34) in man. J Clin Endocrinol Metab 1992;75:417–423.
13. Everhart-Caye M, Inzucchi SE, Guinness-Henry J, Mitnick MA, Stewart AF. Parathyroid hormone (PTH)-related protein(1-36) is equipotent to PTH(1-34) in humans. J Clin Endocrinol Metab 1996;81:199–208.
14. Nutley MT, Parimi SA, Harvey S. Sequence analysis of hypothalamic parathyroid hormone messenger ribonucleic acid. Endocrinology 1995;136:5600–5607.
15. Senior PV, Heath DA, Beck F. Expression of parathyroid hormone-related protein mRNA in the rat before birth: demonstration by hybridization histochemistry. Mol Endocrinol 1991;6:281–290.
16. van de Stolpe A, Karperien M, Löwik CWGM, Jüppner H, Abou-Samra AB, Segre GV, de Laat SW, Defize LHK. Parathyroid hormone-related peptide as an endogenous inducer of parietal endoderm differentiation. J Cell Biol 1993;120:235–243.
17. Jüppner H, Abou-Samra AB, Freeman MW, Kong XF, Schipani E, Richards J, Kolakowski LF Jr, Hock J, Potts JT Jr, Kronenberg HM, Segre GV. A G protein-linked receptor for parathyroid hormone and parathyroid hormone-related peptide. Science 1991;254:1024–1026.

18. Abou-Samra AB, Jüppner H, Force T, Freeman MW, Kong XF, Schipani E, Urena P, Richards J, Bonventre JV, Potts JT Jr, Kronenberg HM, Segre GV. Expression cloning of a common receptor for parathyroid hormone and parathyroid hormone-related peptide from rat osteoblast-like cells: a single receptor stimulates intracellular accumulation of both cAMP and inositol triphosphates and increases intracellular free calcium. Proc Natl Acad Sci USA 1992;89:2732–2736.

19. Schipani E, Karga H, Karaplis AC, Potts JT Jr, Kronenberg HM, Segre GV, Abou-Samra AB, Jüppner H. Identical complementary deoxyribonucleic acids encode a human renal and bone parathyroid hormone (PTH)/PTH-related peptide receptor. Endocrinology 1993;132:2157–2165.

20. Usdin TB, Gruber C, Bonner TI. Identification and functional expression of a receptor selectively recognizing parathyroid hormone, the PTH2 receptor. J Biol Chem 1995;270:15,455–15,458.

21. Gardella TJ, Luck MD, Jensen GS, Usdin TB, Jüppner H. Converting parathyroid hormone-related peptide (PTHrP) into a potent PTH-2 receptor agonist. J Biol Chem 1996;271:19,888–19,893.

22. Vortkamp A, Lee K, Lanske B, Segre GV, Kronenberg HM, Tabin CJ. Regulation of rate of cartilage differentiation by Indian hedgehog and PTH-related protein. Science 1996;273:613–622.

23. Reagan JD. Expression cloning of an insect diuretic hormone receptor. A member of the calcitonin/secretin receptor family. J Biol Chem 1994;269:9–12.

24. Sulston J, Du Z, Thomas K, Wilson R, Hillier L, Staden R, Halloran N, Green P, Thierry-Mieg J, Qiu L, Dear S, Coulson A, Craxton M, Durbin RK, Berks M, Metzstein M, Hawkins T, Inscough RA, Waterston R. The *C. elegans* genome sequencing project: a beginning. Nature 1992;356:37–41.

25. Jüppner H. Molecular cloning and characterization of a parathyroid hormone (PTH)/PTH-related peptide (PTHrP) receptor: a member of an ancient family of G protein-coupled receptors. Curr Opinion Nephrol Hypertens 1994;3:371–378.

26. Bergwitz C, Klein P, Jüppner H. Molecular cloning of complementary DNAs encoding the *Xenopus laevis* (Daudin) PTH/PTHrP receptor. The Comparative Endocrinology of Calcium Regulation. In: Drake C, Dark J, Caple I, Flik G, eds. Journal of Endocrinology Ltd., Bristol, 1996, pp. 97–102.

27. Rubin DA, Bergwitz C, Zon LI, Jüppner H. Cloning of receptors for parathyroid hormone (PTH) and PTH-related protein (PTHRP) in the zebrafish (Danio rerio). J Bone Miner Res 1996;11 (Suppl 1):M483.

28. Karperien M, van Dijk TB, Hoeijmakers T, Cremers F, Abou-Samra AB, Boonstra J, de Laat SW, Defize LHK. Expression pattern of parathyroid hormone/parathyroid hormone related peptide receptor mRNA in mouse postimplantation embryos indicates involvement in multiple developmental processes. Mech Dev 1994;47:29–42.

29. Urena P, Kong XF, Abou-Samra AB, Jüppner H, Kronenberg HM, Potts JT Jr., Segre GV. Parathyroid hormone (PTH)/PTH-related peptide (PTHrP) receptor mRNA are widely distributed in rat tissues. Endocrinology 1993;133:617–623.

30. Tian J, Smorgorzewski M, Kedes L, Massry SG. Parathyroid hormone-parathyroid hormone related protein receptor messenger RNA is present in many tissues besides the kidney. Am J Nephrol 1993;13:210–213.

31. Lee K, Brown D, Urena P, Ardaillou N, Ardaillou R, Deeds J, Segre GV. Localization of parathyroid hormone/parathyroid hormone-related peptide receptor mRNA in kidney. Am. J. Physiol. 1996;270: F186–F191.

32. Lee K, Deeds JD, Chiba S, Un-no M, Bond AT, Segre GV. Parathyroid hormone induces sequential c-*fos* expression in bone cells in vivo: *In situ* localization of its receptor and c-*fos* messenger ribonucleic acids. Endocrinology 1994;134:441–450.

33. Lee K, Deeds JD, Segre GV. Expression of parathyroid hormone-related peptide and its receptor messenger ribonucleic acid during fetal development of rats. Endocrinology 1995;136:453–463.

34. Karaplis AC, Luz A, Glowacki J, Bronson R, Tybulewicz V, Kronenberg HM, Mulligan RC. Lethal skeletal dysplasia from targeted disruption of the parathyroid hormone-related peptide gene. Genes Dev 1994;8:277–289.

35. Amizuka N, Warshawsky H, Henderson JE, Goltzman D, Karaplis AC. Parathyroid hormone-related peptide-depleted mice show abnormal epiphyseal cartilage development and altered endochondreal bone formation. J. Cell. Biol. 1994;126:1611–1623.

36. Alcedo J, Ayzenzon M, von Ohlen T, Noll M, Hooper JE. The Drosophila smoothened gene encodes a seven-pass membrane protein, a putative receptor for the Hedgehog signal. Cell 1996;86:221–232.

37. van den Heuvel M, Ingham PW. smoothened encodes a receptor-like serpentine protein required for hedgehog signalling. Nature 1996;382:547–551.

38. Lanske B, Karaplis AC, Luz A, Vortkamp A, Pirro A, Karperien M, Defize LHK, Ho C, Mulligan RC, Abou-Samra AB, Jüppner H, Segre GV, Kronenberg HM. PTH/PTHrP receptor in early development and Indian hedgehog-regulated bone growth. Science 1996;273:663–666.

39. Jansen M. Über atypische Chondrodystrophie (Achondroplasie) und über eine noch nicht beschriebene angeborene Wachstumsstörung des Knochensystems: Metaphysäre Dysostosis. Zeitschr Orthop Chir 1934;61:253–286.

40. Schipani E, Kruse K, Jüppner H. A constitutively active mutant PTH-PTHrP receptor in Jansen-type metaphyseal chondrodysplasia. Science 1995;268:98–100.

41. Schipani E, Langman CB, Parfitt AM, Jensen GS, Kikuchi S, Kooh SW, Cole WG, Jüppner H. Constitutively activated receptors for parathyroid hormone and parathyroid hormone-related peptide in Jansen's metaphyseal chondrodysplasia. N Engl J Med 1996;335:708–714.

42. Yasuda T, Arakawa K, Minagawa M, Minamitani K, Niimi H. Jansen-type metaphyseal chondrodysplasia: examination of the PTH/PTHrP receptor by the RT-PCR. J Bone Miner Res 1996;11 (Suppl 1):S647.

43. Lenz WD. The First Conference on the Clinical Delineation of Birth Defects. 1969, no. 4, pp. 71, 72.

44. Holthusen W, Holt JF, Stoeckenius M. The skull in metaphyseal chondrodysplasia type Jansen. Pediatr Radiol 1975;3:137–144.

45. Charrow J, Poznanski AK. The Jansen type of metaphyseal chondrodysplasia: conformation of dominant inheritance and review of radiographic manifestations in the newborn and adult. J Med Genet 1984;18:321–327.

46. Kjelsberg MA, Cotecchia S, Ostrowski J, Caron MG, Lefkowitz RJ. Constitutive activation of the α1B-adrenergic receptor by all amino acid substitutions at a single site. J Biol Chem 1992; 1992:1430–1433.

47. Ren Q, Kurose H, Lefkowitz RJ, Cotecchia S. Constitutively active mutants of the α2-adrenergic receptor. J Biol Chem 1993;268:16,483–16,487.

48. Parma J, Duprez L, Van Sande J, Cochaux P, Gervy C, Mockel J, Dumont J, Vassart G. Somatic mutations in the thyrotropin receptor gene cause hyperfunctioning thyroid adenomas. Nature 1993; 365:649–651.

49. Parma J, van Sande J, Swillens S, Tonacchera M, Dumont J, Vassart G. Somatic mutations causing constitutive activity of the thyrotropin receptor are the major cause of hyperfunctioning thyroid adenomas: identification of additional mutations activating both the cyclic adenosine 3′, 5′-monophosphate and inositol phosphate-Ca^{2+} cascades. Mol Endocrinol 1995;9:725–733.

50. Anasti JN, Froehlinch J, Nelson LM, Flack MR. 50th Meeting of the American Fertility Society. Mutations of the third cytostolic loop of the human follicle stimulating hormone receptor (hFsH-R) Canter Constitutive Activation, San Antonio, 1994, pp. 0–145 (abstract).

51. Latronico AC, Anasti J, Arnhold IJP, Mendonca BB, Domenice S, Albano MC, Zachman K, Wajchenberg BL, Tsigos C. A novel mutation of the luteinizing hormone receptor gene causing male gonadotropin-independent precocious puberty. J Clin Endocrinol Metab 1995;80:2490–2494.

52. Gardella TJ, Luck MD, GS GSJ, Schipani E, Potts JT Jr, Jüppner H. Inverse agonism of amino-terminally truncated parathyroid hormone (PTH) and PTH-related peptide (PTHrP) analogs revealed with constitutively active mutant PTH/PTHrP receptors linked to Jansen's metaphyseal chondrodysplasia. Endocrinology 1996;137:3936–3941.

53. Samama P, Pei G, Costa T, Cotecchia S, Lefkowitz RJ. Negative antagonists promote an inactive conformation of the β2-adrenergic receptor. Mol Pharmacol 1994;45:390–394.

54. Spalding T, Burstein E, Brauner-Osborne H, Hill-Eubanks D, Brann M. Pharmacology of a constitutively active muscarinic receptor generated by random mutagenesis. J Pharmacol Exp Ther 1995;275:1274–1279.

55. Goldman ME, Chorev M, Reagan JE, Nutt RF, Levy JJ, Rosenblatt M. Evaluation of novel parathyroid hormone analogs using a bovine renal membrane receptor binding assay. Endocrinology 1988;123:1468–1475.

56. Chorev M, Goldman ME, McKee RL, Roubini E, Levy J, Gay T, Reagan JE, Fisher JE, Caporale LH, Golub EE, Caulfield MP, Nutt RF, Rosenblatt M. Modifications of position 12 in parathyroid hormone and parathyroid hormone related protein: Toward the design of highly potent antagonists. Biochemistry 1990;29:1580–1586.

57. Nutt RF, Caulfield MP, Levy JJ, Gibbons SW, Rosenblatt M, McKee RL. Removal of partial agonism from parathyroid hormone (PTH)-related protein-(7-34)NH$_2$ by substitution of PTH amino acids at positions 10 and 11. Endocrinology 1990;127:491–493.

58. McKee RL, Caulfield MP, Rosenblatt M. Treatment of bone-derived ROS 17/2.8 cells with dexamethasone and pertussis toxin enables detection of partial agonist activity for parathyroid hormone antagonists. Endocrinology 1990;127:76–82.

59. Shenker A, Laue L, Kosugi S, Merendino JJ Jr, Minegishi T, Cutler GB. A Constitutively activating mutation of the luteinizing hormone receptor in familial male precocious puberty. Nature 1993;365:652–654.

60. Pollak MR, Brown EM, Estep HL, McLaine PN, Kifor O, Park J, Hebert SC, Seidman CE, Seidman JG. Autosomal dominant hypocalcaemia caused by a Ca^{2+}-sensing receptor gene mutation. Nature Genet 1994;8:303–307.

61. Parfitt AM, Schipani E, Rao DS, Kupin W, Han Z-H, Jüppner H. Hypercalcemia due to constitutive activity of the PTH/PTHrP receptor. Comparison with primary hyperparathyroidism. J Clin Endocrinol Metab 1996.

62. De Haas WHD, De Boer W, Griffioen F. Metaphysial dysostosis. A late follow-up of the first reported case. J Bone Joint Surg 1969;51B:290–299.

63. Frame B, Poznanski AK. Conditions that may be confused with rickets. In: Pediatric Diseases Related to Calcium. DeLuca HF, Anast CS, eds., Elsevier, New York, 1980, pp. 269–289.

64. Rao DS, Frame B, Reynolds WA, Parfitt AM. Hypercalcemia in metaphyseal chondrodysplasia of Jansen (MCD): an enigma. In: Norman AW, Schaefer K, von Herrath D, Grigoleit HG, Coburn JW, DeLuca HF, Mawer EB, Suda T, eds. Vitamin D, Basic Research and Its Clinical Application. Walter de Gruyter, Berlin, 1979, pp. 1173–1176.

65. Silverthorn KG, Houston CS, Duncan BP. Murk Jansen's metaphyseal chondrodysplasia with long-term followup. Pediatr. Radiol. 1983;17:119–123.

66. Kessel D, Hall CM, Shaw DG. Two unusual cases of nephrocalcinosis in infancy. Pediatr. Radiol. 1992;22:470–471.

67. Kruse K, Schütz C. Calcium metabolism in the Jansen type of metaphyseal dysplasia. Eur J Pediatr 1993;152:912–915.

68. Jüppner H. Jansen's metaphyseal chondrodysplasia: A disorder due to a PTH/PTHrP receptor gene mutation. Trends Endocrinol. Metab. 1996;7:157–162.

69. Cameron JAP, Young WB, Sissons HA. Metaphysial dysostosis. Report of a case. J Bone Joint Surg 1954;36B:622–629.

70. Gram PB, Fleming JL, Frame B, Fine G. Metaphyseal chondrodysplasia of Jansen. J Bone Joint Surg 1959;41A:951–959.

71. Jaffe HL. Certain other anomalies of skeletal development. In: Metabolic, Degenerative, and Inflammatory Diseases of Bones and Joints. Lea and Feibiger, Philadelphia, 1972, pp. 222–226.

72. Weir E, Philbrick W, Neff L, Amling M, Baron R, Broadus A. Targeted overexpression of parathyroid hormone-related peptide in chondrocytes causes skeletal dysplasia and delayed osteogenesis. J Bone Miner Res 1995;10 (Suppl 1):S157.

73. Philbrick WM, Weir EC, Karaplis AC, Dreyer BE, Broadus AE. Rescue of the PTHrP-null mouse reveals multiple developmental defects. J Bone Miner Res 1996;11 (Suppl. 1):P268.

74. Levine MA, Aurbach GD. Pseudohypoparathyroidism. In: DeGroot LJ, ed. Endocrinology. Saunders, Philadelphia, 1989, pp. 1065–1079.

75. Schipani E, Weinstein LS, Bergwitz C, Iida-Klein A, Kong XF, Stuhrmann M, Kruse K, Whyte MP, Murray T, Schmidtke J, van Dop C, Brickman AS, Crawford JD, Potts JT Jr, Kronenberg HM, Abou-Samra AB, Segre GV, Jüppner H. Pseudohypoparathyroidism type Ib is not caused by mutations in the coding exons of the human parathyroid hormone (PTH)/PTH-related peptide receptor gene. J Clin Endocrinol Metab 1995;80:1611–1621.

76. Suarez F, Lebrun JJ, Lecossier D, Escoubet B, Coureau C, Silve C. Expression and modulation of the parathyroid hormone (PTH)/PTH-related peptide receptor messenger ribonucleic acid in skin fibroblasts from patients with type Ib pseudohypoparathyroidism. J Clin Endocrinol Metab 1995;80:965–970.

77. Fukumoto S, Suzawa M, Takeuchi Y, Nakayama K, Kodama Y, Ogata E, Matsumoto T. Absence of mutations in parathyroid hormone (PTH)/PTH-related protein receptor complementary deoxyribonucleic acid in patients with pseudohypoparathyroidism type Ib. J Clin Endocrinol Metab 1996;81:2554–2558.

13 Mutation of the Growth Hormone-Releasing Hormone Receptor in the *little* Mouse

Kelly E. Mayo, PHD, Venita I. DeAlmeida, MS, Kenneth C. Wu, BS, and Paul A. Godfrey, BS

CONTENTS

INTRODUCTION

Growth Hormone-Releasing Hormone (GHRH) and Growth Hormone (GH) Secretion

The peptide hormone GHRH is synthesized in and released from neurosecretory cells in the hypothalamic arcuate nuclei. GHRH acts on pituitary somatotroph cells to stimulate the synthesis and secretion of GH *(1–4)*. The actions of GHRH are opposed by those of somatostatin, a peptide hormone of hypothalamic origin that acts to suppress pituitary growth hormone secretion; together, GHRH and somatostatin are thought to be the predominant mediators of the neural control of GH production *(5,6)*. Although potent synthetic peptide and nonpeptide GH secretagogs have been identified *(7,8)* and a receptor that binds those compounds has been cloned *(9)*, no endogenous ligands that activate growth hormone secretion through this receptor have been identified.

An important role for GHRH in somatic growth has been suggested by clinical studies with tumors that produce GHRH *(3,4)* and by animal studies with transgenic mice that express ectopic GHRH *(10)*. In both models, excessive GHRH leads to pituitary somatotroph hyperplasia, GH hypersecretion, and excessive growth. Thus, in addition to its ability to regulate GH secretion, GHRH modulates the proliferation and/or differentiation of the pituitary somatotroph cells *(11)*.

GHRH belongs to a family of structurally related peptide hormones that includes glucagon, glucagon-like peptide-1 (GLP-1), vasoactive intestinal peptide (VIP), secretin,

From: *Contemporary Endocrinology: G Proteins, Receptors, and Disease*
Edited by: A. M. Spiegel, Humana Press Inc., Totowa, NJ

gastric inhibitory peptide (GIP), peptide with histidine as N terminus and isoleucine as C terminus (PHI), and pituitary adenylate cyclase activating peptide (PACAP) *(12)*. In addition to its expression in the brain, GHRH is produced in the placenta, where it may have paracrine functions or may contribute to fetal growth *(13,14)*, and in the gonads, where it may act as an autocrine or paracrine regulator of ovarian and testicular cell function *(15,16)*.

The Pituitary GHRH Receptor

Binding sites for GHRH have been found on pituitary cell membranes through the use of a variety of radiolabeled GHRH analogs *(17,18)*. GHRH stimulates adenylate cyclase, resulting in increased cyclic adenosine monophosphate (cAMP) production; this indicates that a stimulatory G protein is an intermediate in GHRH action *(19)*. In agreement with the notion that cAMP is an important second messenger for GHRH signaling, both GHRH and cAMP increase the proliferation of pituitary somatotroph cells, stimulate pituitary secretion of GH, and augment GH gene expression *(11,20)*. The pathway by which a GHRH-stimulated cAMP signal leads to increased GH synthesis most likely involves an activation of the transcription factor cAMP response element binding (CREB) by protein kinase A, and targeted expression of a dominant negative form of CREB in somatotrophs results in pituitary hypoplasia and dwarfism *(21)*. Activated CREB is proposed to stimulate expression of the gene for the pituitary-specific regulatory factor Pit-1 or GHF-1, which in turn activates transcription of the GH gene *(22)*.

The structure of the GHRH receptor has been determined by molecular cloning *(23–25)*, and this receptor has many of the conserved structural features of other characterized G-protein-coupled receptors. These features include the seven potential transmembrane domains that are the hallmark of this family, cysteine residues in the first and second extracellular loops that are believed to form a disulfide bond, a cysteine in the cytoplasmic tail that may be palmitoylated, one or more amino-terminal sites for N-linked glycosylation, potential phosphorylation sites in the third cytoplasmic loop, and numerous highly conserved residues within the membrane-spanning domains. The GHRH receptor is homologous to an emerging subfamily of G-protein-coupled receptors that includes the receptors for VIP, GLP-1, secretin, glucagon, GIP, PACAP, calcitonin, parathyroid hormone (PTH), and corticotropin releasing hormone (CRH) *(26–34)*. The GHRH receptor and related receptors have an unusually large amino-terminal domain that includes six conserved cysteine residues and is likely to be extracellular and to participate in ligand binding.

The little *Mouse Mutation*

The study of genetic mutations that cause aberrant growth in mice has provided substantial insight into the regulation of somatic growth. Figure 1 summarizes the characteristics of three mouse mutations that have been studied extensively as models of human growth hormone deficiency. The Snell dwarf mouse (*dw*) *(35)* was found to harbor a mutation in the gene encoding the pituitary-specific transcription factor Pit-1, resulting in a failure of Pit-1-expressing pituitary somatotroph, lactotroph, and thyrotroph cells to differentiate *(36)*. This led to the identification of similar Pit-1 mutations involved in pituitary disease in humans *(37)*. The Ames dwarf mouse (*df*) *(38)* has a pituitary phenotype very similar to that of the Snell dwarf, but the affected gene has not been identified. Both the *dw* and *df* mutations result in severe dwarfism, and the homozygous mutant mice are only one-quarter the size of unaffected animals.

Locus	Year	Chromosome Size		Characteristics	Mutation
Snell Dwarf (*dw*)	1929	16	1/4	Pituitary Hypoplasia, GH Deficiency No Somatotrophs, Lactotrophs, Thyrotrophs	Pit-1
Ames Dwarf (*df*)	1961	11	1/4	Pituitary Hypoplasia, GH Deficiency No Somatotrophs, Lactotrophs, Thyrotrophs	Unknown
Little (*lit*)	1976	6	1/2	Pituitary Hypoplasia, GH Deficiency Reduced Somatotrophs/Lactotrophs?	GHRH-R

Fig. 1. Characteristics of mouse mutations affecting GH secretion and somatic growth. References to the Snell and Ames dwarf mice and the *little* mouse are found in the text. Although *little* exhibits a clear loss of somatotroph cells, reports on the lactotroph cells are somewhat conflicting, and prolactin secretion appears to be nearly normal in these mice.

The *little* mouse *(39)* has been studied intensively as a model for human isolated growth hormone deficiency type 1B. Circulating GH levels and GH mRNA are substantially reduced in these mice, there are fewer pituitary somatotroph cells, and the cells that remain are sparsely granulated *(39–41)*. These mice are not as impaired in growth as are the *dw* or *df* mice and reach an adult size that is 50–60% of normal. Somatotroph cells from *little* mice do not release GH after GHRH treatment in culture but do secrete GH in response to cAMP or agents that elevate intracellular cAMP levels, suggesting that the defect in the *little* mouse is related to an inability of somatotrophs to bind to or respond to GHRH *(42)*. Studies from our laboratory *(43)* and others *(44)* have revealed that the *little* mouse harbors a mutation in the GHRH receptor gene, although the mechanisms by which this mutation leads to the dwarf phenotype have not been uncovered. This chapter presents our studies on an inactivating mutation in the GHRH receptor of the *little* mouse and discusses recent results from other laboratories indicating that similar mutations in the GHRH receptor are associated with human disease. Finally, we speculate on the potential involvement of activating mutations in the pituitary GHRH receptor in human growth disorders.

A MUTATION IN THE GHRH RECEPTOR OF THE *little* MOUSE

Chromosomal Mapping of the Mouse GHRH Receptor

As was described, substantial evidence indicated that the dwarfism observed in the *little* mouse results from a deficiency in some aspect of GHRH signal transduction. We had earlier cloned a cDNA for the mouse GHRH precursor protein *(45)* and used it as a probe to establish that the GHRH gene is on mouse chromosome 2 *(43)* and is therefore not a candidate for the *little* mutation on mouse chromosome 6. After the characterization of GHRH receptor cDNAs, we utilized a mouse probe to establish the chromosomal location of the mouse GHRH receptor gene, in collaboration with N. Jenkins and N. Copeland of the Frederick Cancer Research Institute (Frederick, MD *[43]*). Using interspecific backcross analysis, the GHRH receptor gene was localized to the central region of mouse chromosome 6, very close to the *little* mutation. The GHRH receptor locus is within a region syntenic with human chromosome 7, and the human gene was subsequently mapped to human chromosome 7p14 *(46)*. These findings indicated that the GHRH receptor was a likely candidate gene for the *little* mutation, and we therefore undertook molecular cloning experiments to test this hypothesis.

Identification of the little *Mouse Mutation*

GHRH receptor cDNAs were cloned from the pituitary glands of wild-type (+/+), heterozygous (+/*lit*), and mutant (*lit/lit*) mice provided by W. Beamer of the Jackson Laboratory (Bar Harbor, ME). DNA sequencing of many such clones identified a point mutation within the GHRH receptor coding region that changes an aspartic acid at amino acid position 60 of the protein to a glycine. The mutation was found in both pituitary cDNA clones and partial genomic DNA clones isolated using polymerase chain reaction (PCR) amplification with primers flanking the region of the mutation; it was represented in approximately half the clones from heterozygous mice.

Figure 2 shows the schematic structure of the 423 amino acid mouse GHRH receptor and indicates the location of the *little* mutation within the presumed extracellular domain of the protein. Aspartic acid 60 resides in a conserved domain of the receptor that includes several of the invariant cysteines characteristic of the GHRH receptor subfamily. Two potential sites for N-linked glycosylation are located nearby at residues 49 and 50. Aspartic acid 60 is conserved in the human and rat GHRH receptors.

Functional Consequences of the little *Mutation*

We predicted that the change in the GHRH receptor from aspartic acid 60 to glycine would lead to its functional inactivation, explaining the deficiency in GH secretion and growth observed in the *little* mouse. To test this, expression constructs for the wild-type and *little* mouse GHRH receptors were prepared and transfected into COS monkey kidney cells, after which we measured the ability of those cells to respond to GHRH. As shown in Fig. 3, cells expressing the wild-type receptor show a large, dose-dependent increase in intracellular cAMP levels after GHRH treatment, whereas cells expressing the *little* mouse receptor show no increase in cAMP accumulation. Both cell populations respond robustly to the direct adenylyl cyclase activator forskolin. Subsequent studies with clonal lines of HEK-293S human kidney cells that stably express the wild-type or mutant receptor forms have confirmed this loss of hormone binding and/or signal transduction by the *little* mouse GHRH receptor.

The inability of the *little* mutant GHRH receptor to mediate GHRH-stimulated cAMP accumulation suggests that the receptor is incapable of binding GHRH or is unable to transduce a signal effectively to the Gs protein. An additional possibility is that the mutant receptor is unstable, is rapidly degraded, or is not efficiently transported to the cell surface and therefore cannot interact with the ligand. To allow receptor protein amounts to be assessed independently of receptor GHRH binding or signaling properties, a peptide epitope from the influenza virus hemagglutinin protein (HA) was introduced into the carboxy-terminal cytoplasmic tail of the wild-type and *little* mouse GHRH receptors as well as the human GHRH receptor used as a control. The HA-tagged human GHRH receptor was found to bind GHRH and signal cAMP production in a manner similar to that of the untagged receptor, using a vaccinia virus–bacteriophage T7 polymerase transient expression system in HeLa cells *(47)*. As shown in Fig. 4, HA-tagged versions of the wild-type and *little* mouse GHRH receptors were found to be expressed at similar levels, using immunoprecipitation of metabolically labeled proteins, and to be appropriately localized to the cell surface, using indirect immunofluorescence. These

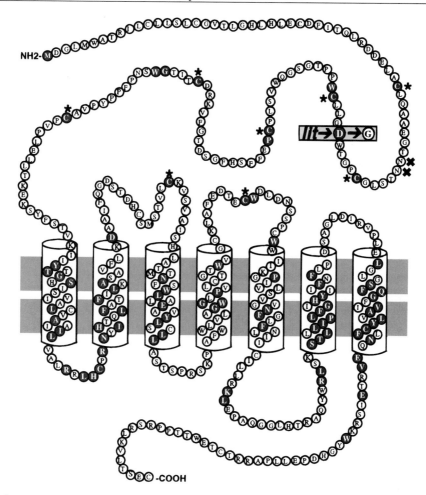

Fig. 2. Structure of the mouse GHRH receptor protein and the location of the *little* mutation. The amino acid sequence of the mouse GHRH receptor (423 amino acids) is shown in one-letter code. The seven potential membrane-spanning domains are shown as cylinders crossing the cell membrane. The circles that are shaded represent amino acids that are conserved completely in the related receptors for the hormones secretin, glucagon, GLP-1, GIP, VIP, and PACAP. The asterisks indicate eight conserved cysteine residues in the presumed extracellular domain of the receptor. The symbol ✖ designates the location of two consensus sites for N-linked glycosylation of the receptor protein. *lit* indicates aspartic acid at position 60, which is mutated to a glycine in the *little* mouse GHRH receptor.

results indicate that the activity rather than the expression of the GHRH receptor is deficient in the *little* mouse *(48)*.

In preliminary studies performed in collaboration with Gaylinn et al. *(49)*, it appeared that the *little* mutant GHRH receptor is unable to bind its ligand in that membranes from HEK-293S cells stably expressing the *little* GHRH receptor failed to bind radiolabeled mouse GHRH, whereas membranes from cells expressing the wild-type receptor exhibited high-affinity binding to this ligand. Thus, it appears likely that mutation of aspartic acid 60 results in a structural alteration of the GHRH receptor that renders it incapable of productive interaction with its ligand, GHRH.

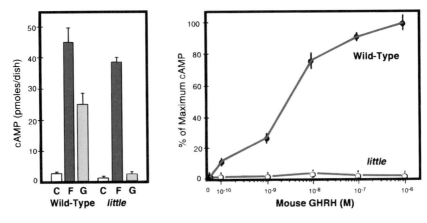

Fig. 3. Signal transduction by wild-type and *little* mutant mouse GHRH receptor proteins. The left panel shows intracellular cAMP levels after treatment of COS monkey kidney cells expressing the wild-type mouse GHRH receptor or the *little* mutant with control medium (C), forskolin at $10^{-5}\,M$ (F), or mouse GHRH at $10^{-7}\,M$ (G). The right panel shows a dose–response to mouse GHRH, measured as intracellular cAMP accumulation, for cells transfected with the wild-type or *little* mouse GHRH receptors. The responses observed with the *little* mutant receptors are at the background level observed in nontransfected COS cells. (Data adapted from ref. *43*.)

DISCUSSION

Mechanism of Receptor Inactivation in the little Mouse

These data indicate that the growth-deficient phenotype of the *little* mouse is caused by an inactivating mutation in the pituitary receptor for GHRH. The left panel of Fig. 5 summarizes current ideas about GHRH signaling in pituitary somatotroph cells and highlights steps that may be affected by the GHRH receptor mutation identified in the *little* mouse. Hormone binding (step 1), receptor signal transduction (step 2), and receptor synthesis, stability, or transport (step 3) are potential sites at which the mutation may lead to inactivation of GHRH receptor function. The precise mechanism by which alteration of aspartic acid 60 to glycine in this receptor leads to its inactivation is under investigation, but the results thus far indicate that hormone binding is the step most likely to be affected.

Interestingly, the aspartic acid that is altered in the *little* mutant receptor is absolutely conserved in all the receptors related to the GHRH receptor, including the ones that bind ligands related to GHRH (e.g., the secretin, glucagon, VIP, and PACAP receptors) as well as the ones that bind ligands unrelated to GHRH (such as the calcitonin, PTH, and CRH receptors). This conservation indicates that aspartic acid 60 plays a critical role in receptor function and further suggests that whatever the function of this residue is, it is unlikely to be involved in establishing the specificity of the GHRH receptor for its ligand. Consistent with this finding, site-directed mutation of the analogous aspartic acid residues in the related glucagon and VIP receptors abolishes their ability to bind these hormones *(50,51)*. Several laboratories have attempted to map hormone-binding determinants within this subfamily of receptors, and several studies indicate that the membrane-proximal part of the amino-terminal extracellular domain (downstream of the *little* mutation) and the first extracellular loop are particularly important *(52,53)*. Thus, aspartic acid 60 seems most likely to play a general structural role in the GHRH receptor and related receptors.

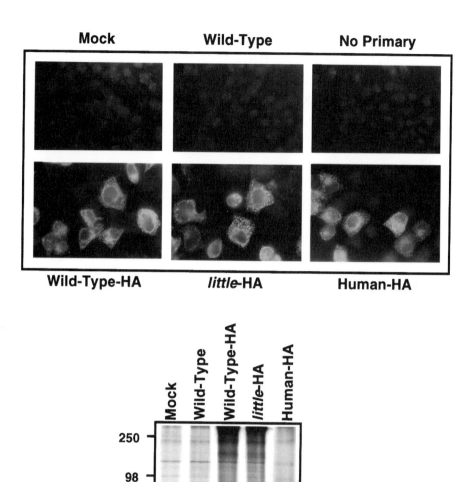

Fig. 4. Expression and localization of wild-type and *little* mutant mouse GHRH receptor proteins. The wild-type or *little* mutant mouse GHRH receptors, or the human GHRH receptor as a control, were tagged at the carboxy-terminals with a peptide epitope from the influenza virus hemagglutinin protein for subsequent detection, using a monoclonal antibody specific to this epitope. cDNA constructs were transiently expressed in HeLa T4 cells, using a vaccinia virus system *(47)*. The top panel shows the use of indirect immunofluorescence of permeabilized cells to localize the receptor proteins. Mock, wild-type, and no primary are all controls that are expected to be negative. The lower part of the panel shows a very similar cellular location of the wild-type and *little* mouse receptors as well as the human GHRH receptor. The protein is distributed both on the cell surface and intracellularly, with the latter presumably representing receptor protein being transported to the cell surface. The bottom panel shows immunoprecipitation to determine the relative amounts of the GHRH receptor proteins. The GHRH receptor protein migrates at approx 50 kDa. Approximately equivalent amounts of ^{35}S-cysteine/methionine-labeled receptor protein are detected in cells expressing the wild-type or *little* mutant mouse GHRH receptors or the human GHRH receptor.

Involvement of the GHRH Receptor in Somatotroph
Proliferation or Differentiation

GHRH is believed to be important for the proliferation or differentiation of pituitary somatotroph cells. In situations of GHRH excess, including ectopic secretion of GHRH by tumors in humans (3,4) and ectopic production of GHRH from transgenes in mice (10), pituitary somatotroph hyperplasia generally is observed. In addition, GHRH directly stimulates the proliferation of pituitary somatotroph cells in primary culture (11). This suggests that inactivation of the GHRH receptor in *little* mice will result in diminished proliferation of somatotroph cells, contributing to the observed diminution in growth hormone secretion.

In elegant developmental studies, Lin and coworkers (44) showed that in the fetal pituitary, on embryonic d 17.5, somatotroph numbers (assessed by GH and GHRH receptor mRNA expression) were indistinguishable between wild-type and *little* mice. However, in the mature pituitary, on postnatal d 60, there was a severe hypoplasia, reflecting a loss of somatotrophs from the *little* pituitary. The remaining somatotrophs were preferentially localized to the anterolateral aspects of the *little* pituitary, while few somatotrophs were found in the caudomedial portion of the gland. Lactotrophs were found to be evenly distributed throughout the *little* pituitary gland. Those investigators proposed a model for somatotroph proliferation that was based on these data, in which an initial population of GHRH-independent somatotroph stem cells found in the anterolateral aspect of the pituitary subsequently proliferated into the caudomedial portions of the gland in a GHRH-dependent fashion. In the *little* pituitary, the caudomedial proliferation of the somatotroph cells would not be expected to occur in the absence of a functional GHRH receptor, leaving a small population of somatotrophs in the anterolateral portions of the mature gland. This model is represented in the right panel of Fig. 5. Thus, it appears likely that mutation of the GHRH receptor in the *little* mouse affects both the population of somatotroph cells in the pituitary gland and the ability of individual somatotrophs to synthesize and secrete GH in response to GHRH.

Related Inactivating Mutations in the Human GHRH Receptor

The demonstration of an inactivating mutation in the GHRH receptor in the *little* mouse, a model for human isolated GH deficiency, suggested that similar alterations in receptor function may play a role in some human growth disorders. This has been shown to be the case, and two groups have reported mutations that truncate and inactivate the GHRH receptor in patients with severe growth hormone deficiency. Wajnrajch and coworkers (54) evaluated two children in a kindred with profound GH deficiency that did not have mutations in the GH gene and failed to produce GH in response to short-term or chronic stimulation with GHRH. These patients were considered to be candidates for a deficiency in GHRH receptor function and therefore were screened for mutations within the extracellular domain of the GHRH receptor. Both patients were found to be homozygous for a nonsense mutation, glutamate 72 to stop, that is near the site of the *little* mutation in the mouse receptor but predicts a severely truncated protein that lacks all seven of the potential membrane-spanning domains. These patients responded well to standard GH replacement therapy, as would be expected since the mutation is upstream of GH production. The GHRH receptor therefore joins an expanding list of mutations in G-protein-coupled receptors in human endocrine disease.

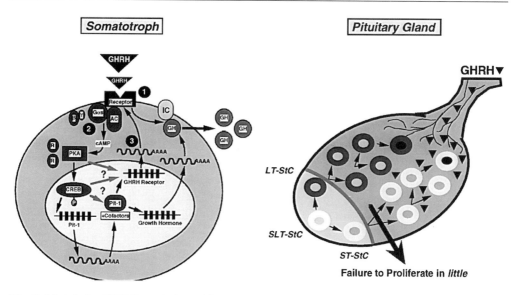

Fig. 5. Models for GHRH regulation of GH synthesis and secretion and proliferation by the pituitary somatotroph cell, illustrating potential defects in the *little* mutant mouse. The left diagram indicates a somatotroph cell in which GHRH interaction with the receptor leads to rapid GH secretion, most likely through the receptor-induced interaction of a G-protein with ion channels (IC) or through ion channel phosphorylation. Stimulation of adenylyl cyclase (AC) by the Gs-protein leads to increased intracellular cAMP accumulation and activation of the catalytic subunit of protein kinase A (PKA). PKA phosphorylates the CREB, resulting in CREB activation and enhanced transcription of the gene for Pit-1, a CREB target. Pit-1 is also subject to phosphorylation, although this may not affect its transcriptional activity. Pit-1 and accessory cofactors activate transcription of the growth hormone gene, resulting in increased growth hormone mRNA and protein. Pit-1 also stimulates transcription of the GHRH receptor gene, perhaps leading to increased GHRH receptors on the somatotroph cell *(24)*. The numbered circles indicate points at which this pathway may be disrupted in the *little* mouse somatotroph: ❶ GHRH receptor is unable to bind its hormone ligand, ❷ GHRH receptor is unable to productively couple to its G protein and stimulate adeylate cyclase activity, and ❸ GHRH receptor protein is unstable or is not correctly localized to the cell surface. The right diagram shows the responses of the developing pituitary gland to GHRH. SLT-StC indicates a somatotroph-lactotroph stem cell. It gives rise to lactotroph stem cells (LT-StC) and somatotroph stem cells (ST-StC) in the anterolateral region of the gland. The latter cells proliferate into the caudomedial portion of the gland in response to GHRH of hypothalamic origin, thus generating the pituitary's complement of somatotrophs. In the GHRH receptor-deficient *little* mouse, this GHRH-dependent proliferative step is proposed to be blocked. (Right diagram adapted from ref. *44*.)

In a second study reported in preliminary form, Maheshwari and coworkers *(55)* identified 18 individuals in a kindred with severe dwarfism and demonstrated linkage of this phenotype with the GHRH receptor gene on human chromosome 7p14. These individuals appear to have the same glutamate 72 to stop mutation described by Wajnrajch et al. *(54)*; it remains unclear whether these two mutations (the former in a Indian Moslem family and the latter in a Pakistani population) arose independently. It will be important to establish the prevalence of such mutations in the GHRH receptor in patients with severe GH deficiency and to determine the spectrum and phenotypes of the mutations that may occur. Such information should have practical applications in establishing appropriate hormone replacement therapy for such patients.

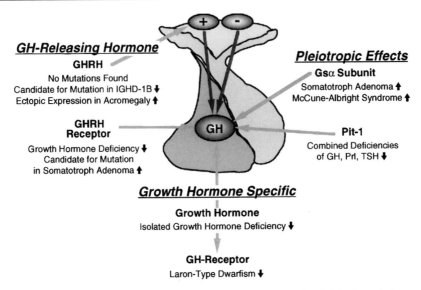

Fig. 6. Summary of the regulation of pituitary GH synthesis and secretion by the hypothalamic peptides GHRH and somatostatin. Genes that are known or speculated targets for mutation in diseases affecting GH production or action are indicated, along with brief comments. Mutations are classified as pleiotropic in nature, specific to growth hormone and its receptor, or involving the GHRH system. Mutations in all the genes shown, with the exception of GHRH, have been identified in human disease. An inactivating mutation of the GHRH receptor in growth hormone deficiency is the focus of this chapter. The arrows indicate either activating (↑) or inactivating (↓) mutations, effects, or predicted changes in function.

Potential for Activating Mutations in the GHRH Receptor

In addition to the established involvement of inactivating mutations in the GHRH receptor in GH deficiency, there is reason to assume that activating mutations in this receptor can be found in growth hormone excess and play a role in pituitary tumorigenesis. Nearly 40% of pituitary tumors from acromegalic patients have activating mutations in the stimulatory G-protein α-subunit to which the GHRH receptor is functionally coupled *(56)*. Furthermore, chronic activation of the GHRH receptor in transgenic mice that overexpress GHRH results in somatotroph hyperplasia and pituitary tumorigenesis *(10)*, and inhibition of the activity of a downstream effector of the GHRH pathway, the cAMP-responsive transcription factor CREB, in transgenic mice leads to somatotroph hypoplasia and dwarfism *(21)*.

These findings suggest that mutations of the GHRH receptor that mimic the activated state might similarly result in growth hormone excess, somatotroph hyperplasia, and possibly pituitary tumorigenesis. The many recent examples of activating mutations in related G-protein-coupled receptors in human disease discussed in this book provide ample precedents for the importance of such mutations. However, it must be noted that despite efforts in several laboratories to identify such activating mutations in the GHRH receptor in human disease, none have been reported.

Summary of Mutations Affecting the GH Axis

Diseases or disorders of the GH axis in both the mouse and the human have revealed much about the normal mechanisms of GH gene regulation, GH secretion, and GH action on target cells. Some of the genes that are known or speculated targets for mutation in disorders of the GH axis are illustrated in Fig. 6. Several different genetic lesions lead to pleiotropic effects within the pituitary gland that involve alterations in GH secretion and in growth. These include activating mutations in the stimulatory G-protein α-subunit in pituitary adenoma *(56)* or McCune-Albright syndrome *(57)* and inactivating mutations in the transcription factor Pit-1/GHF-1 in the Snell and Jackson dwarf mice *(36)* and in human panhypopituitary dwarfism *(37)*. Other mutations directly target the GH structural gene *(58)*, or the GH receptor/binding protein in the case of Laron-type dwarfism *(59)*.

Despite the finding that ectopic production of GHRH by tumors is causative in rare cases of acromegaly *(3,4)* and evidence that many GH–deficient children respond to treatment with exogenous GHRH *(60)*, suggesting that they produce insufficient amounts of GHRH, no mutations in the GHRH gene have been identified. Thus, the GHRH receptor has become an important candidate gene for mutation in disorders of GH secretion. The studies described here in the *little* mouse and recent complementary studies in humans *(54,55)* reveal that the GHRH receptor is a target for mutation in severe forms of GH deficiency and support an important role for GHRH in the regulation of somatic growth in vertebrate organisms. Further investigation will be necessary to establish the frequency of mutations affecting this key signaling step and to determine whether activating mutations in the GHRH receptor exist. In addition, the newly characterized receptor for the synthetic GH secretagogs *(9)* provides another candidate gene for mutations that affect the GH axis.

It is an exciting time for basic and clinical investigations into the molecular and cellular mechanisms that modulate pituitary somatotroph differentiation, GH secretion, and growth regulation. The lessons learned from mouse mutations affecting growth, such as the Snell dwarf and *little*, have been translated rapidly to the clinic so that similar mutations in the human population can be identified. The current challenge is to use this wealth of new genetic information to enhance the diagnosis and treatment of syndromes of GH deficiency and GH excess.

REFERENCES

1. Guillemin R, Brazeau P, Bohlen P, Esch F, Ling N, Wehrenberg WB. Growth hormone-releasing factor from a human pancreatic tumor that caused acromegaly. Science 1982;218:585–587.
2. Rivier J, Spiess J, Thorner M, Vale W. Characterization of a growth hormone-releasing factor from a human pancreatic islet tumour. Nature 1982;300:276–278.
3. Frohman L, Jansson J-O. Growth hormone-releasing hormone. Endocr Rev 1982;7:223–253.
4. Cronin MJ, Thorner MO. Growth hormone-releasing hormone: basic physiology and clinical implications. In: DeGroot LJ, ed. Endocrinology. Saunders, Philadelphia, 1994, pp. 280–302.
5. Brazeau P, Vale W, Burgus R, Ling N, Butcher M, Rivier J, Guillemin R. Hypothalamic polypeptide that inhibits the secretion of immunoreactive pituitary growth hormone. Science 1973;179:77–79.
6. Tannenbaum GS, Ling N. The interrelationship of growth hormone (GH)-releasing factor and somatostatin in generation of the ultradian rhythm of GH secretion. Endocrinology 1984;115:1952–1957.
7. Bowers CY, Momany FA, Reynolds GA, Hong A. On the in vitro and in vivo activity of a new synthetic hexapeptide that acts on the pituitary to specifically release growth hormone. Endocrinology 1984;114:1537–1545.
8. Smith RG, Cheng K, Schoen WR, Pong S-S, Hickey G, Jacks T, Butler B, Chan WW-S, Chaung L-YP, Judith F, Taylor J, Wyvratt MJ, Fisher MH. A nonpeptidyl growth hormone secretagogue. Science 1993;260:1640–1643.
9. Howard AD, Feighner SD, Cully DF, et al. A receptor in pituitary and hypothalamus that functions in growth hormone release. Science 1996;273:974–977.
10. Mayo KE, Hammer RE, Swanson LW, Brinster RL, Rosenfeld MG, Evans RM. Dramatic pituitary hyperplasia in transgenic mice expressing a human growth hormone-releasing factor gene. Mol Endocrinol 1988;2:606–612.
11. Billestrup N, Swanson LW, Vale W. Growth hormone-releasing factor stimulates proliferation of somatotrophs in vitro. Proc Natl Acad Sci USA 1986;83:6854–6857.

12. Campbell RM, Scanes CG. Evolution of the growth hormone-releasing factor (GRF) family of peptides. Growth Regul 1992;2:175–191.

13. Margioris AN, Brockman G, Bohler HLC, Grino M, Vamvakopoulos N, Chrousos GP. Expression and localization of growth hormone-releasing hormone messenger ribonucleic acid in the rat placenta: in vitro secretion and regulation of its peptide product. Endocrinology 1990;126:151–158.

14. Endo H, Yamaguchi M, Farnsworth R, Thordarson G, Ogren L, Alonso FJ, Sakata M, Hirota K, Talamantes F. Mouse placental cells secrete immunoreactive growth hormone-releasing factor. Biol Reprod 1994;51:1206–1212.

15. Bagnato A, Moretti C, Ohnishi J, Frajese G, Catt K. Expression of the growth hormone-releasing hormone gene and its peptide product in the rat ovary. Endocrinology 1992;130:1097–1102.

16. Srivastava CH, Breyer PR, Rothrock JK, Peredo MJ, Pescovitz OH. A new target for growth hormone releasing-hormone in the rat: the Sertoli cell. Endocrinology 1993;133:1478–1481.

17. Seifert H, Perrin M, Rivier J, Vale W. Binding sites for growth hormone releasing factor on rat anterior pituitary cells. Nature 1985;313:487–489.

18. Velicelebi G, Santacroce T, Harpold M. Specific binding of human pancreatic growth hormone releasing factor (1-40-OH) to bovine anterior pituitaries. Biochem Biophys Res Commun 1985;126:33–39.

19. Labrie F, Gagne B, Lefevre G. Growth hormone-releasing factor stimulates adenylate cyclase activity in the anterior pituitary gland. Life Sci 1983;33:2229–2233.

20. Barinaga M, Yamamoto G, Rivier C, Vale W, Evans R, Rosenfeld MG. Transcriptional regulation of growth hormone gene expression by growth hormone-releasing factor. Nature 1983;306:84,85.

21. Struthers RS, Vale WW, Arias C, Sawchenko PE, Montminy MR. Somatotroph hypoplasia and dwarfism in transgenic mice expressing a non-phosphorylatable CREB mutant. Nature 1991;350:622–624.

22. McCormick A, Brady H, Theill LE, Karin M. Regulation of the pituitary-specific homeobox gene *GHF1* by cell-autonomous and environmental cues. Nature 1990;345:829–832.

23. Mayo KE. Molecular cloning and expression of a pituitary-specific receptor for growth hormone-releasing hormone. Mol Endocrinol 1992;6:1734–1744.

24. Lin C, Lin S-C, Chang C-P, Rosenfeld MG. Pit-1 dependent expression of the receptor for growth hormone releasing factor mediates pituitary cell growth. Nature 1992;360:765–768.

25. Gaylinn BD, Harrison JK, Zysk JR, Lyons CE, Lynch KR, Thorner MO. Molecular cloning and expression of a human anterior pituitary receptor for growth hormone-releasing hormone. Mol Endocrinol 1993;7:77–84.

26. Lin H, Tonja H, Flannery M, Aruffo A, Kaji E, Gorn A, Kolakowski LJ, Lodish HF, Goldring S. Expression cloning of an adenylate cyclase-coupled calcitonin receptor. Science 1991;254:1022–1024.

27. Juppner H, Abdul-Badi A-S, Freeman M, Kong X, Schipani E, Richards J, Kolakowski LJ, Hock J, Potts JT, Kronenberg H, Segre G. A G-protein-linked receptor for parathyroid hormone and parathyroid hormone-related peptide. Science 1991;254:1024–1026.

28. Ishihara T, Nakamura S, Toro Y, Takahashi T, Takahashi K, Nagata S. Molecular cloning and expression of a cDNA encoding the secretin receptor. EMBO J 1991;10:1635–1641.

29. Ishihara T, Shigemoto R, Mori K, Takahashi K, Nagata S. Functional expression and tissue distribution of a novel receptor for vasoactive intestinal peptide. Neuron 1992;8:811–819.

30. Thorens, B. Expression cloning of the pancreatic β cell receptor for the gluco-incretin hormone glucagon-like peptide 1. Proc Natl Acad Sci USA 1992;89:8641–8645.

31. Jelinek L, Lok S, Rosenberg GB, Smith RA, Grant FJ, Biggs S, Bensch PA, Kuijer JL, Sheppard PO, Sprecher CA, O'Hara PJ, Foster D, Walker KM, Chen LHJ, McKernan PA, Kindsvogel W. Expression cloning and signaling properties of the rat glucagon receptor. Science 1993;259:1614–1616.

32. Usdan TB, Mezey E, Button DC, Brownstein MJ, Bonner TI. Gastric inhibitory polypeptide receptor, a member of the secretin-vasoactive intestinal peptide receptor family, is widely distributed in peripheral organs and the brain. J Biol Chem 1993;133:2861–2870.

33. Pisegna JP, Wank SA. Molecular cloning and functional expression of the pituitary adenylate cyclase activating polypeptide type I receptor. Proc Natl Acad Sci USA 1993;90:6345–6349.

34. Perrin MH, Donaldson CJ, Chen R, Lewis KA, Vale WW. Cloning and functional expression of a rat brain corticotropin releasing factor (CRF) receptor. Endocrinology 1993;133:3058–3061.

35. Snell, GD. "Dwarf," a new Mendelian recessive character of the house mouse. Proc Natl Acad Sci USA 1929;15:733, 734.

36. Li S, Crenshaw EB III, Rawson EJ, Simmons DM, Swanson LW, Rosenfeld MG. Dwarf locus mutants lacking three pituitary cell types result from mutations in the POU-domain gene pit-1. Nature 1990;347:528–533.

37. Radovick S, Nations M, Du Y, Berg LA, Weintraub BD, Wondisford FE. A mutation in the POU-homeodomain of pit-1 responsible for combined pituitary hormone deficiency. Science 1992;257: 1115–1118.
38. Schaible R, Gowen JW. A new dwarf mouse. Genetics 1961;46:896.
39. Eicher EM, Beamer WG. Inherited ateliotic dwarfism in mice: characterization of the mutation, little, on chromosome 6. J Hered 1976;67:87–91.
40. Cheng TC, Beamer WG, Phillips JA III, Bartke A, Mallonee RL, Dowling C. Etiology of growth hormone deficiency in *little*, Ames, and Snell dwarf mice. Endocrinology 1983;133:1669–1678.
41. Wilson DB, Wyatt DP, Gadler RM, Baker CA. Quantitative aspects of growth hormone cell maturation in the normal and *little* mutant mouse. Acta Anat (Basel) 1988;131:150–155.
42. Jansson J-O, Downs TR, Beamer WG, Frohman LA. Receptor-associated resistance to growth hormone-releasing factor in dwarf "little" mice. Science 1986;232:511, 512.
43. Godfrey PG, Rahal JO, Beamer WG, Copeland NG, Jenkins NA, Mayo KE. GHRH receptor of *little* mice contains a missense mutation in the extracellular domain that disrupts receptor function. Nat Genet 1993;4:227–232.
44. Lin S-C, Lin CR, Gukovsky I, Lusis AJ, Sawchenko PE, Rosenfeld MG. Molecular basis of the *little* mouse phenotype and implications for cell-type specific growth. Nature 1993;364:208–213.
45. Suhr ST, Rahal JO, Mayo KE. Mouse growth hormone-releasing hormone: precursor structure and expression in brain and placenta. Mol Endocrinol 1989;3:1693–1700.
46. Gaylinn BD, von Kap-Herr C, Golden WL, Thorner MO. Assignment of the human growth hormone-releasing hormone receptor gene (GHRHR) to 7p14 by in situ hybridization. Genomics 1994;19:193–195.
47. Fuerst TR, Niles EG, Studier FW, Moss B. Eukaryotic transient expression system based on recombinant vaccinia virus that synthesizes bacteriophage T7 RNA polymerase. Proc Natl Acad Sci USA 1986;83:8122–8126.
48. DeAlmeida VI, Wu KC, Mayo KE. Expression and activity of wild-type, mutant and chimeric GHRH receptors. 10th Int Congress Endocrinol San Francisco, Abst 1996; P1-617.
49. Gaylinn BD, Lyons CE, Mayo KE, Thorner MO. The *little* mouse GHRH receptor mutation (D60 to G) prevents GHRH binding. 76th Ann Meet Endocrine Soc Anaheim, CA, Abstract 1994; 667.
50. Carruthers CJL, Unson CG, Kim HN, Sakmar TP. Synthesis and expression of a gene for the rat glucagon receptor: replacement of an aspartic acid in the extracellular domain prevents glucagon binding. J Biol Chem 1994;269:29,321–29,328.
51. Couvineua A, Gaudin P, Maoret JJ, Rouyer FC, Nicole P, Laburthe M. Highly conserved aspartate 68, tryptophan 73 and glycine 109 in the N-terminal extracellular domain of the human VIP receptor are essential for its ability to bind VIP. Biochem Biophys Res Commun 1995;206:246–252.
52. Holtmann MH, Hadac EM, Miller LJ. Critical contributions of amino-terminal extracellular domains on agonist binding and activation of secretin and vasoactive intestinal peptide receptors. J Biol Chem 1995;270:14,394–14,398.
53. Buggy JJ, Livingston JN, Rabin DU, Yoo-Warren H. Glucagon-glucagon-like peptide I receptor chimeras reveal domains that determine specificity of glucagon binding. J Biol Chem 1995;270:7474–7478.
54. Wajnrajch MP, Gertner JM, Harbison MD, Chua SC Jr, Leibel RL. Nonsense mutation in the human growth hormone-releasing hormone receptor causes growth failure analogous to the *little* mouse. Nat Genet 1996;12:88–90.
55. Maheshwari H, Silverman BL, Dupuis J, Baumann G. Dwarfism of Sindh: a novel form of familial isolated GH deficiency linked to the locus for the GH releasing hormone receptor. 10th International Congress of Endocrinology, San Francisco, Abstract 1996; OR46-2.
56. Landis C, Masters S, Spada A, Pace A, Bourne H, Vallar L. GTPase inhibiting mutations activate the α chain of Gs and stimulate adenyl cyclase in human pituitary tumours. Nature 1989;340:692–696.
57. Weinstein LS, Shenker A, Gejman PV, Merino MJ, Friedman E, Spiegel AM. Activating mutations of the stimulatory G protein in the McCune-Albright syndrome. N Engl J Med 1991;325:1688–1695.
58. Phillips JA, Cogan JD. Molecular basis of familial human growth hormone deficiency. J Clin Endocrinol Metab 1994;78:11–16.
59. Amselem S, Duquesnoy P, Duriez B, Dastot F, Sobrier ML, Valleix S, Goossens M. Spectrum of growth hormone receptor mutations and associated haplotypes in Laron syndrome. Hum Mol Genet 1993;2:355–359.
60. Thorner MO, Rogol AD, Blizzard RM, Klingensmith GJ, Najjar J, Misra R, Burr I, Chao G, Martha P, McDonald J, et al. Acceleration of growth rate in growth hormone-deficient children treated with human growth hormone-releasing hormone. Pediatr Res 1988;24:145–151.

14 Functional Variants of the MSH Receptor (MC1-R), *Agouti*, and Their Effects on Mammalian Pigmentation

Dongsi Lu, PhD, Carrie Haskell-Luevano, PhD, Dag Inge Vage, PhD, and Roger D. Cone, PhD

Contents

ROLE OF THE MC1-R IN MAMMALIAN PIGMENTATION

The melanocyte-stimulating hormone (MSH) receptor, recently renamed the MC1-R, is a seven transmembrane domain receptor in the rhodopsin superfamily that plays an important role in the regulation of mammalian pigmentation. No diseases and in fact no pigmentation phenotypes in humans have been definitively linked to this receptor. Nevertheless, the study of the MC1-R has introduced at least two novel paradigms to the G-protein signaling field: functionally variant receptors *(1)* and endogenous receptor antagonists *(2)*. To elaborate on these findings, it is first necessary to review briefly mammalian pigmentation and the role of the MC1-R in its regulation.

The Melanocyte

The complex biopolymer known as melanin is the key determinant of mammalian pigmentation. Melanin in skin and hair is produced by neural crest-derived melanocytes, which migrate from the neural crest to populate the epidermis and hair follicles early during gestation. The melanocytes act as unicellular exocrine glands, since melanin is secreted via specialized endoplasmic reticulum (ER)-derived vesicles known as melanosomes. The absorption of melanin by surrounding keratinocytes or by the growing hair shaft is what causes the pigmentation of hair and skin.

From: *Contemporary Endocrinology: G Proteins, Receptors, and Disease*
Edited by: A. M. Spiegel, Humana Press Inc., Totowa, NJ

Genetics has long played an important role in the study of pigmentation and melanocyte function. Since the beginning of animal husbandry, humans have bred animals for the retention of identifiable traits, and pigmentation has, naturally, been one of the most common traits analyzed. In the mouse, an animal long bred both by hobbyists and scientists alike, there are now more than 60 genes identified that affect pigmentation (for reviews, *see* refs. *3–5*). Classically, these have been divided into three *(6)*, and more recently six *(5)* categories of genes, affecting:

1. Melanocyte development and migration (*steel, piebald*);
2. Melanocyte gene expression (*microphthalmia*);
3. Melanocyte morphology (*dilute, leaden*);
4. Melanosome structure and function (*silver, pink-eyed dilution*);
5. Melanogenic enymes (*albino, brown, slaty*); and
6. Regulators of melanogenesis (*extension, agouti, mahogany, mahoganoid, umbrous*).

The MC1-R, encoded by the *extension* locus *(1)*, falls into this last category and is the focus of this chapter.

Biochemistry of Melanin Synthesis

The complex melanin polymers synthesized by the melanocyte can be divided into two major categories, the sulfur-containing yellow-red pheomelanins, and the brown-black eumelanins (Fig. 1). The synthesis of both classes is completely dependent on the rate-limiting enzyme, tyrosinase, which catalyzes two steps in the conversion of tyrosine to the common precursor dopaquinone. Albinism, or the absence of any melanin pigment, results when tyrosinase activity is lacking. DOPAquinone can spontaneously form high-mol-wt melanins, although many enzymatic activities are also known to catalyze reactions downstream from the formation of DOPAquinone. For example, tyrosinase also has dihydroxyindole (DHI) oxidase activity, specifically required for the synthesis of black eumelanins.

Less is known about the synthesis of phaeomelanins, and no enzymes specific to this pathway have yet been identified. The only requirements that are understood for phaeomelanin synthesis are tyrosinase and a thiol donor for the conversion of DOPAquinone to cysteinylDOPA. It is likely that there are multiple enzymes operating along this branch of the melanin synthetic pathway given the diversity of pigment seen in animals lacking eumelanin—from the red coat of the Irish Setter to the cream or bright yellow colors of the Labrador Retriever, to the orange of the calico cat.

In addition to tyrosinase, three other melanogenic enzymes are known, DHICA oxidase (tyrosinase-related protein, TRP1), DOPAchrome tautomerase (TRP 2), and DHICA polymerase (Pmel17). The TRP1 and TRP2 proteins are highly related to tyrosinase, and are encoded by the pigmentation loci *brown (7)* and *slaty (8)*. Pmel 17 has some limited homology to tyrosinase, and maps to a pigmentation locus known as *silver (9)*. Less is known regarding the enzymatic activities of this protein. All three enzymes appear to be primarily involved in eumelanogenesis, and as their associated genetic names imply, these enzymes are modulatory of eumelanin synthesis.

The Eumelanin/Phaeomelanin Switch

The switch regulating the mode of melanin synthesis seems to be linked to the rate-limiting enzyme tyrosinase. The level of tyrosinase expression is significantly lower

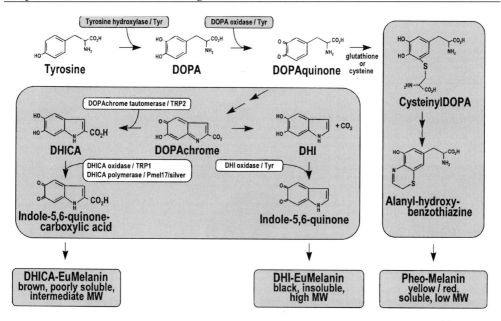

Fig. 1. The melanogenic pathway. Characterized enzymes are indicated, followed by the genetic locus encoding the enzyme. Figure kindly provided by Vincent Hearing (National Institutes of Health).

during phaeomelanogenesis vs eumelanogenesis *(10,11)*, and stimulation of tyrosinase with a variety of treatments leads to eumelanogenesis *(12,13)*. Thus, low basal levels of tyrosinase lead to default synthesis of phaeomelanin, whereas higher levels lead to eumelanin production; the mechanism by which substrate is routed along one pathway or another on the basis of the levels of expression of the common rate-limiting enzyme is not understood. Other enzymes involved specifically in eumelanogenesis, TRP1, TRP2, and Pmel 17, are undetectable in phaeomelanic hair bulbs *(14)*. Tyrosinase, in turn, is regulated both transcriptionally *(15,16)*, and posttranslationally *(17,18)* by cAMP. The primary hormonal stimulator of tyrosinase is α-melanocyte-stimulating hormone, which potently elevates intracellular cyclic adenosine monophosphate (cAMP) in the melanocyte via its $G\alpha_s$-coupled receptor, the MC1-R *(19)*.

Genetic investigations of pigmentation in the mouse (for review, *see* refs. *3* and *5*) and a large number of other mammalian species (for review, *see* ref. *6*) have led to the identification primarily of two loci specifically involved in regulation of the eumelanin/phaeomelanin switch, *agouti* and *extension*. (Fig. 2). These loci have diametrically opposed actions. Recessive *extension* alleles result in phaeomelanization, or yellow-red coat colors, and dominant alleles result in the "extension" of dark black across the coat of the animal; dominant *agouti* alleles cause yellow-red coats, whereas homozygosity for null alleles causes dark black coat colors. As mentioned, the *extension* locus encodes the MC1-R, whereas cloning of *agouti* demonstrated the locus to encode a 108 amino acid secreted peptide *(22,23)*, subsequently demonstrated to be a high-affinity antagonist of the MC1-R *(2)*. *Extension* alleles act within the hair follicle melanocyte to regulate the eumelanin/phaeomelanin switch *(24–26)*, whereas the *agouti* gene product is made by the surrounding hair follicle cells to regulate the switch both temporally and spatially *(27,28)*. The wild-type allele of *agouti* induces a temporary supression of

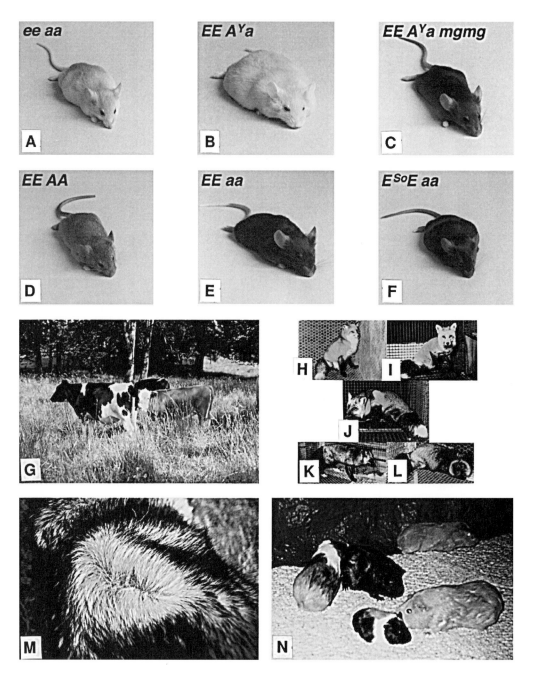

Fig. 2. Mammalian *extension* and *agouti* phenotypes. **(A–F)** Phenotypic effects of *agouti*, *extension*, and *mahogany* genes in the C57B1/6J mouse. When homozygous, *mahogany* suppresses both the coat color and obesity phenotypes of the dominant A^y allele of *agouti (20)*. **(G)** Dominant black (E^D) and recessive red (*ee*) coat colors seen in Holstein and Hereford cattle. **(H–L)** Coat colors resulting from the nonepistatic interaction of *extension* and *agouti* in the fox, *V. vulpes*. In order, animals are the Red (*EEAA*), Smoky Red (*EEAa*), Gold Cross (*EE^AAA*), Silver Cross (*EE^AAa*), and Silver fox (*EEaa*, E^AEaa, E^AE^Aaa, E^AE^AAa, or E^AE^AAA). **(M)** My dog, Coda. She is not pure-bred, but has a marked agouti banding pattern indicative of the wild-type A allele. **(N)** Black (*E*), red (*ee*), and tricolor (e^p) coat patterns in the guinea pig, *(20) Cavia porcellus*. Portions **(H–L)** of this figure reprinted with permission from *Nature Genetics (21)*.

eumelanin synthesis during hair growth to produce the subterminal phaeomelanin band resulting in the "*agouti*" pigmentation pattern seen in most mammalian coats.

Structure and Function of the MC1-R

α-Melanocyte-stimulating hormone and other proopiomelanocortin (POMC)-derived melanotropic peptides stimulate eumelanogenesis by binding to a single class of membrane receptor of approx 45 kDa found specifically on the surface of the melanocyte *(29,30)*. Cloning of the murine and human MC1-Rs demonstrated that this receptor is a member of the large superfamily of seven membrane-spanning receptors *(29–32)*. MC1-R sequences are now known from the fox *(21)*, cow *(33,34)*, chicken *(35)*, sheep (D. I. V., unpublished), and panther (R. D. Cone, unpublished) as well (Fig. 3). The MC1 receptor also shares 39–61% amino acid identity with a family of G-protein-coupled receptors that all bind melanocortin peptides. This family includes the MC2-R adreno-corticotropic hormone receptor [ACTH-R]) *(31)*, MC3-R *(36,37)*, MC4-R *(38,39)*, and MC5-R *(40–44)*. The MC1-R and related melanocortin receptors do not appear to be closely related to any other particular G-protein-coupled receptors, although an initial alignment study suggested some distant relationship with the cannabinoid receptors *(31)*.

The MC1-R is somewhat unusual from a structural point of view in that hydrophobicity analysis suggests the absence of the second extracellular loop. Furthermore, the disulfide bond present in many G-protein-coupled receptors (GPCRs) between the first and second extracellular loops *(45,46)* is absent owing to the loss of the relevant cysteines residues. A structural model of the MC1-R, based on:

1. Primary sequence;
2. Naturally occuring functional variants;
3. Studies of the α-MSH pharmacophore; and
4. In vitro mutagenesis studies

is described in structure of MC1-R.

An extensive body of work exists describing the pharmacological properties of the MC1-R, and has been reviewed elsewhere *(47,48)*. A key component for recognition of the MC1-R by a peptide ligand is the core pharmacophore His-Phe-Arg-Trp. The MC1-Rs bind most melanocortin peptides containing this pharmacophore, but generally do not recognize γ-MSH-derived peptides cleaved from the amino-terminal portion of the POMC precursor. There can be significant pharmacological variation in the MC1-R from species to species. For example, the relative preference for α-MSH over ACTH, a 39 amino acid peptide containing α-MSH$_{1-13}$ at its amino-terminus, varies widely. ACTH and α-MSH are equipotent at the human MC1-R *(49–51)*, whereas α-MSH is fivefold more potent in activation of the mouse MC1-R (Fig. 4) and 1000-fold more potent in activation of the MC1-R from *Rana pipiens* and *Anolis carolinensis (48,52)*.

It is interesting to speculate that the increase in ACTH sensitivity of the human MC1-R may be owing to the altered biology of the processing of ACTH to α-MSH in humans. In most mammals, ACTH is known to be processed to α-MSH in the intermediate lobe of the pituitary, from where it is then secreted. Humans lack this division of the pituitary and, hence, have undectable levels of circulating α-MSH in the serum. Of course, this highlights the troublesome issue of the source of melanotropic peptide involved in the regulation of melanogenesis in dermal and follicular melanocytes.

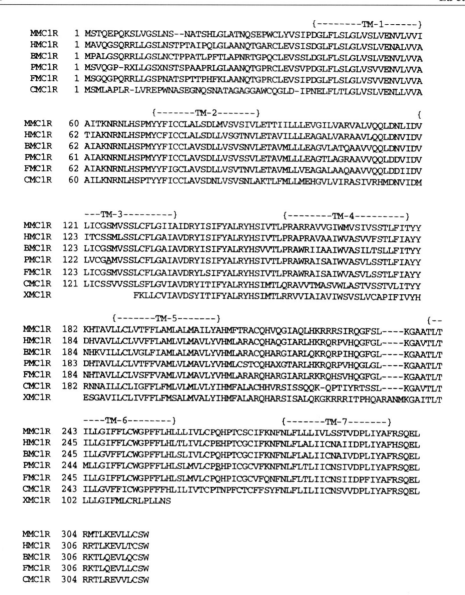

Fig. 3. Alignment of known MC1-R sequences. Amino acid sequences are from the mouse, human, bovine, fox, and chicken receptors (references indicated in the text), or from *Xenopus laevis* and *P. pardus* (R. D. C., unpublished).

High circulating melanotropins clearly induce euMmelanogenesis. Injection of α-MSH into mice induces the synthesis of dark black hair *(24,25)*, whereas injection of α-MSH in humans results in eumelanization, or tanning, of the skin *(53,54)*. Furthermore, elevation of endogenous circulating ACTH in endocrine disorders, such as Cushing's or Addison's disease, can often result in hyperpigmentation *(55)*. Despite the fact that high circulating melanotropins induce eumelanogenesis in skin and hair, it has been clearly demonstrated that the pituitary is unneccesary for maintenance of eumelanogenesis. For example, hypophysectomy in the mouse does not affect resynthesis of the dark black coat in the C57B1/6J mouse *(25)*. POMC expression has now been demonstrated in a

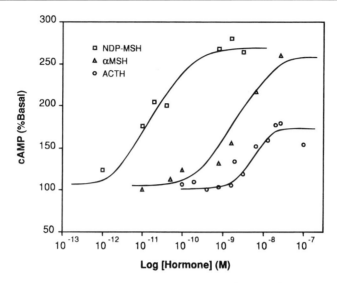

Fig. 4. Pharmacology of the murine MC1-R. Curves show the increase in intracellular concentration of cAMP in cells transfected with an MSH-R expression vector in response to increasing concentrations of the three melanotropic peptides NDP-α-MSH, αMSH, and ACTH. The abscissa indicates the concentration of each hormone, and the ordinate indicates the percent of basal concentrations of intracellular cAMP measured after each treatment. Points indicate the mean of duplicate incubations, and the standard error did not exceed 15% for any data points. Human 293 cells were transfected with vector alone, or vector plus the 2.1-kb MSH-R cDNA with a calcium phosphate procedure, and stable populations of transfected cells were selected in medium containing G418 (Gibco, Gaithersburg, MD). Cells (~1 × 10^6) were plated in six-well dishes, washed once with Dulbecco's Modified Eagle's Medium containing BSA (0.1%) and 0.5 mM IBMX, and then incubated for 45 min at 37°C with the various concentrations of the melanotropic peptides shown. After hormone treatment, the cells were washed twice with phosphate-buffered saline (PBS), and intracellular cAMP was extracted. The cells were lysed with 60% ethanol (1 mL), centrifuged to remove cellular debris, and the supernatant was lyophilized. Intracellular cAMP concentrations were determined with an assay that measures displacement of [8-^{3}H] cAMP from a high-affinity cAMP binding protein. No increase in the amount of cAMP was detected after the same treatment of cells transfected with the vector lacking the MSH-R cDNA. Reprinted with permission from *Science (31)*.

number of sites, such as keratinocytes *(56)*, and it is possible that this cell type and perhaps the hair follicle cell is the primary site of melanotropin synthesis for the regulation of dermal and hair pigmentation.

Structure and Function of Agouti

Classic genetic studies have demonstrated in a number of species that *agouti* and *extension* alleles interact to produce the final distribution of eumelanin and phaeomelanin pigments both spatially, across the coat of the animal, as well as temporally across the length of each individual hair shaft (Fig. 2M). For example, the *agouti* banding pattern results from temporary inhibition of the wild-type allele of *extension*, but the action of *agouti* can be overridden in most species by the presence of dominant *extension* alleles. In most species, *extension* is epistatic to *agouti* (e.g., in the mouse *see* ref. *57*), meaning that when an animal contains a dominant *agouti* and a dominant *extension* allele, the *extension* phenotype prevails, implying that *extension* acts downstream of *agouti*. Another example familiar to most is the coat color variation seen in the German Shepherd dog, where the variable distribution of tan and black results from the interaction of at least two *extension* alleles (*E, e*), and three *agouti* alleles (*a^y*, *a^w*, and *a^+*) *(58)*.

Agouti has long been studied in the mouse, where approx 20 alleles have been identified, beginning with non-agouti (*a*) and dominant yellow mutations (*A^y*) first identified by mouse fanciers (for review, *see* ref. *5*). Genetic evidence led to the hypothesis that *agouti* was an antagonist of α-MSH or α-MSH signaling; identification of the MC1-R as *extension* and the cloning of the *agouti* gene supported and allowed a direct test of the hypothesis. Cloning of *agouti* demonstrated the gene to encode a 131 amino acid peptide with a putative 22 amino acid signal peptide *(22,23)* (Fig. 5). Furthermore, the gene encoding the wild-type allele was shown to be expressed in a developmentally regulated fashion peaking at posnatal day three, corresponding well to the time period during which the phaeomelanin band begins to be deposited in the developing hair shaft in the mouse. Subsequent analysis of additional alleles has demonstrated that the variable distribution of phaeomelanin owing to those alleles results from various promoter mutations that restrict *agouti* gene expression to the phaeomelanized regions (for review, *see* ref. *5*).

As mentioned, the cloning of *agouti* and the MC1-R allowed a direct test of the hypothesis that *agouti signaling protein (ASP)*, is an antagonist of α-MSH. Indeed, a 108 amino acid recombinant *agouti* protein, produced in insect cells, was demonstrated to be a high-affinity competitive antagonist ($K_i = 6.6 \times 10^{-10}$) of the MC1-R *(2)* (Fig. 6). Parenthetically, the mechanism of *agouti* action held interest for those outside the pigmentation field, because ectopic expression of *agouti* resulting from some dominant alleles (*A^y*, *A^w*; for review, *see* refs. *62* and *63*) produces one of the five monogenic obesity syndromes known in the mouse (compare the mouse in Fig. 2B with that in Fig. 2E).

Initial characterization of baculovirus-produced *agouti signaling protein* demonstrated that the peptide was also a high-affinity antagonist of a related melanocortin receptor in the hypothalamus, called the MC4-R *(2)*. This receptor had been demonstrated to be present in brain regions known to be involved in the regulation of feeding and metabolism *(39)*. However, a number of groups hypothesized that a unique ASP receptor must exist, and could potentially contribute to the action of ASP both in obesity and pigmentation, arguing that endogenous peptide antagonists of the G-protein-coupled receptors were not known to exist *(64)*, and that ASP also has effects on intracellular Ca^{2+} that are not likely to be mediated via melanocortin receptors *(65,66)*. At least in the case of *agouti*-induced obesity, this issue seems to have been resolved. A small peptide antagonist of the MC4-R Ac-Nle^4-c[Asp^5, *D*-Nal(2')^7, lys^{10}]α-MSH(4-10)-NH$_2$ *(67)* that mimics ASP pharmacologically at the MC4-R has been demonstrated to stimulate feeding on intracerebroventricular administration *(68)*. This finding demonstrates that melanocortinergic neurons exert an inhibitory tone on feeding behavior. Furthermore, ablation of the MC4-R by gene knockout produces an animal that virtually duplicates the obesity phenotype seen in the *A^y* mouse *(69)*. Together, these studies strongly argue that inhibition of MC4-R signaling is the only alteration required for the *agouti* obesity syndrome.

Although it is now generally agreed on that ASP blocks MSH binding to the MC1-R *(70–72)*, there is still some debate concerning a target for ASP action on the melanocyte in addition to the MC1-R. This derives first from a simple observation: the quality of the phaeomelanic pigment in the *A^y* and *ee* animals, though both have a disruption of MC1-R signaling, is not the same. In the same C57B1/6J background, the *A^y* animal has a bright yellow coat whereas the *ee* animal has a more dusty yellow coat (compare the mouse in Fig. 2A with that shown in Fig. 2B). Second, several more recent studies have

```
                          SIGNAL PEPTIDE


          MOUSE    MDVTRLLLATLVSFLCFFTVHS
          HUMAN    MDVTRLLLATLLVFLCFFTANS
            FOX    MNIFRLLLATLLVFLCFLTAYS




                          BASIC DOMAIN


   HLALEETLGDDRSLRSNSSMNSLDFSSVSIVALNKKSKKISRKEAEKRKRSSKKKASMKK
   HLPPEEKLRDDRSLRSNSSVNLLDVPSVSIVALNKKSKQIGRKAAEK-KRSSKKEASMKK
   HLA-EEKPKDDRSLRSNSSVNLLDFPSVSIVALNKKSKKISRKEAEK-KRSSKKKASMKN




                       PEPTIDE TOXIN DOMAIN


      VA--RPPPPS--PCVATRDSCKPPAPACCDPCASCQCRFFGSACTCRVLNPNC
      VV--RPRTPLSAPCVATRNSCKPPAPACCDPCASCQCRFFRSACSCRVLSLNC
      VARPRPPPPN--PCVATRNSCKSPAPACCDPCASCQCRFFRSACTCRXXXXXX
```

Fig. 5. Amino acid sequence of the *agouti* signaling protein from mouse *(22,23)*, human *(59,60)*, and the fox, *V. vulpes (31)*.

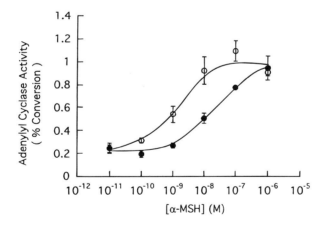

Fig. 6. Functional antagonism of the mMC1-R by the ASP. ASP inhibits activation of the mMC1-R by α-MSH in stably transfected 293 cells as monitored by stimulation of adenylyl cyclase activity. Measurement of adenylyl cyclase activity was performed as described *(61)*. Data represent means and standard deviations from triplicate data points. Reprinted with permission from *Nature (2)*. ○, α = MSH, ●, α = MSH + 0.7 n*M agouri*.

argued that ASP has various actions on melanocytes in the absence of α-MSH. For example, recombinant ASP has been demonstrated not only to block α-MSH-stimulated melanogenesis, but also to reduce further basal melanogenesis in B16 F1 murine melanoma cells in the absence of exogenous α-MSH *(72)*. ASP has also been demonstrated to inhibit forskolin- and dbc AMP-stimulated proliferation and tyrosinase activity in primary human melanocytes *(73)*. Finally, as mentioned previously, long-term exposure to ASP has been demonstrated to produce a rise in intracellular Ca^{2+} in a skeletal muscle cell line *(66)*, and the homology of ASP to the agatoxin/conotoxin family of proteins *(65)* has been used to argue that ASP must interact with a Ca^{2+} channel. Of course, this family of proteins is known to bind to many different proteins other than Ca^{2+} channels *(74)*, and in any event, when they do interact with Ca^{2+} channels, they generally act as channel blockers, inhibiting Ca^{2+} entry.

There are, additionally, several flaws inherent in these experiments. First, all of these experiments have used recombinant baculovirus ASP that is only 60–90% pure. No controls for the effects of the 10–40% component comprised of various insect cell proteins were included. Second, these experiments use a recombinant form of the protein that can only be inferred to resemble the mammalian protein in vivo. No biochemical analysis of the native protein has been reported yet, and it is quite possible that the native form is cleaved at one or more of the many dibasic residues found in the amino-terminal half of the protein. An equally likely hypothesis to explain the action of ASP on basal melanogenesis is that ASP is an inverse agonist of the MC1-R, binding to the receptor in the absence of ligand and downregulating its basal signaling activity *(75,76)*. Support for this hypothesis comes from a recent study with the B16-F1 melanoma cell line, and a subclone, G4F, lacking MC1-R expression *(77)*. The inhibition of cell growth induced by recombinant ASP in the absence of α-MSH was shown to occur in the B16 line, but not the MC1-R minus subclone *(70)*.

ALLELIC VARIANTS OF THE MC1-R

The possibility that the *extension* locus might encode an α-MC1-R was posited in 1984 *(12)*, when Tamate and Takeuchi showed that "the *e* locus controls a mechanism that determines the function of an α-MSH-R." This elegant study demonstrated that dbcAMP could induce eumelanin synthesis in hairbulbs from both A^y and ee mice, whereas α-MSH could only do so in A^y mice, demonstrating a primary defect in the α-MSH response mapping to the *e* locus.

The cloned MC1-Rs were used to map the chromosomal location of the receptors in humans and mouse to determine if the receptors mapped to a known pigmentation locus, such as *extension*, or possibly a melanoma susceptibility locus. Fluorescent *in situ* hybridization to metaphase chromosomes demonstrated that the human receptor maps to 16q2 *(78,79)*, a region not linked to melanoma susceptibility. The murine *extension* locus was previously mapped near the distal end of chromosome 8 in the mouse *(80–82)*, and an intersubspecific mapping panel was used to place the MC1-R near the *Es-11* locus, in this same region *(83)*.

Definitive evidence that *extension* encoded the MC1-R came from a study by Robbins et al. in which the MC1-R was cloned from mice containing five different *extension* locus alleles, *e, E^+, E^{so}, E^{so-3J}*, and *E^{tob}* *(1)*. At the time of this finding, no functional variants of the G-protein-coupled receptors had yet been reported. The possible existence of literally hundreds of functionally variant *extension* locus alleles, identified in most domesticated mammals during the past century by classical breeding, raised some exciting research possibilities. First, the data suggested the possibility of finding among the dominant alleles receptors that had been constitutively activated

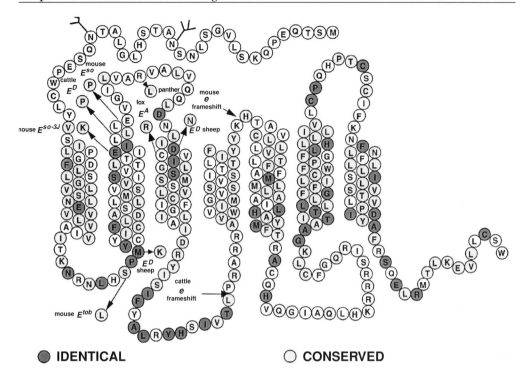

● IDENTICAL　　　　　　　　　　**○ CONSERVED**

Fig. 7. Naturally occurring functional variants of the MC1-R. Functional mutations are illustrated using the sequence of the mouse MC1-R for reference. Dark shading (●) indicates residues identical among all melanocortin receptor sequences and unique to this receptor family. Light shading (○) indicates all conserved residues. References provided in the text, except for changes seen in the panther (R. D. C., unpublished), and the sheep (D. I. V., unpublished).

by naturally occurring mutations, and second, suggested that perhaps the best in vitro mutagenesis studies of MC1-R structure and function had already been laboriously performed by Mother Nature. The functional variants that are known as of this writing can be seen in Fig. 7.

Mouse

Four *extension* phenotypes are found in the mouse. Wild-type (E^+), sombre (encoded by two independently occurring alleles, E^{so} and E^{so-3J}, tobacco (E^{tob}), and recessive yellow (*e*). *Recessive yellow* (*e*) arose spontaneously in the C57BL inbred strain and is almost entirely yellow because an absence of eumelanin synthesis in the hair follicles *(84)*. A small number of dark hairs can be found dorsally in *e/e* animals, and the animals have black eyes as well. E^{tob} is a naturally occurring *extension* allele present in the tobacco mouse, *Mus poschiavinus (85)*. This wild mouse is confined primarily to the Val Poschiavo region of southeastern Switzerland. The E^{tob} allele in the *M. poschiavinus* background produces a darkening of the back, which is only visible after the eighth week when the flanks become *agouti*. The E^{tob} allele is epistatic to *agouti* producing a darkened back when crossed with yellow (A^y) or black (*aa*) mice. Consequently, unlike the *sombre* phenotype described below, the dominant melanizing effect of E^{tob} is incompletely expressed. The E^{so} allele arose spontaneously in 1961 in the C3H strain *(57)*. E^{so}

homozygotes are, with the exception of a few yellow hairs, entirely black and have darkened skin as well, resembling extreme non-*agouti* mice (a^e/a^e). As heterozygous E^{so}/+ animals mature, yellow hairs appear on the flanks and the bellies become gray, clearly distinguishing them from homozygotes, and resembling the non-*agouti* mouse (a/a). Like E^{tob}, the E^{so}, allele is also epistatic to *agouti*. E^{so-3J} arose spontaneously in 1985 at the Jackson Laboratory in the CBA/J strain and is phenotypically similar to the original E^{so} allele. No evidence has been presented for phenotypic effects of variant *extension* alleles, outside of their effects on pigmentation.

Robbins et al. demonstrated that the murine *extension* locus encodes the MC1-R, and the different pigmentation phenotypes of these alleles result from point mutations in the receptor that alters its functional properties *(1)*. In the *recessive yellow* mouse, a frameshift mutation at position 183 between the fourth and the fifth transmembrane domains, results in a prematurely terminated nonfunctional MC1-R. In the *sombre* mice, there is a glu-to-lys change at position 92 in the E^{so-3J} allele and a leu-to-pro change at position 98 in the E^{so} allele, with both of these mutations located in the putative exterior portion of the second transmembrane domain of the receptor. When expressed in the heterologous 293 cell line, both *sombre-3J* and *sombre* receptors are constitutively activated up to 30–50% of the maximal stimulation levels of the wild-type receptor, even in the absence of the α-MSH (Fig. 8). The receptor is not further stimulated by higher concentrations of α-MSH. However, the superpotent melanocortin analog Nle^4-D-Phe^7-α-MSH (NDP-α-MSH) is capable of fully activating the *sombre* receptor *(1,87)*. Though the phenotypes of the *tobacco* and the *sombre* mice are similar, the receptor of the tobacco allele, which has a ser-to-leu change at position 69 of the first intracellular loop of the receptor, has different pharmacological features from the *sombre* receptor (Fig. 9). The *tobacco* receptor only has a slightly elevated basal activity, but can be further stimulated by α-MSH and has a much higher maximal adenylyl cyclase level than the wild-type receptor *(1)*.

Cattle

Three *extension* alleles were postulated in the cattle based on the genetic studies, E^D for dominate black, *e* for recessive red, and E^+, the only allele in cattle and mice that allows phenotypic expression of *agouti (88)*. A leu-to-pro change at position 99, homologous to position 97 of the mouse, has been found in the E^D allele, and a frameshift mutation resulting from a single base deletion at position 104 has been found in the *e* allele of the cattle *(33)*. The red and black pigments that result are represented by the colors seen, for example, in the Hereford and Holstein breeds (Fig. 2G). The E^D allele has not yet been pharmacologically characterized, but is likely to have functionally similar consequences to the leu98pro change that occurs just two amino acids away in the mouse. This change constitutively activates the MC1-R similarly to the glu92lys change; all three mutations are predicted to operate via the same mechanism, the glu92lys change directly disrupting a molecular interaction, and the leu99pro (bovine) and leu98pro (mouse) changes indirectly disrupting the same interaction by altering the α-helical structure of the second membrane-spanning domain.

Fox

As mentioned above, in many species, including the mouse, dominant alleles at *extension* are epistatic to *agouti*. On the molecular level, this translates to the observation

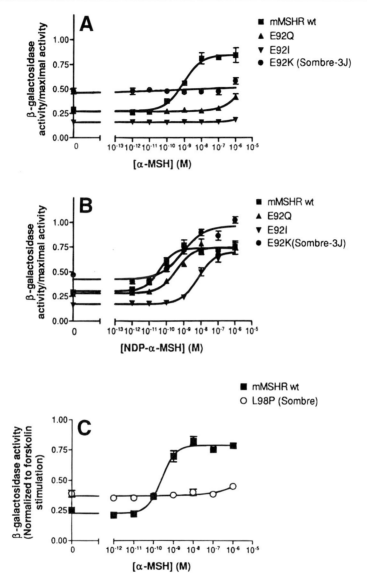

Fig. 8. Pharmacology of the mouse *sombre* and *sombre-3J* receptors. The wild-type MC1-R, E^{so-3J} allele, in vitro-generated E92Q and E92I mutants, and E^{so} alleles were cloned into the pcDNA Neo expression vector (Invitrogen), and transfected stably into the HEK 293 cell line. G418^r cell populations were selected and assayed for intracellular cAMP levels following hormone stimulation using a cAMP-dependent β-galactosidase reporter construct as described previously *(86)*. Data points are the average of triplicate determination with error bars indicating the standard deviation. Data are normalized to cell number and presented as % maximal activity (μ*M* forskolin-stimulated) for each individual cell population. The forskolin-stimulated activities did not vary significantly among cell populations. Panels show data from stimulations with α-MSH (**A** and **C**) and NDP-MSH (**B**). Reprinted with permission from the *Endocrine Society (87)*. Portions of associated text were reprinted with permission from *Cell (1)*.

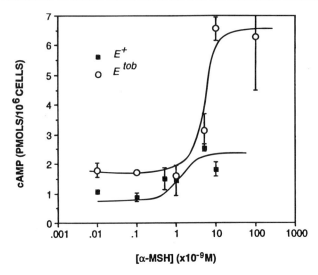

Fig. 9. Pharmacology of the mouse *tobacco* receptor. Curves show the accumulation of intracellular cAMP in 293 cells transfected with the E^{tob} or the $E+$ allele in response to increasing concentrations of α-MSH. RIA for intracellular cAMP performed as described in Fig. 4. Points indicate the mean of two independent experiments, and bars indicate the standard deviations. Reprinted with permission from *Cell (1)*.

that once receptors have been made constitutively active by mutation, they can no longer be inhibited by ASP. However, in the fox, *Vulpes vulpes*, the proposed *extension* locus is not epistatic to the *agouti* locus *(89,90)*. Both the MC1-R and *agouti* genes were recently cloned from this species to attempt to understand this novel relationship between the receptor and its antagonist *(21)*.

A constitutively activating cys125arg mutation in the MC1-R was found specifically in darkly pigmented animals carrying the Alaska Silver allele (E^A). This mutation was introduced by in vitro mutagenesis into the homologous position (aa123) of the highly conserved mouse MC1 receptor (85% amino acid identity) for pharmacological analysis. MC1-R (cys123arg), when expressed in the 293-cell system, was found to activate adenylyl cyclase from 25–90% maximal levels, in the absence of any hormone stimulation (Fig. 10). The full-length wild-type fox MC1-R was transiently expressed in Cos-1 cells, and appeared to couple normally to adenylyl cyclase, as measured by analysis of intracellular cAMP concentrations, with an EC_{50} of $1.6 \times 10^{-9}M$ (not shown), comparable to the value reported for the mouse MC1-R (*[31]*, $2.0 \times 10^{-9}M$).

A deletion in the first coding exon of the *agouti* gene was found associated with the proposed recessive allele of *agouti* in the darkly pigmented Standard Silver fox *(aa)*. This deletion removes the start codon and the signal sequence, and thus is likely to ablate the production of functional ASP. Thus, as in the mouse, dark pigmentation can be caused by a constitutively active MC1-R or homozygous recessive status at the *agouti* locus.

These findings allow a detailed interpretation of fox coat color phenotypes resulting from *extension* and *agouti*. Red coat color in cattle and the red guinea pig (*see* Fig. 2G and 2N) result from homozygosity of defective alleles of the MC1-R. In contrast, no deletions or deleterious mutations in the MC1-R were observed in DNA from the Red fox *(EEAA)*. This allele of the receptor appeared normal in functional expression assays

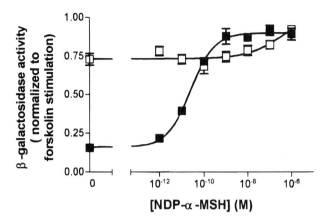

Fig. 10. Constitutive activation of adenylyl cyclase by a mouse MC1-R containing the *Alaska Silver fox* (cys125arg) mutation. Wild-type and mutant MC1 receptors were assayed by analyzing their ability to activate expression of a cAMP-responsive β-galactosidase fusion gene, as described in Fig. 8. Cells stably expressing each receptor were stimulated for 6 h with medium alone or with medium containing increasing concentrations of α-MSH, and β-galactosidase concentrations determined. Data points are the mean of triplicate determinations divided by maximal levels achieved by forskolin stimulation to normalize for transfection efficiency, and error bars represent standard deviation. Reprinted, along with associated portions of the text, with permission from *Nature Genetics (21)*. ■, mMC1-R (wt); □, mMC1-R (C123R).

in tissue culture (not shown), demonstrating that, in this species, red coat color results from inhibition of the MC1-R by the product of the *A* allele of *agouti*.

When two constitutively active MC1-Rs are found, such as in the Alaskan Silver fox ($E^A E^A AA$), primarily eumelanin is found. In striking contrast to the mouse, however, heterozygosity of the dominant *extension* allele E^A is not sufficient to override inhibition of eumelanin production by *agouti*. One wild-type *agouti* allele produces significant red pigment around the flanks, midsection, and neck in the Blended Cross fox ($E^A E Aa$; Fig. 2K). This strongly suggests an interaction between *extension* and *agouti* distinct from the epistasis seen in the mouse. One possible model to explain this interaction is that in the fox, the ASP is an inverse agonist of the MC1-R.

In the recently proposed allosteric ternary complex model *(75)*, G-protein-coupled receptors are in equilibrium between the inactive (R) and active (R*) states, even in the absence of ligand. In contrast to the classical competitive antagonist, which binds equally well to R and R* and acts by blocking ligand binding, inverse agonists, recently verified experimentally *(76)*, bind preferentially to R and thus shift the receptor equilibrium in the direction of the inactive state. Although the mouse ASP behaves like a classical competitive antagonist, it is possible that the fox protein is an inverse agonist and can inhibit the constitutively active E^A allele of the MC1-R.

Guinea Pig

Variegated pigment patterns, that is, coats containing an irregular patchwork of two or more colors, have often been associated with heterozygosity of X-linked pigment genes in the female animal. A classic example is the orange locus (*O*) in the cat, resulting from X chromosome inactivation in the female as proposed by Lyon *(91)*. Males and homozygous females containing this allele are yellow-orange, whereas heterozygous females (+/O) have the tortoiseshell or calico coat consisting of irregularly distributed patches of yellow and brown pigment. However, variegated brindle and tortoiseshell coat color patterns map to the autosomal *extension* locus in a variety of mammals, including the rabbit, dog, cattle, pig, and guinea pig *(6)*.

Preliminary results are available from a study of the *extension* in the guinea pig, in which an allele, e^p, produces the tortoiseshell coat pattern in homozygous male or female animals. Our initial hypothesis was that such a phenotype might result from variable MC1-R gene expression that could be easily detectable as a gene rearrangement. Analysis of the MC1-R gene locus by Southern hybridization has not confirmed this, and additional work needs to be done *(87)*. Interestingly, however, after probing DNA from the black, tortoiseshell, and red guinea pig with a small coding sequence fragment of the mouse MC1-R a large deletion in this gene was observed in the red guinea pig. This confirms the observations in the mouse and in cattle that absence of functional MC1 receptor does not affect melanocyte development or migration into the skin and hair follicle, but simply ablates expression of eumelanin in the coat of the animal. Further work will be required to understand the mechanism of variegated function of the MC1-R in tortoiseshell and brindle animals.

Panther

A coat color phenotype that has always fascinated viewers is the melanized coat seen in a number of the large felines. In the leopard, *Panthera pardus*, the classic spotting seen in the wild-type tan and brown animal can actually still be seen beneath the sleek black coat of the eumelanic variant. Unfortunately, it is obviously difficult to imagine accumulating a sufficient number of samples to perform a linkage analysis in this species. Furthermore, attempting to collect even small tissue samples from this species in the wild is not recommended, even if it were legal. The absence of a defined *extension* locus in domestic felines further compounds the problem of analyzing the role of the MC1-R in feline pigmentation. Nonetheless, the gene that produces the dark black coat in several of the large cats is reported to be dominant acting, and this laboratory was fortunate to obtain blood samples from Chewy and Boltar, tan and black *P. pardus*, respectively, residing at the Octagon Wildlife Sanctuary in Florida. These animals have been bred twice, throwing both black and tan offspring. Cloning and sequence analysis of the MC1-R from both animals demonstrated Boltar to be heterozygous for a arg106leu change, whereas Chewy was arg106 at both alleles. Given the proximity of this mutation to the constitutively activating mutations in the mouse, cow, and fox, it is tempting to speculate that this change represents a dominant allele of the MC1-R in *P. pardus*. The allele has not yet been characterized pharmacologically.

Human

Tremendous polymorphism of skin, hair, and eye color is seen in humans, and it would be interesting to determine if any of this results from functional variants of the MC1-R. Furthermore, homozygous recessive inheritance of red hair is often seen in humans *(92)*, and a reasonable hypothesis would be that this derives from a defective MC1-R. In further support of the hypothesis, the specific response to α-MSH has been shown to be defective in 88% of primary melanocyte cultures from red-haired individuals, but only 11% of melanocyte cultures from dark-haired Caucasians *(93)*.

The entire human MC1-R gene was examined from 30 unrelated British or Irish individuals with different shades of red hair and a poor tanning response, and from another

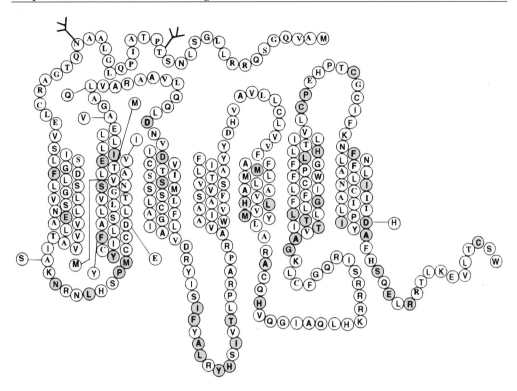

Fig. 11. Allelic variants of the human MC1-R. Coding polymorphisms in the human MC1-R. Shading indicates residues identical among all the melanocortin receptors and unique to this receptor family.

30 unrelated British or Irish control individuals with brown or black hair with a good tanning response *(94)*. Several amino acid changes were found, with most clustered around the second transmembrane domain, except the most commonly observed variant, asp294his (Fig. 11). The other variants were all conservative changes, as shown.

A second study was conducted with samples from patients attending dermatology clinic at Oregon Health Sciences University *(95)*. In this study, samples resulted from dermatologic procedures on patients characterized with regard to hair and eye color, and skin type. This latter characteristic was determined according to the method of Fitzpatrick *(96)*, and is a general indicator of the degree of melanization of the skin. MC1 receptor coding fragments were isolated from these samples by polymerase chain reaction and sequenced following subcloning. Two coding polymorphisms of the MC1-R were identified, val92met and asp84glu. Individuals were found that were both heterozygous and homozygous for val92met, and the one asp84glu allele was found in an individual that was a compound heterozygote, also containing the val92met allele.

Remarkably, in both studies, there was a very significant concentration of variant alleles in the red-haired or fair-skinned individuals. In the British study, 80% of red-haired, fair-skinned individuals had one or more MC1-R variants, compared to 20% of the control group. In the US study, the val92met allele was found at a frequency of 0.11 in individuals with type I skin, compared with an allele frequency of 0.02 in individuals with type II skin. Nevertheless, the data at this time do not support a direct role for the variant MC1-R alleles in the phaeomelanic phenotype: very few individuals were homozygous or even compound heterozygotes for the variant forms. The majority of the variants result from conservative amino acid changes, and preliminary pharmacological characterization of the val92met allele failed to indicate any defect in this variant form of the receptor *(95)*. Interestingly, there is an unusually high frequency of double mutations, suggesting that the MC1-R (and TMII in particular) may be a hot spot for mutation. Additional work will be required to determine if the MC1-R is directly involved in the determination of the monogenic red-haired trait or the polygenic trait of skin type *(97,98)*. Valverde and colleagues *(99)* also pointed out that since melanoma frequency is much greater in fair-skinned individuals, the variant MC1-R alleles are, as expected, associated with melanoma.

STRUCTURE OF THE MC1-R

In addition to studies of naturally occurring variants of the MC1-R, other approaches have been taken to understand better the structure and function of this receptor. Two discussed here include in vitro mutagenesis studies and computer modeling of the receptor.

In Vitro Mutagenesis Studies

To understand further the structure and function of the MC1-R, in vitro mutagenesis studies have been performed on both murine and human MC1-R. Only limited data are available thus far. Based on residues conserved across the entire melanocortin receptor family, several residues, including asp117, phe179, his209, and his260, were mutated to alanine in the human MC1-R *(100)*. These mutants were examined for binding of both α-MSH and NDP-α-MSH. For NDP-α-MSH, binding affinities were all similar to the wild type, but for α-MSH, binding affinities were significantly altered in some cases. Affinities were reduced about 267-fold for asp117ala, about 132-fold for his260ala, and similar to the wild type for phe179ala and his209ala. Though the data clearly show a different interaction of NDP-α-MSH with the receptor compared to the native ligand, it is likely to result from variations on binding to the same binding pocket, with the mutations either directly or indirectly affecting the specific NDP-α-MSH contacts only.

The charged residues in the extracellular loop of the human MC1-R, including ser6, glu102, arg109, asp184, glu269, and thr272, were also mutated to alanine to investigate whether these residues are involved in ligand binding to the receptor *(101)*. The binding affinity to either α-MSH or NDP-α-MSH was reduced for ser6, asp184, glu269, and thr272, but similar to the wild type for glu102 and arg109. These results demonstrated that certain extracellular residues are important in the ligand–receptor interaction. It has been known for some time that the residues of α-MSH flanking the core H-F-R-W pharmacophore contribute importantly to the affinity of the interaction between ligand and receptor; these flanking sequences are not necessary for full agonist activity and are perhaps the residues interacting with extracellular residues to enhance ligand affinity (for review, *see* refs. *47* and *48*.)

Computer Modeling of the Receptor

Identification of chemical and structural ligand interactions with receptor proteins may provide insights to designing receptor subtype-selective agonists and antagonists and understanding naturally occurring mutations. Determination of true 3-D structure at high resolution requires X-ray diffraction techniques. Unfortunately, the members of the

GPCR superfamily are resistant thus far to crystallization techniques. Lacking this direct structural information, computer-assisted molecular modeling of these receptors has become a common approach to try to predict receptor structure and probable ligand-receptor interactions. This approach is based on the low-resolution electron-microscopy structure of the non-G-protein-coupled seven transmembrane-spanning protein, bacterio-rhodopsin *(102,103)*, with further refinements that include the footprint of the mammalian G-protein-coupled rhodopsin receptor *(104)*.

Transmembrane region alignment of the sequences that constitute the α-helical regions may be determined by hydrophobicity plots, such as Kyte-Doolittle analysis *(105)*, or more consistently using the "Baldwin" alignment *(106)*, which accommodates similar positioning of the GPCR superfamily conserved amino acid residues.

Several melanocortin receptor models have been developed by different groups *(87,107,108)* to propose receptor residues that may be interacting with regions of the melanotropin ligands. Figure 12 illustrates the mMC1R interacting with the NDP-α-MSH peptide. Figure 12A shows a side view of the ligand-docked receptor with flanking residues of the ligand proposed to increase affinity via interaction with extracellular loops shown in yellow. Residues of the pharmacophore are labeled, with charged residues shown in red and blue, and hydrophobic residues in other colors. Examination of the receptor (Fig. 12B) shows two domains that are proposed to interact with the charged and hydrophobic domains of the ligand. A highly charged domain, shown in red and blue, is made of the residues in TM II and TM III, glu92, asp115, and asp119, whereas a domain containing multiple phenylalanines and a tyrosine residue is proposed to interact via the aromatic phenylalanine and histidine residues of the pharmacophore. Figure 12C illustrates a view of NDP-α-MSH docked with the mMC1-R looking down on the surface of the membrane. Specific residues proposed to interact between ligand and the mouse MC1R are illustrated in Fig. 13 for the melanocortin pharmacophore residues His-DPhe-Arg-Trp of NDP-α-MSH. These interactions for the mMC1-R are predicted based on structural and functional homology, although with minor differences *(51)* with the hMC1-R, which has been extensively studied and modeled *(108)*.

Additionally, based on this type of receptor molecular modeling, we can propose specific residue interactions that may explain the basis for the constitutive activation observed for naturally occurring mutations and can be extrapolated to a general mechanism for melanocortin receptor activation. Figure 14 illustrates a possible mechanism that accounts for the *Somber-3J* mutation *(1)*. For this glu92lys mutation, an acidic negatively charged residue in TM II, is replaced by a longer basic positively charged residue. The Arg residue of the pharmacophore is proposed to interact with complementary negatively charged receptor residues (Fig. 13) *(87,108)*. With this in mind, it can be postulated that the lys92 residue can possess similar functional properties as the ligand arg residue and, therefore, mimic the ligand-induced receptor conformation in the absence of ligand. A report of point mutations of the hMC1-R identified asp117ala (Asp115 in the mouse MC1R) as significantly (267-fold) decreasing α-MSH binding affinity *(100)*. Thus, with this supporting information, the lys92 residue (TM II) can be proposed to interact with the conserved Asp residue(s) illustrated in Figs. 12–14. Specifically, these interactions may include complementary electrostatic (charge–charge) interactions and up to two hydrogen bonds, as illustrated. In a hydrophobic environment, a salt bridge such as this may generate up to 10 kcal/mol stabilization energy

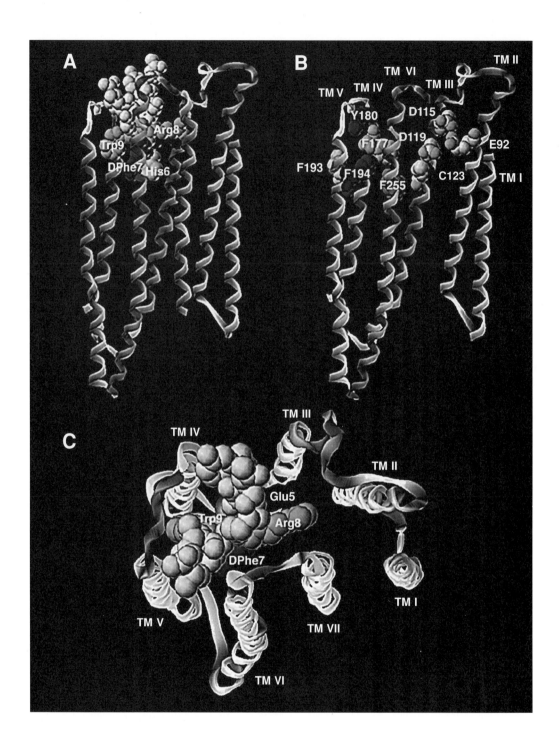

Fig. 12. Molecular model of NDP-α-MSH docked into the mMC1R. The α-helical backbone of the receptor is denoted in various shades of gray. The ligand residues highlighted in yellow consist of the regions of NDP-MSH that flank the "message" residues. The "message" residues His[6] (orange), DPhe[7] (aqua), Arg[8] (red), and Trp[9] (magenta) are docked into the putative binding pocket of the receptor, and labeled in **(A)**. **(A, B)** represent side on views of the ligand–receptor complex, with TM I

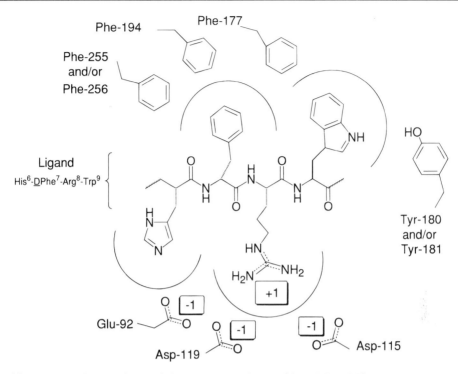

Fig. 13. Proposed interactions of the melanocortin peptide NDP-α-MSH message sequence, His-DPhe-Arg-Trp, interacting with specific mMC1R residues. The aromatic ligand residues DPhe and Trp are postulated to interact within an aromatic hydrophobic pocket consisting primarily of TMs IV, V, and VI, whereas the Arg residue is interacting within a network of charged receptor residues in TMs II and III.

(109). Furthermore, asp115, located one helical turn above asp119, is also conserved within the melanocortin receptor family. Rotation around the lys side chain torsion angles, as illustrated in Fig. 13, would allow for nearly identical interactions with asp115 as proposed for asp119. This is important since some ambiguity is present regarding which particular Asp residue, or combination of, may be an acceptable complementary acidic residue. Once these interactions have formed, a receptor conformation may be formed in which the highly conserved DRY sequence in TM III, proposed to be important for signal transduction *(110,111)*, can obtain the necessary conformational and spatial orientation important for signal transduction. The exact mechanism may involve a change in TM spanning α-helical packing of TMs II and III, thus modifying the packing orientation of the entire receptor.

Two mutations of the MC1R, leu98pro (E^{so}) in the mouse *(1)* and leu99pro in bovine *(33)*, resulted in constitutive activation and black coat color. Interestingly, both mutations

Fig. 12. *(continued)* located on the far right, and TM V located on the far left. mMC1R receptor residues, which are proposed to interact with the ligand "message" residues, are labeled in B. (C) A space-filled model of NDP-α-MSH docked into mMC1R looking down toward the intracellular portion of the ligand–receptor complex. This model was generated based originally on the bacteriorhodopsin structure (BR1) obtained from the Protein Data Bank *(103)*, modified manually to fit the helical packing arrangement of rhodopsin *(104)*, and based on homology with the hMC1R *(108)*.

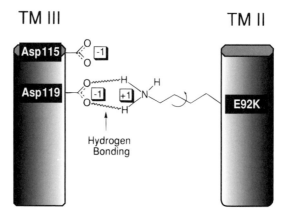

Fig. 14. An illustration of the proposed glu92lys *somber-3J* mutation in TM II, which results in constitutive activation of the mMC1R *(1)*. Mutation of the homologous residue of asp119 in the human MC1R was identified as being important for ligand binding *(100)*. This information provided a complementary receptor residue in which the lys92 residue could interact both by up to two hydrogen bonds, as indicated, and electrostatic interactions. Rotation of lys side chain torsion angles, indicated by the arrow, would allow for identical interactions with the asp115 residue one helical turn above asp119.

are at the borderline of the transmembrane-spanning helical interface of TM II on the extracellular surface. As alluded to previously, proline residues possess a variety of structural implications in transmembrane helices. This particular amino acid can modify α-helices 20–30° from helices lacking the proline residue at the interface between the extracellular surface and TM regions, and can affect the packing of entire transmembrane helical spanning regions *(112)*. The hydrophobicity of the wild-type region (mouse, Ile-Ile-Leu-Leu-Leu) is modified dramatically by the leu to pro mutation. Leu possess a value of 3.8 on the hydropathy index, whereas pro possesses a value of −1.6 *(100)*. Therefore, this particular modification, at this location in the receptor, may not only modify helical packing of TM II, but also modify the position of the helical secondary structure and orientation in the membrane, thus likely disrupting the interaction(s) glu92 normally participates in.

A mutation found in the fox TM III, cys125arg, has also been demonstrated to result in a constitutively active melanocortin receptor *(21)*. This arg residue is likely to interact electrostatically with the asp residues one and two turns above it on the helix, and an interaction with glu92 of TM II is also probable. In the latter interaction, a similar mechanism described for the glu92lys mutation may be applicable in that these ionic interactions modify the helical packing arrangement in TMs II and III and, therefore, generate a receptor population that can couple to the G protein in the absence of ligand.

The E^{tob} mutation, ser69leu *(1)*, which is located in the cytoplasmic region of TM II and adjacent to a structurally important proline residue *(112)*, may function by decreasing hydrogen bonding interactions collectively with neighboring asn66 and his68 with TM VII and C-terminal intracellular residues gln301, glu302 (Fig. 15), or a variety of other possibilities in the C-terminus intracellular region. Notably, the leu residue is also one of the 20 amino acids with highest propensity of being involved with α-helical structures and may function as a nucleation center, whereas ser has a

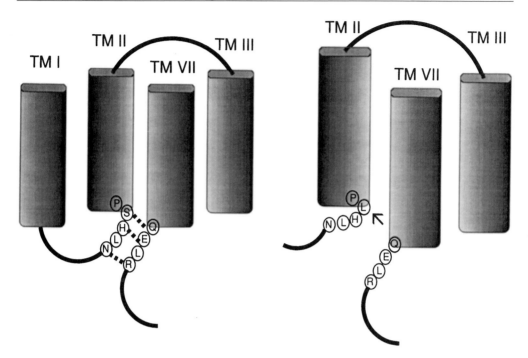

Fig. 15. Illustration of the mouse MC1R TMs I–III and VII, which may be involved in helical packing alterations by the ser69leu E^{tob} mutation *(1)*. The mechanism proposed for the resulting increased basal activity and increased cAMP stimulation on ligand binding may involve specific disruptions of proposed electrostatic interactions between TMs II and VII. Since leu has a high propensity for being involved in α-helices, this ser to leu mutation may modify the local secondary structure and disrupt the proposed interactions, therefore modifying receptor populations that interact with the G protein.

low propensity for being involved with α-helical structure *(113)*. Interestingly, one of the notable differences between the initial bacteriorhodopsin structure used for initial GPCR modeling *(103)* and the low-resolution structure of rhodopsin *(104)* was the positioning of TM I. The rhodopsin and refined bacteriorhodopsin *(102)* structures both position TM I out of the "binding pocket" region and position TM II and TM VII in closer proximity. Thus, it can be speculated that by replacing the hydrophobic ser residue with a sterically larger, α-helical structural biased, and hydrophobic leu residue, that resulting modifications in structure, electrostatic, and steric (Van der Waals) interactions may disrupt local helical packing of the receptor in this region (TM II, Fig. 15), therefore modifying the mutated receptor's activity. Support for helical interactions between TM II and TM VII being important for signal transduction comes from a report in which complementary charged residues were mutated (arg in TM II and gln in TM VII) and resulted in defective receptor signaling *(114)*. Additionally, the structural motif in TMVII, N/D-XX-Y, highly conserved within the entire GPCR superfamily *(115)*, modified G-protein coupling when mutated in the Angiotensin II receptor *(116)*.

Interestingly, all the constitutively activating mutations identified to date for the melanocortin receptors are located in the TM II and TM III region. This concentration of mutations and resulting constitutively active receptors allows us to propose a general mechanism for this biological phenomenon for the melanocortin receptors. The direct structural changes, in the case of ser69leu, leu98pro, and leu99pro, or indirect changes in the case of glu92lys and cys125arg, resulted in modifying the overall helical packing of the receptor by possibly modifying important interactions among TM II, TM III, and TM VII (discussed above) and led to a shift in receptor population that was able to couple to the G protein in the absence of ligand, resulting in a dark color skin coat. Although these speculations remain to be experimentally confirmed, molecular modeling has provided new hypotheses that may account for the constitutive activities that result from naturally occurring melanocortin mutations, and can be tested experimentally.

CONCLUSIONS AND FUTURE PROSPECTS

A good deal has been learned over the past few years regarding the MC1-R and the regulation of mammalian pigmentation. Thus far, it appears that normal variation in the eumelanin/phaeomelanin switch directly involving the MC1-R results primarily from genetic variation in the coding sequence of this receptor. Interestingly, in contrast to many of the constitutively activating mutations in other G-protein-coupled receptors, activating mutations of the MC1-R are localized to TM II and TM III, and appear in some way to mimic ligand binding. Alterations in the expression levels of the receptor or its ligand as a mechanism for genetic diversity remain to be demonstrated. As an alternative mechanism, the eumelanin/phaeomelanin switch may also be regulated by the novel G-GPCR antagonist, ASP. In this case, nearly all variation characterized thus far in the mouse, fox, and cow results from alterations in temporal, spatial, or quantitative aspects of expression of the *agouti* gene. Naturally occurring pharmacological variants of ASP do not appear to be common.

Thus far, no definitive link between human skin and hair pigmentation and the MC1-R or *agouti* has been demonstrated. The high frequency of MC1-R variants, their regional localization in the receptor coding sequence, and their association with red hair and fair skin remain a mystery. Additional work will be required to determine the value of these polymorphisms in relation to melanoma and other disorders of pigment cells or the pigmentation process. Likewise, the role of the conserved human ASP in pigmentation, or other physiological processes, remains to be determined.

REFERENCES

1. Robbins LS, Nadeau JH, Johnson KR, Kelly MA, Roselli-Rehfuss L, Baack E, Mountjoy KG, Cone RD. Pigmentation phenotypes of variant *extension* locus alleles result from point mutations that alter MSH receptor function. Cell 1993;72:827–834.
2. Lu D, Willard D, Patel IR, Kadwell S, Overton L, Kost T, Luther M, Chen W, Woychik RP, Wilkison WO, Cone RD. Agouti protein is an antagonist of the melanocyte-stimulating hormone receptor. Nature 1994;371:799–802.
3. Silvers WK. The Coat Colors of Mice: A Model for Mammalian Gene Action and Interaction. Springer-Verlag, New York 1979.
4. Barsh GS. The genetics of pigmentation: from fancy genes to complex traits. TIG 1996;12:299–305.
5. Jackson IJ. Molecular and developmental genetics of mouse coat color. Annu Rev Genet 1994; 28:189–217.
6. Searle AG. Comparative Genetics of Coat Colors in Mammals. Logos, London, 1968.
7. Jackson IJ. A cDNA encoding tyrosinase-related protein maps to the mouse brown locus. Proc Natl Acad Sci USA 1988;85:4392–4396.
8. Jackson IJ, Chambers DM, Tsukamoto K, Copeland NG, Jenkins NA, Hearing V. A second tyrosinase-related protein, TRP-2, maps to and is mutated at the mouse *slaty* locus. EMBO J 1992;11:527–535.

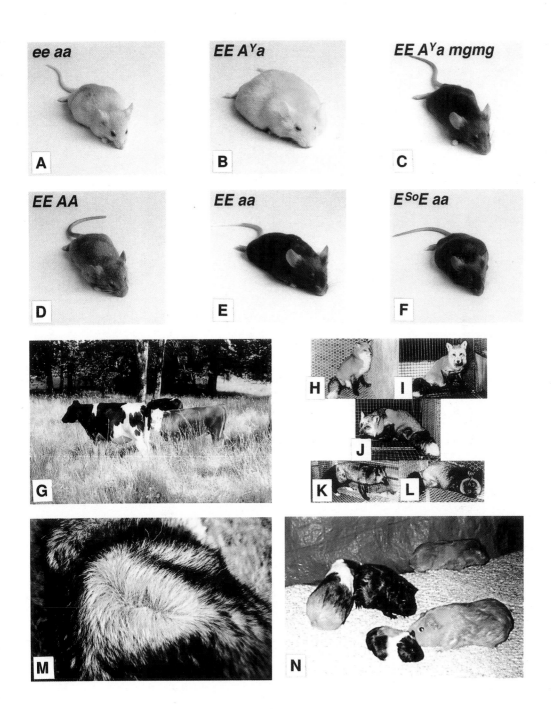

Fig. 2.

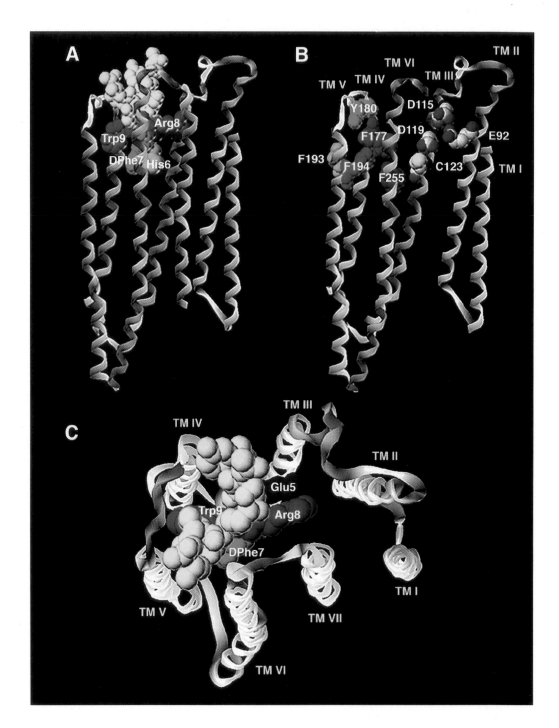

Fig. 12.

9. Kwon BS, Chintamaneni CD, Kozak CA, Copeland NG, Gilbert DJ, Jenkins NA, Barton DE, Francke U, Kobayashi Y, Kim KK. A melanocyte-specific gene, Pmel 17, maps near the silver coat color locus on mouse chromosome 10, and is a syntenic region on human chromosome 12. Proc Natl Acad Sci USA 1991;88:9228–9232.

10. Burchill SA, Thody AJ, Ito S. Melanocyte-stimulating hormone, tyrosinase activity and the regulation of eumelanogenesis and phaeomelanogenesis in the hair follicular melanocytes of the mouse. J Endocrinol 1986;109:15–21.

11. Burchill SA, Virden R, Thody AJ. Regulation of tyrosinase synthesis and its processing in the hair follicular melanocytes of the mouse during eumelanogenesis and phaeomelanogenesis. J Invest Dermatol 1989;93:236–240.

12. Tamate HB, Takeuchi T. Action of the *e* locus of mice in the response of phaeomelanic hair follicles to alpha-melanocyte stimulating hormone in vitro. Science 1984;224:1241–1242.

13. Takeuchi T, Kobunai T, Yamamoto H. Genetic control of signal transduction in mouse melanocytes. Soc Invest Dermatol 1989;92:239-S-242S.

14. Kobayashi T, Vieira WD, Potterf B, Saka C, Imokawa G, Hearing V. Modulation of melanogenic protein expression during the switch from eumelanogenesis. J Cell Sci 1995;108:2301–2309.

15. Kwon BS, Wakulchik M, Haq AQ, Halaban R, Kestler D. Sequence analysis of mouse tyrosinase cDNA and the effect of melanotropin on its gene expression. Biochem Biophys Res Commun 1988;153:1301–1309.

16. Hoganson GE, Ledwitz-Rigby F, Davidson RL, Fuller BB. Regulation of tyrosinase mRNA levels in mouse melanoma cell clones by melanocyte-stimulating hormone and cyclic AMP. Som Cell Mol Genet 1989; 15:255–263.

17. Halaban R, Pomerantz SH, Marshall S, Lerner AB. Tyrosinase activity and abundance in cloudman melanoma cells. Arch Biochem Biophys 1984;230:383–387.

18. Wong G, Pawelek J. Melanocyte stimulating hormone promotes activation of preexisting tyrosinase molecules in Cloudman S91 melanoma cells. Nature 1975;255:644–646.

19. Pawelek J. Factors regulating growth and pigmentation of melanoma cells. J Invest Dermatol 1976;66:201–209.

20. Lane PW, Green MC. *Mahogany*, a recessive color mutation in linkage group V of the mouse. J Heredity 1960;51:228–230.

21. Vage DI, Lu, D, Klungland, H, Lien, S, Adalsteinsson, S, and Cone, RD. A non-epistatic interaction of *agouti* and *extension* in the fox, *Vulpes vulpes*. Nature & Genet, 1997;15:311–315.

22. Bultman SJ, Michaud EJ, Woychik RP. Molecular characterization of the mouse *agouti* locus. Cell 1992;71:1195–1204.

23. Miller MW, Duhl DMJ, Vrieling H, Cordes SP, Ollmann MM, Winkes BM, Barsh GS. Cloning of the mouse *agouti* gene predicts a novel secreted protein ubiquitously expressed in mice carrying the *lethal yellow* (*A^y*) mutation. Genes Dev 1993;7:454–467.

24. Geschwind II. Change in hair color in mice induced by injection of α-MSH. 1966;79:1165–1167.

25. Geschwind II, Huseby RA, Nishioka R. The effect of melanocyte-stimulating hormone on coat color in the mouse. Rec Prog Horm Res 1972;28:91–130.

26. Lamoreux ML, Mayer TC. Site of gene action in the development of hair pigment in *recessive yellow* (*e/e*) mice. Dev Biol 1975;46:160–166.

27. Silvers WK, Russel ES. An experimental approach to action of genes at the *agouti* locus in the mouse. J Exp Zool 1955;130:199–220.

28. Silvers WK. An experimental approach to action of genes at the agouti locus in the mouse. III. Transplants of newborn *A^w*-, *A*-, and *a^t*- skin to *A^Y*, *A^w*, *A*-, and *aa* hosts. J Exp Zool 1958;137:189–196.

29. Gerst JE, Sole J, Hazum E, Salomon Y. Identification and characterization of melanotropin binding proteins from M2R melanoma cells by covalent photoaffinity labeling. Endocrinology 1988; 123:1792–1797.

30. Solca F, Siegrist W, Drozdz R, Girard J, Eberle AN. The receptor for α-melanotropin of mouse and human melanoma cells. J Biol Chem 1989;264:14,277–14,280.

31. Mountjoy KG, Robbins LS, Mortrud MT, Cone RD. The cloning of a family of genes that encode the melanocortin receptors. Science 1992;257:543–546.

32. Chhajlani V, Wikberg JES. Molecular cloning and expression of the human melanocyte stimulating hormone receptor cDNA. FEBS Lett 1992;309:417–420.

33. Klungland H, Vage DI, Gomez-Raya L, Adelsteinsson S, Lien S. The role of melanocyte-stimulating hormone (MSH) receptor in bovine coat color determination. Mammalian Genome 1995;6:636–639.

34. Vanetti M, Schonrock, C, Meyerhof, W, Hollt, V. Molecular cloning of a bovine MSH receptor which is highly expressed in the testis. FEBS Lett 1994;348:268–272.

35. Takeuchi S, Suzuki S, Hirose S, Yabuuchi M, Sato C, Yamamoto H, Takahashi S. Molecular cloning and sequence analysis of the chick melanocortin 1-receptor gene. Biochem Biophys Acta 1996;1306:122–126.

36. Gantz I, Konda Y, Tashiro T, Shimoto Y, Miwa H, Munzert G, Watson SJ, DelValle J, Yamada T. Molecular cloning of a novel melanocortin receptor. J Biol Chem 1993;268:8246–8250.

37. Roselli-Rehfuss L, Mountjoy KG, Robbins LS, Mortrud MT, Low MJ, Tatro JB, Entwistle ML, Simerly R, Cone RD. Identification of a receptor for γ-MSH and other proopiomelanocortin peptides in the hypothalamus and limbic system. Proc Natl Acad Sci USA 1993;90:8856–8860.

38. Gantz I, Miwa H, Konda Y, Shimoto Y, Tashiro T, Watson SJ, DelValle J, Yamada T. Molecular cloning, expression, and gene localization of a fourth melanocortin receptor. J Biol Chem 1993;268:15,174–15,179.

39. Mountjoy KG, Mortrud MT, Low MJ, Simerly RB, Cone RD. Localization of the melanocortin-4 receptor (MC4-R) in neuroendocrine and autonomic control circuits in the brain. Mol Endocrinol 1994;8:1298–1308.

40. Chhajlani V, Muceniece R, Wikberg JES. Molecular cloning of a novel human melanocortin receptor. Biochem Biophys Res Commun 1993;195:866–873.

41. Labbe O, Desarnaud F, Eggerickx D, Vassart G, Parmentier M. Molecular cloning of a mouse melanocortin 5 receptor gene widely expressed in peripheral tissues. Biochemistry 1994;33:4543–4549.

42. Gantz I, Shimoto Y, Konda Y, Miwa H, Dickinson CJ, Yamada T. Molecular cloning, expression, and characterization of a fifth melanocortin receptor. Biochem Biophys Res Commun 1994;200:1214–1220.

43. Griffon N, Mignon V, Facchinetti P, Diaz J, Schwartz J-C, Sokoloff P. Molecular cloning and characterization of the rat fifth melanocortin receptor. Biochem Biophys Res Commun 1994;200:1007–1014.

44. Barret P, MacDonald A, Helliwell R, Davidson G, Morgan P. Cloning and expression of a new member of the melanocyte-stimulating hormone receptor family. J Mol Endocrinol 1994;12:203–213.

45. Dixon RAF, Sigal IS, Candelore MR, Register RB, Scatergood A, Rands E, Strader CD. Structural features required for ligand binding to the β-adrenergic receptor. EMBO J 1987;6:3269–3275.

46. Karnik SS, Sakmann JP, Chen HB, Khorana HG. Cysteine residues 110 and 187 are essential for the formation of correct structure in bovine rhodopsin. Proc Natl Acad Sci USA 1988;85:8459–8463.

47. Hadley ME, Hruby VJ, Jiang J, Sharma SD, Fink JL, Haskell-Leuvano C, Bentley DL, Al-Obeidi F, Sawyer TK 1996 Melanocortin receptors: Identification and characterization by melanotropic peptide agonists and antagonists. Pigment Cell Res, 1996;9:213–234.

48. Eberle AN. The melanotropins. Chemistry, Physiology and Mechanisms of Action. S. Karger, Basel, 1988.

49. Abdel-Malek Z, Swope VB, Suzuki I, Akcali C, Harriger MD, Boyce ST, Urabe K, Hearing VJ. The mitogenic and melanogenic stimulation of normal human melanocytes by melanotropic peptides. Proc Natl Acad Sci USA 1995;92:1789–1793.

50. Hunt G, Todd C, Kyne S, Thody AJ. ACTH stimulates melanogenesis in cultured human melanocytes. J Endocrinol 1994;140:R1–R3.

51. Mountjoy KG. The human melanocyte stimulating hormone receptor has evolved to become "supersensitive" to melanocortin peptides. Mol Cell Endocrinol 1994;102:R7–R11.

52. Eberle AN, de Graan PNE, Baumann JB, Girard J, van Hees G, van de Veerdonk FCG. Structural requirements of α-MSH for the stimulation of MSH receptors on different pigment cells. Yale J Biol Med 1984;57:353–354.

53. Lerner AB, McGuire JS. Effect of alpha- and beta-melanocyte stimulating hormones on the skin color of man. Nature 1961;189:176–177.

54. Levine N, Sheftel SN, Eytan T, Dorr RT, Hadley ME, Weinrach JC, Ertl GA, Toth K, McGee DL, Hruby VJ. Induction of skin tanning by subcataneous administration of a potent synthetic melanotropin JAMA 1991;266:2730–2736.

55. Orth DN, Kovacs WJ, DeBold CR. The adrenal cortex. In: Wilson JD, Foster DW, eds. Williams Textbook of Endocrinology, 8th ed. Saunders, Philadelphia, 1992, p. 523.

56. Schauer E, Trautinger F, Kock A, Schwarz A, Bhardwaj R, Simon M, Ansel JC, Schwarz T, Luger TA. Proopiomelanocortin-derived peptides are synthesized and released by human keratinocytes. J Clin Invest 1994;93:2258–2262.

57. Bateman N. *Sombre*, a viable dominant mutant in the house mouse. J Heredity 1961;52:186–189.

58. Carver EA. Coat color genetics of the German shepherd dog. J Hered 1984;75:247–252.

59. Kwon HY, Bultman SJ, Loffler C, Chen W-J, Furdon PJ, Powell JG, Usala A-L, Wilkison W, Hansmann I, Woychik RP. Molecular structure and chromosomal mapping of the human homolog of the *agouti* gene. Proc Natl Acad Sci, USA 1994;91:9760–9764.

60. Wilson BD, Ollmann MM, Kang L, Stoffel M, Bell GI, Barsh GS. Structure and function of ASP, the human human homologue of the mouse *agouti* gene. Hum Mol Genet 1995;4:223–230.

61. Johnson RA, Salomon Y. Assay of adenylyl cyclase catalytic activity. Methods Enzymol 1991; 195:3–21.

62. Siracusa LD. The *agouti* gene: turned on to yellow. TIG 1994;10:423–428.

63. Yen TT, Gill AM, Frigeri LG, Barsh GS, Wolff GL. Obesity, diabetes, and neoplasia in yellow A^{vy}/- mice: ectopic expression of the *agouti* gene. FASEB 1994;8:479–488.

64. Conklin BR, Bourne HR. Mouse coat color reconsidered. Nature 1993;364:110.

65. Manne J, Argeson Ac, Siracusa LD. Mechanisms for the pleiotropic effects of the *agouti* gene. Proc Natl Acad Sci USA 1995;92:4721–4724.

66. Zemel MB, Kim JH, Woychik RP, Michaud EJ, Kadwell SH, Patel IR, Wilkison WO. *Agouti* regulation of intracellular calcium: role in the insulin resistance of viable yellow mice. Proc Natl Acad Sci USA 1995;92:4733–4737.

67. Hruby VJ, Lu D, Sharma SD, Castrucci AL, Kesterson RA, Al-Obeidi FA, Hadley ME, Cone RD. Cyclic lactam α-melanotropin analogues of Ac-Nle^4-c[Asp^4,D-Phe^7,Lys^{10}]α-MSH(4–10)-NH$_2$ with bulky aromatic amino acids at position 7 show high antagonist potency and selectivity at specific melanocortin receptors. J Med Chem 1995;38:3454–3461.

68. Fan W, Boston BA, Kesterson RA, Hruby VJ, Cone RD 1997 Role of melanocortinergic neurons in feeding and the *agouti* obesity syndrome. Nature, 1997;385:165–168.

69. Huszar D, Lynch CA, Fairchild-Huntress V, Dunmore JH, Fang Q, Berkemeier LR, Gu W, Kesterson RA, Boston BA, Cone RD, Smith FJ, Campfield LA, Burn D, Lee F. Targeted disruption of the melanocortin-4 receptor results in obesity in mice. Cell 1997;88:131–141.

70. Siegrist W, Willard DH, Wilkison WO, Eberle AN. *Agouti* protein inhibits growth of B16 melanoma cells in vitro by acting through melanocortin receptors. Biochem Biophys Res Commun 1996; 218:171–175.

71. Blanchard SG, Harris CO, Ittoop ORR, Nichols JS, Parks DJ, Truesdale AT, Wilkison WO. *Agouti* antagonism of melanocortin binding and action in the B16F10 murine melanoma cell line. Biochemistry 1995;34:10,406–10,411.

72. Hunt G, Thody AJ. *Agouti* protein can act independently of melanocyte-stimulating hormone to inhibit melanogenesis. J Endocrinol 1995;147:R1–R4.

73. Suzuki I, Tada A, Ollmann M, Barsh GS, Im S, Lamoreux ML, Hearing VJ, Nordlund JJ, Abdel-Malek Z. 1996 *Agouti* signalling protein inhibits melanogenesis and the response of human melanocytes to α-melanotropin. J Invest Dermatol 1997;108:838–842.

74. Olivera BM, Miljanich GP, Ramachandran J, Adams ME. Calcium channel diversity and neurotransmitter release: The ω-Conotoxins and ω-Agatoxins. Annu Rev Biochem 1994;63:823–867.

75. Lefkowitz RJ, Cotecchia S, Samama P, Costa T. Constitutive activity of receptors coupled to guanine nucleotide regulatory proteins. TIPS 1993;14:303–308.

76. Samama P, Pei G, Costa T, Cotecchia S, Lefkowitz RJ. Negative antagonists promote an inactive conformation of the β$_2$-adrenergic receptor. Mol Pharm 1994;45:390–394.

77. Solca FF, Chluba-de Tapia J, Iwata K, Eberle AN. B16-G4F mouse melanoma cells: an MSH receptor-deficient clone. FEBS Lett 1993;322:177–180.

78. Gantz I, Yamada T, Tashiro T, Konda Y, Shimoto Y, Miwa H, Trent JM. Mapping of the gene encoding the melanocortin-1 (alpha-melanocyte stimulating hormone receptor (MC1-R) to human chromosome 16q24.3 by fluoresence in situ hybridization. Genomics 1994;19:394, 395.

79. Magenis RE, Smith L, Nadeau JH, Johnson KR, Mountjoy KG, Cone RD. Mapping of the ACTH, MSH, and neural (MC3 and MC4) melanocortin receptors in the mouse and human. Mammalian Genome 1994;5:503–508.

80. Falconer DS. *Sombre (So)* on LG XVIII. Mouse News Lett 1962;27:30.

81. Meredith R. Linkage of *am* and *e*. Mouse News Lett 1971;45:31.

82. Searle AG, Beechey CV. Linkage of *Os* and *E^{SO}*. Mouse News Lett 1970;42:27.

83. Cone RD, Mountjoy KG, Robbins LS, Nadeau JH, Johnson KR, Roselli-Rehfuss L, Mortrud MT. Cloning and functional characterization of a family of receptors for the melanotropic peptides. Ann NY Acad Sci 1993;680:342–363.

84. Hauschka TS, Jacobs BB, Holdridge BA. Recessive yellow and its interaction with belted in the mouse. J Heredity 1968;59:339–341.

85. von Lehmann E. Coat color genetics of the *tobacco*-mouse (*Mus poschiavinus Fatio*). Mouse News Lett 1973;48:23.

86. Chen W, Shields TS, Stork PJS, Cone RD. A colorimetric assay for measuring activation of Gs and Gq coupled signaling pathways. Anal Biochem 1995;226:349–354.

87. Cone RD, Lu D, Chen W, Koppula S, Vage DI, Klungland H, Boston B, Orth DN, Pouton C, Kesterson RA. The melanocortin receptors: agonists, antagonists, and the hormonal control of pigmentation. Rec Prog Horm Res 1996;51:287–318.

88. Adalsteinsson S, Bjarnadottir S, Vage DI, Jonmundsson JV. Brown coat color in Icelandic cattle produced by the loci *agouti* and *extension*. J Heredity 1995;86:395–398.

89. Adalsteinsson S, Hersteinsson P, Gunnarsson E. Fox colors in relation to colors in mice and sheep. J Heredity 1987;78:235–237.

90. Ashbrook FG. The Breeding of fur animals. Yearbook of Agriculture U.S. Dept. of Agriculture, Washington D.C. 1379–1395, 1937.

91. Lyon MF. Gene action in the X-chromosome of the mouse (*Mus musculus L.*). Nature 1961; 190:372–373.

92. Reed TE. Red hair colour as a genetical character. Ann Eugen Lond 1952;17:115–139.

93. Hunt G, Todd C, Thody AJ. Unresponsiveness of human epidermal melanocytes to melanocyte-stimulating hormone and its association with red hair. Mol Cell Endocrinol 1996;116:131–136.

94. Valverde P, Healy E, Jackson I, Rees JL, Thody AJ. Variants of the melanocyte-stimulating hormone receptor gene are associated with red hair and fair skin in humans. Nature Genetics 1995;11:328–330

95. Koppula SV, Robbins LS, Lu D, Baack E, White CR, Swanson NA, Cone RD. 1997 Identification of common polymorphisms in the coding sequence of the human MSH receptor (MC1-R). Hum Mutation;9:30–36.

96. Pathak MA, Fitzpatrick TB, Greiter F, Kraus EW. Preventive treatment of sunburn, dermatoheliosis, and skin cancer with sun-protective agents. In: Fitzpatrick TB, Eizen AZ, Wolff K, Freeberg IM, Austen KF, eds. Dermatology in General Medicine, 3rd ed. McGraw-Hill, New York, 1987, p. 1507.

97. Stern C. Model estimates of the number of gene pairs involved in pigmentation variability of the Negro-American. Hum Heredity 1970;20:165.

98. Harrison GA. Differences in human pigmentation: Measurement, geographic variation, and causes. J Invest Dermatol 1973;60:418.

99. Valverde P, Healy E, Sikkink S, Haldane F, Thody AJ, Carothers A, Jackson IJ, Rees JL. The Asp84Glu variant of the melanocortin 1 receptor (MC1R) is associated with melanoma. Hum Mol Genet 1996;5:1663–1666.

100. Frändberg P-A, Muceniece R, Prusis P, Wikberg J, Chhajlani V. Evidence for alternate points of attachment for α-MSH and its stereoisomer [Nle^4, D-Phe^7]-α-MSH at the melanocortin-1 receptor. Biochem Biophys Res Commun 1994;202:1266–1271.

101. Chhajlani V, Xu X, Blauw J, Sudarshi S. Identification of ligand binding residues in extracellular loops of the melanocortin 1 receptor. Biochem Biophys Res Commun 1996;219:521–525.

102. Grigorieff N, Ceska TA, Downing KH, Baldwin JM, Henderson R. Electron-crystallographic refinement of the structure of bacteriorhodopsin. J Mol Biol 1996;259:393–421.

103. Henderson R, Baldwin JM, Ceska TA, Zemlin F, Beckmann E, Downing KH. Model for the structure of bacteriorhodopsin based on high-resolution electron cryo-microscopy. J Mol Biol 1990;213: 899–929.

104. Schertler GFX, Villa C, Henderson R. Projection structure of rhodopsin. Nature 1993;362:770–772.

105. Kyte J, Doolittle RF. A simple method for displaying the hydrophobic character of a protein. J Mol Biol 1982;157:105–132.

106. Baldwin J. The probable arrangement of helices in the G protein-coupled receptors. EMBO J 1993;12:1693–1703.

107. Prusis P, Frändberg P-A, Muceniece R, Kalvinsh I, Wikberg JES. A three dimensional model for the interaction of MSH with the melanocortin-1 receptor. Biochem Biophys Res Commun 1995;210:205–210.

108. Haskell-Luevano C, Sawyer TK, Trumpp-Kallmeyer S, Bikker J, Humblet C, Gantz I, Hruby VJ. Three-dimensional molecular models of the hMC1R melanocortin receptor: Complexes with melanotropin peptide agonists. Drug Design Discovery 1996;14:197–211.

109. Strader CD, Fong TM, Tota MR, Underwood D, Dixon RAF. Structure and function of G protein-coupled receptors. Annu Rev Biochem 1994;63:101–132.

110. Savarese TM, Fraser CM. In vitro mutagenesis and the search for structure-function relationships among G protein-coupled receptors. Biochem J 1992;283:1–19.

111. Zhu SZ, Wang SZ, Hu J, El-Fakahany EE. An arginine residue conserved in most G protein-coupled receptors is essential for the function of the m1 muscarinic receptor. Mol Pharm 1994;45:517–523.

112. Williams KA, Deber CM. Proline residues in transmembrane helices: Structural or dynamic role? Biochemistry 1991;30:8919–8923.

113. Chou PY, Fasman GD. Empirical predictions of protein conformation Ann Rev Biochem 1978;47:251–276.

114. Gardella TJ, Luck MD, Fan M-H, Lee CW. Transmembrane residues of the parathyroid hormone (PTH)/PTH-related peptide receptor that specifically affect binding and signaling by agonist ligands. J Biol Chem 1996;271:12,820–12,825.

115. Berlose J-P, Convert O, Brunissen A, Chassaing G, La Vielle S. Three-dimensional structure of the highly conserved seventh transmembrane domain of G-protein-coupled receptors. Eur J Biochem 1994;225:827–843.

116. Hunyady L, Bor M, Baukal AJ, Balla T, Catt KJ. A conserved NPLFY sequence contributes to agonist binding and signal trandsuction but is not an internalization signal for the type 1 angiotensin II receptor. J Biol Chem 1996;270:16,602–16,609.

15 ACTH Resistance Syndromes

Constantine Tsigos, MD, PhD
and George P. Chrousos, MD

Contents

The adrenocorticotrophic hormone (ACTH) receptor controls adrenal steroidogenesis in response to circulating ACTH. The recent cloning of the receptor has opened a new understanding of the normal and pathologic functioning of the adrenal cortex. This chapter will focus on the clinical forms of hereditary ACTH resistance syndromes and their association with abnormalities of the ACTH receptor gene.

ACTH RECEPTOR—BIOLOGY

The ACTH receptor together with the other melanocortin receptors form a distinct subfamily of the canonical G-protein-coupled receptors, sharing among themselves some unique structural characteristics *(1–3)*. Thus, they are the smallest members of the G-protein-coupled receptor superfamily, the ACTH receptor having 297 amino acid residues, and are encoded by intronless genes. They also lack several amino acid residues present in most of the other members of this superfamily, such as the proline residues in the fourth and fifth transmembrane domains, which introduce bends in the α-helical structure, and one or both cysteine residues thought to form disulfide bonds between the first and second extracellular loops. In addition, the melanocortin receptors have somewhat unusual transmembrane topology. Their second extracellular loop is quite short and hydrophobic, so that no extracellular domain may exist. The recent 3-DS modeling of the skin melanocortin receptor suggested that the binding pocket for the ligand is located between the second, third, and sixth transmembrane domains, with several points of interaction. All melanocortin receptors, including the ACTH receptor, are coupled to G_s.

From: *Contemporary Endocrinology: G Proteins, Receptors, and Disease*
Edited by: A. M. Spiegel Humana Press Inc., Totowa, NJ

The expression of the ACTH receptor, assessed by Northern blot analysis, is characteristically limited to the adrenal cortex *(1)*. *In situ* hybridization has actually demonstrated that the receptor is expressed in all three adrenocortical *zonae (1)*. Thus, it appears that the reported actions of ACTH in a spectrum of extra-adrenal, tissues and cells, most notably peripheral blood leukocytes *(5)*, adipocytes *(6,7)*, and the brain *(8,9)* are mediated by other melanocortin receptors, which bind ACTH. A typical example is the ability to ACTH to stimulate melanin synthesis by melanocytes through the skin MSH receptor *(1,10)*. Thus, in the human, circulating ACTH, in the absence of circulating αMSH, serves a dual role: regulation of adrenal steroidogenesis and pigmentation *(11)*.

ACTH RECEPTOR—SIGNALING CASCADE

ACTH, a 39 amino acid peptide, is the major circulating proteolytic product of proopiomelanocortin (POMC). The adrenal cortex is the principal target organ of circulating ACTH *(12)*. ACTH regulates glucocorticoid and adrenal androgen secretion by the *zonae fasciculata* and *reticularis*, respectively. ACTH also participates in the control of aldosterone secretion by the *zona glomerulosa (13)*. ACTH receptors mediate all these actions of ACTH.

The biologic activity of ACTH resides in the N-terminal portion of its molecule, with the first 24 amino acids being necessary for maximal activity. On binding with ACTH, the receptors are activated and, in turn, activate the heterotrimeric G-protein complex, which subsequently activates adenylyl cyclase *(14)*. This enzyme catalyzes cyclic adenosine monophosphate (cAMP) generation, which results in activation of protein kinase A. This, in turn, stimulates cholesterol ester hydrolase, the enzyme responsible for the conversion of cholesterol esters to cholesterol, which is then transported inside the mitochondria for side chain cleavage and the subsequent steroidogenesis steps. In addition to the direct effect on steroidogenesis, ACTH also increases the uptake of cholesterol from plasma lipoproteins and has a trophic effect on the adrenal cortices *(15)*. Thus, ACTH excess produces adrenal hyperplasia, and conversely, ACTH deficiency causes atrophy. Adrenocortical dysfunction might also result from abnormalities along the ACTH signaling cascade, from the membrane receptor to the kinases stimulating steroidogenesis.

ACTH RECEPTOR—REGULATION

The cloning of the ACTH receptor gene has also allowed a more detailed analysis of the physiological regulation of this receptor. Thus, in contrast to the commonly observed homologous downregulation of target tissue receptors by their own hormone ligands, ACTH apparently upregulates its own receptors and results in an increase in their numbers in the cells of the *zonae fasciculata* and *reticularis (16–18)*. In addition, ACTH produces dose- and time-dependent increases in the transcription rate of the ACTH receptor and in the ACTH receptor mRNA longevity. It could be argued that teleologically this represents an advantage for the hypothalamic–pituitary–adrenal axis, one of the two principal effector limbs of the stress system. It also suggests that the exaggerated glucocorticoid secretion observed during continuous or intermittent treatment with ACTH, as well as in patients with ACTH-secreting tumors, is caused not only by the positive trophic effect of ACTH on adrenocortical cells and the stimulation of the steroidogenesis enzymes, but also by the positive effects of the hormone on its own receptors. Interestingly, angiotensin II also appears to dose-dependently increase the

ACTH receptor mRNA in the same cells, primarily a transcriptional effect *(17,18)*. Since angiotensin II acts mainly by causing elevations of Ca^{2+} and diacylglycerol, it is likely that the ACTH receptor gene is regulated by multiple signal transduction pathways, including those of Protein kinase A and Protein kinase C.

ACTH RESISTANCE SYNDROMES

Clinical Presentation and Diagnosis

Hereditary unresponsivenes to ACTH or isolated glucocorticoid deficiency is a rare autosomal-recessive disorder that manifests as primary adrenal insufficiency, usually without mineralocorticoid deficiency. This disorder was first described in 1959 by Shepard et al. *(19)*, since when many cases, including childhood deaths, have been described *(20–26)*. Affected children commonly present with hyperpigmentation, recurrent hypoglycemia that can lead to convulsions or coma, chronic asthenia, and failure to thrive. Typically, plasma cortisol levels are undetectable and do not respond to exogenous ACTH, whereas endogenous plasma ACTH concentrations are very high, consistent with resistance to ACTH action. Aldosterone and adrenal androgen responses to ACTH are also lost in these patients. However, renin and aldosterone levels are usually normal, and respond appropriately to activation of the renin–angiotensin axis by salt restriction, orthostasis, and furosemide-induced diuresis. Evidence of congenital adrenal hyperplasia in the form of excessive steroid precursors and evidence of adrenoleukodystrophy in the form of excess very long-chain fatty acids is lacking.

In keeping with the biochemical studies, histological examination of the adrenal glands from patients who died from the disease has revealed that the ACTH-dependent *zonae fasciculata* and *reticularis* are extremely atrophic, reduced to a narrow band of fibrous tissue, whereas the angiotensin II–dependent *zona glomerulosa* is relatively well preserved *(19,21)*. This has led to the suggestions that the disorder might reflect a defect in the ACTH receptor, in ACTH signal tranduction, or in adrenocortical development. The isolated nature of the defect, however, which appears to be limited to the ACTH-dependent *zonae* of the adrenal cortex, pointed toward a receptor abnormality as the locus of the disease, and the cloning of the ACTH receptor has permitted a test of this hypothesis.

A subset of the patients with hereditary ACTH resistance, however, in addition to hypocortisolism, develops alacrima (lack of tears) and achalasia of the esophagus (leading to difficulty in swallowing), suggesting potential heterogeneity in the etiology of this syndrome *(27–31)*. The latter constellation of symptoms is referred to as triple A or Allgrove's syndrome, first described in 1978 *(27)*. Low tear production may be confirmed with the Shirmer's test, whereas esophageal dysmotility can be demonstrated by barium swallow and/or endoscopic examination. These patients may also develop variable degrees of mineralocorticoid deficiency. Histologic examination of the adrenals reveals an appearance very similar to that in isolated glucocorticoid deficiency, with atrophic inner zones of the cortex. More recently, it has become apparent that progressive and variable neurologic impairment, which might include autonomic and peripheral neuropathy, ataxia, and mental retardation, is also frequently associated with the triple A syndrome, which can thus be quite debilitating *(30,31)*.

Treatment for both ACTH resistance syndromes, the isolated glucocorticoid deficiency, and the triple A syndrome consists of glucocorticoid replacement therapy and, when appropriate, additional mineralocorticoid replacement. Patients with isolated glucocorticoid deficiency achieve normal growth and development with steroid replacement and live an otherwise normal life. For the patients with the triple A syndrome, however, the quality of life depends on the severity and course of esophageal dysmotility and neurological impairment that develops. The former can effectively be treated with surgical intervention (Heller's myotomy), but there is no known means to prevent or influence the latter.

Molecular Pathophysiology

The cloning of the ACTH receptor gene enabled us to amplify by PCR its entire coding region from leukocyte DNA from individuals affected with isolated glucocorticoid deficiency. DNA sequencing revealed that our initial patient, an African-American boy, was a compound heterozygote for two different point mutations in the ACTH receptor gene *(32)*. One allele contained a stop codon at amino acid 201 of the third cytosolic loop (Fig. 1), resulting in a truncated receptor protein, lacking a major part of the third cytosolic loop, the sixth and seventh transmembrane domains, as well as the third extracellular loop and the cytosolic carboxy-tail. Thus, the mutant receptor, even in the unlikely event that it was expressed, should be unable to transduce the signal. In the other allele, neutral Ser[120] within the apolar third transmembrane domain was replaced by the basic Arg, which would be expected to disrupt receptor structure and ligand binding, since this domain is important for the formation of the binding pocket of the receptor. Furthermore, by performing a standard 3-h ovine CRH test in the parents and grandparents of the proband, we demonstrated that heterozygosity for either of the mutations was associated with exaggerated and prolonged ACTH responses to ovine CRH. This suggested subclinical resistance to ACTH in these individuals, and also provided in vivo evidence for a causal relationship between mutations of the ACTH receptor and the ACTH resistance in this family.

In another African-American kindred with isolated glucocorticoid deficiency, we found a homozygote A→G substitution *(33)* changing Tyr[254] to Cys in the third extracellular loop of the receptor protein, probably interfering with disulfide bond formation, and hence, with the tertiary structure of the receptor and its capacity to bind the ligand and/or to couple with appropriate G proteins. Support for the idea that the mutant cysteine renders the ACTH receptor dysfunctional also comes from previous reports of point mutations introducing extra cysteines in the extracellular loops of the V2 vasopressin receptor in kindreds with nephrogenic diabetes insipidus *(34)*.

Six additional point mutations and two frameshift mutations have been reported as homozygote or compound heterozygote mutations in different pedigrees with isolated glucocorticoid deficiency. These mutations are scattered throughout the molecule and affect all aspects of receptor function as outlined in Table 1 and Fig. 1. Clark et al. *(35)* reported a homozygous point mutation that converted Ser[74] to Ile. This mutation, which later was also identified in two additional British families *(36)*, was predicted to induce a modification in the affinity for the ligand and/or in the coupling to adenylyl cyclase of the mutant receptor. It is interesting to note that this mutation is in the second transmembrane domain of the ACTH receptor, where two independent mutations that profoundly affect the function of the skin MSH receptor have also been found *(37)*. In one of these British families, the S74I mutation was in compound heterozygote form with a point mutation converting Arg[128] into a cysteine. Arg[128] is a highly conserved residue on the C-terminal side of the third transmembrane domain (Fig. 1), a very important region

ACTH Receptor

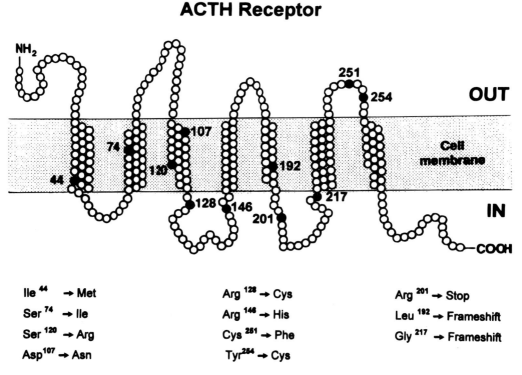

Ile ^{44} → Met	Arg ^{128} → Cys	Arg ^{201} → Stop
Ser ^{74} → Ile	Arg ^{146} → His	Leu ^{192} → Frameshift
Ser ^{120} → Arg	Cys ^{251} → Phe	Gly ^{217} → Frameshift
Asp ^{107} → Asn	Tyr ^{254} → Cys	

Fig. 1. Schematic representation of the ACTH receptor with the characteristic seven transmembrane domain structure, indicating the position of amino acid substitutions thus far identified to be associated with hereditary isolated glucocorticoid deficiency.

for interacting with or activating G_s-protein. Thus, this mutation probably results in diminished or abolished signal transduction.

Weber et al. *(36)* also reported a Finnish pedigree, which combined a point mutation substituting Ile44 by methionine with a frameshift mutation (caused by a 2-bp deletion) after Leu^{192} in the fifth transmembrane domain. The latter mutation results in major disruption of the structure of the ACTH receptor, with most probably complete loss of its function. In contrast, it is not clear how the 144M mutation alters receptor function, if at all, as the hydrophobic Ile44 in the first transmembrane domain is not a conserved residue and is substituted by the relatively hydrophobic Met in the bovine ACTH receptor.

Weber et al. *(36)* also reported two other independent families, one of Pakistani and one of African-American ancestry, which were both homozygous for a mutation changing Arg^{146} to His. In view of the location of Arg^{146} in the C-terminal end of the second intracellular loop, it may have an important role in signal transduction.

Naville et al. *(38)* reported another patient with a homozygote mutation, converting the negatively charged Asp^{107} in the third transmembrane domain to an uncharged Asn residue. They also described a compound heterozygote patient, in whom the paternal allele contained a one-nucleotide insertion at the junction of the third intracellular loop and the sixth transmembrane domain, which modified the reading frame after residue Gly^{217}, eventually leading to a stop codon within the third extracellular loop. The maternal allele of the same patient contained a point mutation converting Cys^{251} to Phe,

Table 1
Mutations of the ACTH Receptor Gene in Patients
with Hereditary Isolated Glucocorticoid Deficiency

Mutation	Probable effect of mutation	Refs.
R201X	Truncated receptor	Tsigos et al. (32)
L192fs	Truncated receptor	Weber et al. (36)
G217fs	Truncated receptor	Naville et al. (38)
S120R	Possible structural disruption	Tsigos et al. (32)
S74I	Possible loss of ligand affinity	Clark et al. (35)
I44M	Possible loss of ligand affinity	Weber et al. (36)
Y254C	Possible structural disruption	Tsigos et al. (33)
R146H	Loss of signal transduction	Weber et al. (36)
R128C	Loss of signal transduction	Weber et al. (36)
D107N	Possible loss of ligand affinity	Naville et al. (38)
C251F	Possible structural disruption	Naville et al. (38)

also in the third extracellular loop. All three mutations were expressed in the M3 cell line, in which no response to physiological ACTH concentrations was detected for either of the mutant receptors. It would, indeed, be expected that the G217 mutation would lead to the production of a truncated receptor protein unable to transduce the signal. The D107 and Cys^{251} mutations must affect amino acids that are important for ligand binding and/or signal transduction. These two residues are conserved in all members of the melanocortin receptor family. Moreover, substitution of Asn for Asp^{107} in the histamine H1 receptor substantially decreased the affinity of the receptor to the ligand owing to disruption of the important ionic interactions of this residue (39). In contrast, substitution by site-directed mutagenesis of the corresponding Asp at position 113 by an Asn in the human β-adrenergic receptor produced a receptor that failed to couple with adenylyl cyclase (40). Interestingly, the ACTH receptor has two more Cys residues, other than Cys^{251}, in its short third extracellular loop, all conserved among the melanocortin receptor family. These residues appear to be important for ligand binding, as studies on homologous Cys residues in other G-protein-coupled receptors (e.g., TSH receptor, type 1 angiotensin II receptor, and the β-adrenergic receptor) have clearly demonstrated (41,42.)

It should be stressed at this point that preparation of functional cell lines that express the ACTH receptor transiently or permanently has proven a very difficult task for many laboratories, since it seems that cells with an endogenous melanocortin receptor are the only ones to express the gene successfully. It might well be that some additional cell machinery component is required for efficient expression of the ACTH receptor. Moreover, ACTH ligand binding studies are quite difficult, further complicating the investigation of the structure/function relationships of the ACTH receptor. Undoubtedly, greater understanding of the relevance of the mutations for ACTH receptor function will have to await further expression and binding studies.

Not all clinically defined cases of hereditary isolated glucocorticoid deficiency, however, are associated with mutations within the coding region of the ACTH receptor gene. Weber and Clark (43) and Naville et al. (38) actually described 4 and

13 such families, respectively, which were clinically indistinguishable from those in whom mutations were identified. In addition. Weber and Clark et al. *(43)*, using a pair of polymorphic dinucleotide repeats that is localized in the same region of chromosome 18, to which the human ACTH receptor has been mapped (18p11.2) *(44)*, demonstrated no apparent linkage between the disease and the ACTH receptor gene in four families. These findings suggest that there may be an abnormality in the promoter region of the gene or that a gene other than that of the ACTH receptor might produce the same phenotype.

It has been proposed that the ACTH receptor may also be defective in the triple A syndrome. We have been unable, however, to find mutations in the entire coding region of this gene in several families with the triple A syndrome *(33,45)*. This syndrome has some features of a contiguous gene defect, since there are clearly cases in whom only two of the three features are present, and there is significant variability in the occurrence and nature of the neurological abnormalities *(29,31,46)*. However, chromosomal abnormalities in these patients have not been described. A developmental defect might, thus, be implicated in this syndrome or, alternatively, an abnormality in the intracellular signaling of ACTH. Reverse genetics and linkage analysis will probably offer the means to resolve this question, which, given the progressive nature of the syndrome, may allow the development of therapeutic approaches that can prevent further deterioration.

Finally, it is interesting, that unlike the occurrence of activating mutations in other G-protein-coupled receptors that cause either tumorigenesis (e.g., mutations of the TSH receptor in functioning thyroid adenomas [47]) or hereditary hormone hypersecretion syndromes (e.g., mutations of the LH receptor in familial male precocious puberty [48,49]), no such mutations have been identified in more than 40 adrenocortical tumors studied so far *(50,51)*. It appears, therefore, that this mechanism could only very rarely be associated with adrenal neoplasia, if at all.

SUMMARY

The syndromes of hereditary isolated glucocorticoid deficiency and triple A syndrome are potentially life-threatening and severely disabling. Clinical awareness of these syndromes is of considerable prognostic and therapeutic importance. The defects in the ACTH receptor causing isolated glucocorticoid deficiency help illuminate the mechanisms of ligand binding and signal transduction by this receptor. Identification of the molecular defect(s) responsible for isolated glucocorticoid deficiency in cases with a normal ACTH receptor gene coding region and for the triple A syndrome remains a challenge. Discovery of these defects will hopefully eventually provide further insight into the mechanisms of adrenocortical function and will allow new therapeutic approaches.

REFERENCES

1. Mountjoy KG, Robbins LS, Mortrud MT, Cone RD. The cloning of a family of genes that encode the melanocortin receptors. Science 1992;257:1248–1251.
2. Cone RD, Mountjoy KG. Molecular genetics of the ACTH and melanocyte-stimulating hormone receptors. Trends Endocrinol Metab 1993;4:242–247.
3. Cone RD, Mountjoy KG, Robbins LS, Nadeau JH, Johnson KR, Roselli-Rehfus L, Mortrud MT. Cloning and functional characterization of a family of receptors for the melanotropin peptides. Ann NY Acad Sci 1993;680:342–363.

4. Prusis P, Frandberg P-A, Muceniece R, Kalvinsh I, Wikberg JES. A three dimentional model for the interaction of MSH with the melanocortin-1 receptor. Biochem Biophys Res Commun 1995;10:205–210.

5. Smith EM, Brosnan P, Meyer WH, Blalock JE. An ACTH receptor on human mononuclear lymphocytes. N Engl J Med 1987;317:1266–1269.

6. Oelofsen W, Ramachandran J. Studies of corticotropin receptors on rat adipocytes. Arch Biochem Biophys 1983;225:414–421.

7. Boston BA, Cone RD. Characterization of melanocortin receptor subtype expression in murine adipose tissues and in the 3T3-L1 cell line. Endocrinology 1996;137:2043–2050.

8. Low MJ, Simerly RB, Cone RD. Receptors for the melanocortin peptides in the central nervous system. Curr Opinion Endocrinol Diabetes 1994;1:79–88.

9. Tatro JB. Melanotropin receptors are differentially distributed and recognize both corticotropin and α-melanocyte stimulating hormone. Brain Res 1990;536:124–132.

10. Hunt G, Todd C, Kyne S, Thody AJ. ACTH stimulates melanogenesis in cultured human melanocytes. J Endocrinol 1994;140:R1–R3.

11. Tsigos C, Arai K, Latronico AC, Weber E, Chrousos GP. Receptors for melanocortin peptides in the hypothalamic-pituitary-adrenal axis and skin. Ann NY Acad Sci 1995;771:352–363.

12. Tsigos C, Chrousos GP. Physiology of the hypothalamic-pituitary adrenal axis in health and dysregulation in psychiatric and autoimmune disorders. Endocrinol Metab Clin North Am 1994;23:451–466.

13. Aguilera G. Factors controlling steroid biosynthesis in the zona glomerulosa of the adrenal. J Biochem Mol Biol 1993;45:147–152.

14. Buckley DL, Ramachandran J. Characterization of corticotropin receptors on adrenocortical cells. Proc Natl Acad Sci USA 1981;78:7431–7435.

15. Kimura T. Effects of hypophysectomy and ACTH administration on the level of adrenal cholesterol side chain desmolase. Endocrinology 1969;85:492–499.

16. Penhoat A, Jaillard C, Saez JM. Corticotropin positively regulates its own receptors and cyclic AMP response in cultured bovine adrenal cells. Proc Natl Acad Sci USA 1989;86:4978–4981.

17. Lebrethon MC, Naville D, Begeot M, Saez JM. Regulation of corticotropin receptor number and messenger RNA in cultured human adrenocortical cells by corticotropin and angiotensin II. J Clin Invest 1994;93:1828–1833.

18. Mountjoy KG, Bird IM, Rainey WE, Cone RD. ACTH induces up-regulation of ACTH receptor mRNA in mouse and human adrenocortical cell lines. Mol Cell Endocrinol 1994;99:R17–R20.

19. Shepard TH, Landing BH, Mason DG. Familial Addison's disease. Case reports of two sisters with corticoid deficiency unassociated with hypoaldosteronism. AMA J Dis Child 1959;97:154–162.

20. Migeon CJ, Kenny FM, Kowarski, Snipes CA, Spaulding JS, Finkelstein JW, Blizzard RM. The syndrome of congenital unresponsiveness to ACTH. Report of six cases. Pediatr Res 1968;2:501–513.

21. Kelch RP, Kaplan SL, Biglieri EG, Daniels GH, Epstein CJ, Grumbach MM. Hereditary adreno-cor-tical unresponsiveness to adrenocorticotropin hormone. J Pediatr 1972;81:726–736.

22. Kershnar AK, Roe TF, Kogut MD. Adrenocorticotropin hormone unresponsiveness: report of a girl with excessive growth and rewiew of 16 reported cases. J Pediatr 1972;80:610–619.

23. Thistletwaite D, Darling JAB, Fraser R, Mason PA, Rees LH, Harkness RA. Familial glucocorticoid deficiency. Studies of diagnosis and pathogenesis. Arch Dis Child 1975;50:291–297.

24. Spark RF, Etzkorn JR. Absent aldosterone response to ACTH in familial glucocorticoid deficiency. N Engl J Med 1977;297:917–920.

25. Davidai G, Kahara L, Hochberg Z. Glomerulosa failure in congenital adrenocortical unresponsiveness to ACTH. Clin Endocrinol (Oxford) 1984;20:515–520.

26. Yamaoka T, Kudo T, Takuwa Y, Kawakami Y, Itakura M, Yamashita K. Hereditary adrenocortical unresponsiveness to adrenocorticotropin with a postreceptor defect. J Clin Endocrinol Metab 1992;75:270–274.

27. Allgrove J, Clayden GS, Grant BD, Macaulay JC. Familial glucocorticoid deficiency with achalasia of the cardia and deficient tear production. Lancet 1978;1:1284–1286.

28. Geffner ME, Lippe BM, Kaplan SA, Berquist WE, Bateman JB, Paterno VI, Seegan R. Selective ACTH insensitivity, achalasia, and alacrima: a multi-system disorder presenting in childhood. Pediatr Res 1983;17:532–536.

29. Moore PSJ, Couch RM, Perry YS, Shuckett EP, Winter JSD. Allgrove syndrome: an autosomal recessive syndrome of ACTH insensitivity, achalasia and alacrima. Clin Endocrinol 1991;34:107–114.

30. Stuckey BG, Mastaglia FL, Reed WD, Pullan PT. Glucocorticoid insufficiency, achalasia, alacrima with autonomic and motor neuropathy. Ann Intern Med 1993;106:62–64.

31. Grant DB, Barnes ND, Dumic M, Ginalska-Malinowska M, Milla PJ, v Petrykowski W, Rowlatt RJ, Steendijk R, Wales JHK, Werder E. Neurological and adrenal dysfunction in the adrenal insufficiency/alacrima/achalasia (3A) syndrome. Arch Dis Child 1993;68:779–782.

32. Tsigos C, Arai K, Hung W, Chrousos GP. Hereditary isoalated glucocorticoid deficiency associated with abnormalities of the adrenocorticotropin receptor gene. J Clin Invest 1993;92:2458–2461.

33. Tsigos C, Arai K, Latronico AC, DiGeorge AM, Rapaport R, Chrousos GP. A novel mutation of the adrenocorticotropin receptor (ACTH-R) gene in a family with the syndrome of isolated glucocorticoid deficiency, but no ACTH-R abnormalities in two families with the triple A syndrome. J Clin Endocrinol Metab 1995;80:875–877.

34. Pan Y, Metzenberg A, Das S, Jing B, Gitschier J. Mutations in the V2 vasopressin receptor gene are associated with X-linked nephrogenic diabetes insipidus. Nature Genet 1992;2:103–106.

35. Clark AJL, McLoughlin L, Grossman A. Familial glucocorticoid deficiency associated with point mutation in the adrenocorticotropin receptor. Lancet 1993;341:461–462.

36. Weber A, Toppari J, Harvey RD, Klann RC, Shaw NJ, Ricker AT, Nanto-Salonen K, Bevan JS, Clark AJL. Adrenocorticotropin receptor gene mutations in familial glucocorticoid deficiency: relationships with clinical features in four families. J Clin Endocrinol Metab 1995;80:65–71.

37. Robbins LS, Nadeau JH, Johnson XR, Kelly MA, Roselli-Rehfuss L, Baack E, Mountjoy KG, Cone RD. Pigmentation phenotypes of variant extension locus alleles result from point mutations that alter MSH receptor function. Cell 1993;72:827–834.

38. Naville D, Barjhoux L, Jaillard C, Fauty D, Despert F, Esteva B, Durand P, Saez JM, Begeot M. Demonstration by tranfection studies that mutations in the adrenocorticotropin receptor gene are one cause of the hereditary syndrome of glucocorticoid deficiency. J Clin Endocrinol Metab 1996;81:1442–1448.

39. Ohta K, Hayashi H, Mizuguchi H, Kagamiyama H, Fujimoto K, Fukui H. Site-directed mutagenesis of histamine H1 receptor: roles of aspartic acid 107, asparagine 198 and threonine 194. Biochem Biophys Res Commun 1994;203:1096–1011.

40. Strader CD, Sigal IS, Register RB, et al. Identification of residues required for ligand-binding to the β-adrenergic receptor. Proc Natl Acad Sci USA 1987;84:4384–4388.

41. Kosugi S, Ban T, Akamizu T, Kohn LD. Role of cysteine residues in the extracellular domain and exoplasmic loops of the transmembrane domain of the TSH receptor: effect of mutation to serine on TSH receptor activity and response to thyroid stimulating autoantibodies. Biochem Biophys Res Commun 1992;189:1754–1762.

42. Fraser CM. Site-directed mutagenesis of b-adrenergic receptors. J Biol Chem 1989;264:9266–9270.

43. Weber A, Clark AJL. Mutations of the ACTH receptor gene are only one cause of familial glucocorticoid deficiency. Hum Mol Genet 1994;358:585–588.

44. Vamvakopoulos NC, Durkin S, Nierman W, Chrousos GP. Mapping of the human adrenocorticotropin hormone receptor (ACTH-R) gene to the small arm of chromosome 18 (18p. 11.21-pter.). Genomics 1993;18:454–455.

45. Heinrichs C, Tsigos C, Deschepper J, Drews R, Collu R, Dugardeyn C, Goyens P, Ghanem G, Bosson D, Chrousos G, Van Vliet G. Familial adrenocorticotropin unresponsiveness associated with alacrima and achalasia: biochemical and molecular studies in two siblings with clinical heterogeneity. Eur J Pediatr 1995;154:191–196.

46. Haverkamp F, Zerres K, Rosskamp R. Three sibs with achalasia and alacrima: a separate entity different from triple-A syndrome. Am J Med Genet 1989;34:289–291.

47. Parma J, Duprez L, Van Sande J, et al. Somatic mutations in the thyrotropin receptor gene cause hyperfunctioning thyroid adenomas. Nature 1993;365:649–651.

48. Shenker A, Laue L, Kosugi S, Merendino JJ Jr, Minegishi T, Cutler Jr GB. A constitutively activating mutation of the luteinizing hormone receptor in familial male precocious puberty. Nature 1993;365:652–654.

49. Latronico AC, Reincke M, Mendonca BB, Arai K, Mora P, Allolio B, Wajchenberg BL, Chrousos GP, Tsigos C. No evidence for oncogenic mutations in the adrenocorticotropin receptor (ACTH-R) gene in human adrenocortical neoplasms. J Clin Endocrinol Metab 1995;80:2490–2494.

50. Latronico AC, Anasti J, Arnhold IJP, Mendonca BB, Domenice S, Albano MCC, Zachman K, Wajchenberg BL, Tsigos C. A novel mutation of the luteinizing hormone receptor gene causing male gonadotropin-independent precocious puberty. J Clin Endocrinol Metab 1995;80:2490–2494.

51. Light K, Jenkins PJ, Weber A, Perrett C, Grossman A, Pistorello M, Asa SL, Clayton RN, Clark AJL. Are activating mutations of the adrenocorticotropin receptor involved in adrenal cortical neoplasia? Life Sci 1995;56:1523–1527.

16 Altering Adrenergic Signaling and Cardiac Function in Transgenic Mice

Walter J. Koch, PhD, and Robert J. Lefkowitz, MD

CONTENTS

INTRODUCTION

The ability to maintain and manipulate mouse embryos in vitro, perfected over the last decade, has launched the expanding field of transgenic experimentation models. With the successful insertion of foreign genes into the mouse genome, important in vivo transgenic models have emerged in several venues of biomedical research, which allows for a broader understanding of pathological conditions. Transgenic mice permit investigation of the consequences of a protein's overexpression in specific tissues. In addition, the loss of function of a protein or enzyme in a given organ can be examined by overexpression of an inhibitor peptide or a dominant-negative mutant. Elimination of a protein from all tissues can also be achieved by gene disruption techniques. These approaches are well suited to study the physiological roles of cellular proteins.

It is apparent that the cutting edge of the field of cardiovascular biology currently centers on the integrative study of genes and physiology. Transgenic models geared toward the study of cardiovascular regulation have recently been described and provide powerful tools to study normal and compromised cardiac physiology. Some of these transgenic models have addressed changes in blood pressure, whereas others examined the consequences of altering apolipoprotein levels *(1)*. Most recently, transgenic mice have been developed in which plasma membrane G-protein-coupled receptor signaling

From: *Contemporary Endocrinology: G Proteins, Receptors, and Disease*
Edited by: A. M. Spiegel Humana Press Inc., Totowa, NJ

has been altered; these animals provide powerful new information regarding the role of signal transduction in cardiac function both under normal and diseased states *(2)*.

Heart disease and its complications are the leading cause of mortality in this country, and its treatment consumes millions of health care dollars. Although the overall mortality rate owing to cardiovascular disease has dropped in the last decade, congestive heart failure continues to be a major cause of morbidity, since hospitalizations have dramatically increased in recent years with 400,000 new cases diagnosed annually in the United States *(3)*. Chronic congestive heart failure is a disease that is characterized by heightened sympathetic nervous system activity and elevated plasma norepinephrine levels with related changes in myocardial adrenergic signaling *(3,4)*. Thus, adrenergic signaling in the heart is of much interest and has recently been a key target of investigation in transgenic animal models. Manipulation of various components of the myocardial adrenergic receptor system has increased our understanding of cardiovascular diseases, such as congestive heart failure in which adrenergic signaling plays a critical role. These transgenic model systems have led to novel agonist-independent approaches to enhance signaling and augment cardiac function.

MYOCARDIAL ADRENERGIC SIGNALING

Probably the most important receptors involved in beat-to-beat cardiac regulation are the adrenergic receptors. These G-protein-coupled receptors modulate cardiomyocyte function by stimulating effector molecules, which give rise to increases in intracellular second messengers like cAMP and diacylglycerol. In the human heart, as stated above, adrenergic receptors are critical regulators of function under both normal and diseased conditions. Myocardial β-adrenergic receptors (β-ARs), for example, mediate increases in heart rate and contractility in response to increases in the levels of both noreprinephrine (NE) and the adrenal medullary hormone epinephrine. These two catecholamines bind selectively to adrenergic receptors, most importantly β-ARs, present on the sarcolemma.

β-ARs in cardiac muscle include both the β_1- and β_2-subtypes. In the human heart, as with most mammals, the β_1-AR is the predominant subtype approaching 75–80% of total β-ARs *(4)*. Classically, β_1- and β_2-ARs selectively couple to the adenylyl cyclase stimulatory G protein, G_s, which triggers the catalysis of cyclic adenosine monophosphate (cAMP) formation. Subsequently, this leads to the activation of cAMP-dependent protein kinase (PKA), which targets and phosphorylates several myocardial proteins involved in the positive chronotropic and inotropic response, such as L-type voltage-dependent calcium channels and the sarcoplasmic reticulum protein phospholamban. Activation of both β_1- and β_2-ARs can lead to increased cardiac contractility *(4)*. However, recent evidence has demonstrated that β_2-ARs elicit qualitatively different signaling mechanisms from those of β_1-ARs within cardiac myocytes *(5)*. cAMP-independent β_2-ARs regulation of cardiac contractile function has been observed in several species including humans *(5,6)*. The nature and significance of β_2-AR function in the myocardium, in light of this new evidence, are not well understood.

In addition to β-ARs, cardiac muscle also contains α_1-ARs, which are expressed at low levels comparable to densities of β_2-ARs *(7)*. Myocytes and myocardial tissue from several species contain both α_{1A}- and α_{1B}-AR subtypes with the predominate subtype varying among mammals *(8)*. The general signaling paradigm for α_1-ARs is that they couple to the G protein, G_q, which stimulates phospholipase C-β (PLC-β), producing the second messengers inositol trisphosphate and diacylglycerol. These messengers, in turn, increase intracellular Ca^{2+} concentrations and activate protein kinase C (PKC), respectively. The exact role of the α_1-AR-G_q-PLC-β pathway in myocardial beat-to-beat regulation is not clear, and the precise function of these receptors is unknown (7,8). In fact, it appears that not all α_1-ARs in the heart are coupled to this Ca^{2+}-mobilization pathway, since other actions of α_1-agonists have been demonstrated in cardiac myocytes, including changes in ionic conductances and intracellular pH, suggesting coupling to other G proteins (8). Recent in vitro studies, however, suggest that activation of α_1-ARs and other G_q-coupled receptors that activate PKC, such as those for endothelin I and angiotension II (AngII), play a critical role in the initiation of myocyte hypertrophy (9).

The regulation of myocardial adrenergic receptors, like most G-protein-coupled receptors involves desensitization mechanisms, which are characterized by a rapid loss of receptor responsiveness despite continued presence of agonist, occurring through phosphorylation of receptors (10). Two types of kinases appear to mediate desensitization: second messenger kinases, such as PKA and PKC, mediate feedback regulation by phosphorylating receptors on cytoplasmic serine and threonine residues, thereby altering conformation and impairing coupling with G proteins; and a second family of kinases, which contains at least six members referred to as G-protein-coupled receptor kinases (GRKs) (11). GRKs initiate a two-step process known as homologous or "agonist-specific" desensitization, by phosphorylating only activated receptors (10,11). Once receptors are phosphorylated by GRKs, they bind inhibitory proteins, called β-arrestins, which sterically inhibit further activation of G proteins (10,11).

The GRKs most abundantly expressed in the heart are βARK1 (GRK2), βARK2 (GRK3), and GRK5. These three GRKs have been shown to phosphorylate and desensitize β_1-ARs in vitro (12), which are the most critical receptors for mediating acute changes in heart function, and recently, through transgenic mouse models, βARK1 and GRK5 have been shown to desensitize myocardial receptors in vivo (13,14).

Unique mechanisms for the cellular regulation of βARK1 and other GRKs have recently been elucidated (11). Like most GRKs, βARK1 is a cytosolic enzyme that must translocate to the membrane in order to phosphorylate its activated receptor substrate. The mechanism for translocation of βARK1 involves the physical interaction between the kinase and the membrane-bound $\beta\gamma$-subunits of G proteins (G$\beta\gamma$) (15). G$\beta\gamma$, anchored to the membrane through a lipid modification on the carboxyl-terminus of the γ-subunit, is available to interact with βARK1 following G protein activation and dissociation. Thus, this conforms to the property of βARK1 phosphorylating agonist-occupied receptors, since G$\beta\gamma$ is free to translocate βARK1 only after receptor-G-protein coupling. The region of βARK1 responsible for binding G$\beta\gamma$ has been mapped to a 125 amino acid domain located within the carboxyl-terminus of the enzyme (16). Peptides derived from the G$\beta\gamma$-binding domain of βARK1 have been shown to act as in vitro βARK1 inhibitors by competing for G$\beta\gamma$ and preventing translocation (16).

In contrast to βARK1, GRK5 does not undergo agonist-dependent translocation, but rather is constitutively membrane-bound (17) and, therefore, G$\beta\gamma$-independent. Exact mechanisms for GRK5 regulation are not well understood. However, recently it has been shown that an integral membrane lipid, phophatidylinositol-4,5-bisphosphate

(PIP2), enhances GRK5-mediated β_2-AR phosphorylation by directly binding to the amino-terminus of this kinase *(18)*. Interestingly, PIP2 also binds to βARK1 (carboxyl-terminus) affecting its activity *(19)*. The precise in vivo roles for βARK1 and GRK5 in myocardial adrenergic signaling are not completely understood. However, their roles may be even more critical during pathophysiological conditions.

ADRENERGIC SIGNALING IN HEART DISEASE

Changes in adrenergic signaling, in particular β-AR signaling, occur in several cardiac disorders, including acute myocardial ischemia, cardiomyopathies, and cardiac transplantation *(4)*. The most well-characterized β-AR signaling alteration occurs in chronic congestive heart failure where there is a loss of β-AR density, apparently limited to the β_1-AR subtype *(20)*. Both β_1-AR mRNA and protein are reduced by approx 50%, which results in a higher percentage of β_2-ARs. High levels of catecholamines during heart failure may also serve to desensitize the remaining β-ARs, probably through a GRK-mediated mechanism. In fact, βARK1 levels have been shown to be markedly elevated in tissue samples taken from the left ventricle (LV) of failing human hearts *(21)*. This is consistent with, and may contribute to, the functional uncoupling of cardiac β-ARs seen in this condition. Myocardial levels of βARK2 and β-arrestins appear to be unchanged in human heart failure *(21)*, whereas levels of GRK5 have yet to be studied. Taken together, this suggests that elevated activity of βARK1 in failing human myocardium may be an important mechanism for β-AR desensitization through enhanced receptor phosphorylation and subsequent receptor uncoupling from G proteins. The consequence of this pathologic process would lead to one of the characteristic observations found in chronic heart failure.

Levels of other adrenergic signaling components may also be altered during heart failure, since there is good evidence for an increase in G_i, an adenylyl cyclase inhibitory protein *(22,23)*, which could also contribute to diminished β-AR responsiveness as seen in chronic heart failure. In contrast, no change in the cyclase stimulatory G protein, G_s, or adenylyl cyclase itself has been documented *(22,23)*.

Adrenergic receptors may also play a role in myocardial hypertrophy. Most cardiac diseases manifest some degree of hypertrophy, which represents an initial compensatory state; frequently, these conditions ultimately progress to heart failure. The biochemical mediators of hypertrophy are poorly understood, but stimulation of α_1-ARs (and other G_q-coupled receptors) in vivo can initiate cardiomyocyte hypertrophy. Thus, the G_q-PLC-PKC pathway may be important in the hypertrophy associated with several cardiac diseases.

TRANSGENIC MANIPULATION OF MYOCARDIAL ADRENERGIC SIGNALING

Despite significant advances in the understanding of β-AR signaling in heart failure, it remains to be determined whether changes in β-AR function can directly promote deterioration of heart function or are just secondary phenomena resulting as a consequence of enhanced local and systemic circulating norepinephrine concentrations. Transgenic technology coupled with the availability of strong cardiac-specific promoters, such as the α-myosin heavy chain (α-MyHC) gene promoter, have made it possible to target adrenergic signaling components directly to the heart, producing alterations in myocardial signal transduction. The targeted, selective overexpression of these molecules provides a powerful approach to understanding how molecular alterations, which are known to occur in a disease, can modify the physiological phenotype without disrupting the normal circulation. Thus, our understanding of the roles of receptors, such as β-ARs, in cardiac function can be increased.

We and others have recently generated and characterized the phenotype of transgenic mice created from several different constructs involving adrenergic signaling components, including β-ARs, GRKs, and G proteins. The detailed molecular, biochemical, and physiologic analyses that have been performed provide important insight into the in vivo function of β-AR signaling in the heart (Table 1).

Myocardial Overexpression of β_2-ARs

To determine whether increasing the number of receptors would lead to greater G protein coupling, transgenic mice were generated by overexpressing the human β_2-AR *(24–26)*. The murine α-MyHC promoter was utilized to target specifically the β_2-AR to the myocardium. Since α-MyHC is not expressed during embryonic development, this strategy results in a progressive increase in β_2-AR expression into adulthood. Several lines of mice were generated, and one line had unexpectedly robust expression approaching 40 pmol/mg membrane protein, which is higher than the levels of receptors reached in cell-culture transfection experiments *(24)*. This β-AR density represents well over 100-fold overexpression of myocardial β-ARs, and these animals represent a model where the heart is under β_2-AR control in contrast to the normal heart where myocardial β-AR signaling occurs via the β_1-subtype.

Surprisingly, in these β_2-AR overexpressing animals, β-AR signaling in the heart was maximal even in the absence of exogenous agonist, as assessed by the measurement of several biochemical and physiological parameters. Baseline membrane adenylyl cyclase activity from transgenic hearts was increased twofold over baseline control activity and equaled maximal, isoproterenol-stimulated activity of control nontransgenic mouse hearts. Consistent with this biochemical phenotype, isometric tension studies using isolated atria from these animals demonstrated maximal tension in the absence of a β-agonist *(24)*.

To assess the cardiac phenotype in the intact animal, in vivo contractile function was measured using a 2-Fr high-fidelity micromanometer catheter inserted into the LV. Overexpression of the human β_2-AR resulted in marked enhancement of LV contractility as assessed by the maximal first derivative of LV pressure, dP/dt max, compared to negative littermate controls. LV relaxation, as assessed by peak negative dP/dt, and the time constant of isovolumic pressure decay (Tau) was also enhanced in the transgenic mice *(24,26)*. With infusion of isoproterenol, no increase in dP/dtmax or Tau occurred.

The lack of response to isoproterenol in this well-defined preparation suggests that in vivo the β-AR signaling pathway is maximally activated. Myocardial receptors are hypothesized to exist in an equilibrium between R, the predominant inactive conformation, and R*, an activated conformation that couples to G proteins. The presence of an agonist, which binds to R*, effects a shift toward this active conformation (Fig. 1). Thus, the maximal signaling seen in the β_2-AR-overexpressing transgenic animals is likely owing to the significant increase in spontaneously isomerized receptors present in the active conformation, in the absence of agonist. With 200-fold overexpression, even the minor fraction of receptors thought to be naturally undergoing this agonist-independent

Table 1
Various Transgenic Mouse Models That Have Been Generated with Alterations in the β-AR System[a]

Mouse	Transgene	Biochemistry	Physiological phenotype	Principle
TG4 (24–26)	α-MyHC-human β$_2$-AR	↑200-fold β-AR density ↑AC activity	↑Contractility ↑Myocardial relaxation ↑Heart rate	β-AR can couple to G proteins and stimulate AC in absence of agonist Supports in vivo existence of inverse agonists
TGβARK12 (13,14)	α-MyHC-bovine βARK1	↓High-affinity coupling of β-ARs ↓AC activity	↓Inotropic and chronotropic response to β-AR stimulation ↓Inotropic response to AngII	In vivo, β$_1$- and β$_2$-ARs and AT$_1$ receptors are targets for βARK1-induced desensitization ↑Expression of βARK in heart failure contributes to blunted catecholamine responsiveness
TGMini27 (13)	α-MyHC-carboxyl-terminal 194 aa of βARK1	Peptide inhibitor competes for Gβγ binding to βARK1	↑Basal contractility ↑Myocardial relaxation	↓Desensitization of β-ARs with βARK inhibition

276

	↓Agonist-dependent GRK phosphorylation of rhodopsin and β_2-AR in vitro	Preserved isoproterenol responsiveness	βARK1 is a critical in vivo modulator of cardiac function
TGGRK5-45 (14) α-MyHC–bovine GRK5	↓AC activity basally, and in response to isoproterenol	↓Basal contractility and inotropic responses to β-AR stimulation No change in response to AngII	In vivo, β_1- and β_2-ARs are targets for GRK5-induced desensitization, whereas AT$_1$ receptors are not targets for GRK5 action
TG line 39 (31,32) α-MyHC–canine/human Gα_s.	No alteration in AC activity ↑High-affinity coupling of β-ARs	No change in basal contractility ↑Chronotropic and inotropic response to catecholamine infusion	Increased expression of cardiac Gα_s can enhance β-AR-G$_s$ coupling and signaling in response to β-agonists

[a]Adapted from ref. *33* with permission. Abbreviations: AC, Adenylyl cyclase; α-MyHC, α-myosin heavy chain; AngII, angiotensin II; AT$_1$, angiotensin II type 1 receptor; β-AR, β-adrenergic receptor; βARK, β-adrenergic receptor kinase; GRK, G-protein-coupled receptor kinase.

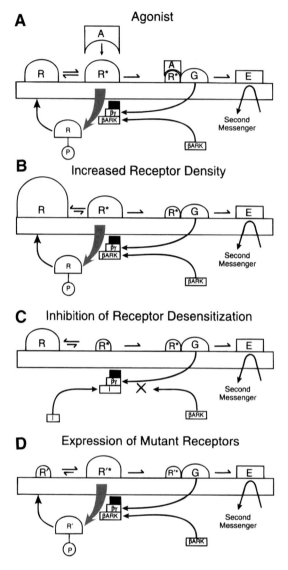

Fig. 1. Potential mechanisms for activation of myocardial receptor systems. **(A)** Traditionally, myocardial receptor systems are activated by the presence of agonist **(A)**. Receptors exist in an equilibrium between the predominant R conformation and R* (activated conformation). Agonist binds and thereby shifts the equilibrium toward R*, which unlike R is able to bind the heterotrimeric G protein (G). The G protein then dissociated into Gα-GTP and βγ-subunits, leading to activation of effector enzymes (e.g., adenylyl cyclase), which catalyze the formation of second messenger (e.g., cAMP). βγ-subunits enable a translocation of myocardial βARK to the membrane compartment, allowing for phosphorylation of R* and subsequent interruption of the interaction with G protein (a process known as desensitization). **(B)** In the absence of agonist, large increases in receptor density result in increases of both the R and R* conformation. Although the equilibrium remains in favor of R, the absolute amount of R* may equal that which occurs at lower receptor densities when agonist is present. Subsequent interaction with G protein and activation of the effector enzyme occur in an identical fashion. **(C)** In the presence of an inhibitor (I) that binds βγ-subunits, myocardial βARK does not translocate and R* subsequently does not undergo phosphorylation. Even in the absence of agonist, baseline concentrations of R* go on to interact with the G protein, and the effector enzyme is activated. **(D)** Constitutively activated mutant receptors (R′) exist mainly as the activated conformation (R′*), and can couple to and activate G proteins in the absence of agonist. (Reprinted with permission from 2).

conformational change (R to R*) becomes significant and results in maximal signaling *(24–26)*. Thus, when wild-type receptors are overexpressed at this extraordinary level, the resultant phenotype seen is what would be expected from expression of mutant adrenergic receptors, which have been shown to be constitutively activated. These mutant adrenergic receptors, which have been described in detail *(27)*, result from point mutations within the third intracellular domain of the receptor protein. These mutations apparently alleviate certain structural constraints that result in a much greater proportion of receptors spontaneously in the R* conformation. Thus, two different mechanisms account for the activated phenotype seen with overexpression of wild-type vs mutated, constitutively active receptors. For the wild-type receptors, the increase in R* is a consequence of the sheer overexpression of the receptors, whereas for the constitutively active mutant receptors, it is a consequence of an increase in the fraction of receptors in the R* state. These two scenarios where signaling is enhanced in the absence of agonist are illustrated along with normal agonist-driven signal transduction in Fig. 1.

The increased cellular concentration of the R* conformation present in the β_2-AR overexpressing mice allows for the study of receptor signaling in the absence of an agonist. This model has been utilized for the further characterization of the class of receptor ligands known as inverse agonists *(25)*. Inverse agonists, unlike agonists that prefer R*, bind preferentially to R, driving the equilibrium further toward R, thus decreasing signaling. Inverse agonists are also distinct from neutral antagonists that bind with equal affinity to either R or R* and do not perturb the equilibrium. The phenomenon of increased R* present in the hearts of β_2-AR overexpressing mice has been demonstrated by the administration of the inverse agonist ICI-118, 551, which caused a reduction of all the elevated basal biochemical and physiological parameters, including basal contractility *(24,25)*.

Myocardial Overexpression of a Constitutively Active α_1-AR

As mentioned earlier, and illustrated in Fig. 1, another potential way to increase the number of receptors in the R* conformation is to transfer constitutively activated mutant receptors to the myocardium. This has been accomplished in mice by the α-MyHC-targeted expression of a transgene encoding a constitutively activated mutant of the α_{1B}-AR *(28)*. Thus mutant receptor has been shown to evoke agonist-independent activation of the G_q-PLC signaling pathway *(27)*. It has been hypothesized that this pathway may be involved in pressure or volume-overload-induced hypertrophy. However, this has been difficult to test, since administration of α-agonists evokes peripheral vascular effects, which secondarily induce myocardial hypertrophy. In mice with cardiac overexpression of the α_{1B}-AR mutant, hearts were significantly larger, and ventricular myocyte size was increased *(28)*. Other properties associated with ventricular hypertrophy were also seen, including the ventricular expression of atrial natriuretic factor. These mutant α_1-AR mice contrast with the β_2-AR overexpressing animals, which featured marked functional changes without myocardial hypertrophy *(see above)*. These mice, overexpressing a constitutively active α_{1B}-AR (for which R* is the predominant conformation, Fig. 1), demonstrate that continuous activation of the G_q-coupled pathway can induce ventricular hypertrophy.

Transgenic Manipulation of Myocardial GRK Activity

An alternative means to alter adrenergic signaling in the heart is to overexpress transgenes that affect desensitization. With the recent finding that βARK1 levels are elevated in chronic heart failure (21), which may contribute to diminished β-AR signaling, βARK1 and other myocardial GRKs have become important targets of study. Inhibition of GRK-mediated β-AR phosphorylation and desensitization is a potentially novel way to increase myocardial signaling.

βARK1 activity can be inhibited in vitro by peptides derived from its Gβγ binding domain (16). Therefore, we have recently created transgenic mice with cardiac-specific targeting of the Gβγ binding domain of βARK1, to test the hypothesis that a βARK1 inhibitor may enhance β-AR signaling (13). In addition, mice were generated with cardiac-targeted overexpression of βARK1 itself to study the effects of enhanced GRK activity on myocardial function (13). Paralleling expression of the respective transgenes, myocardial signaling and function were reciprocally altered in these two types of transgenic mice.

Mice overexpressing the βARK1 inhibitor in their hearts had increased basal in vivo LV contractility and enhanced responses to administered isoproterenol (13). These results indicate that βARK1 may exert a tonic inhibitory effect on myocardial β_1-ARs, even in the absence of agonist. The cardiac phenotype demonstrated in these mice further supports the hypothesis that isomerization of receptors to R* occurs under "basal" conditions, since this conformation is the only substrate for GRK phosphorylation. As illustrated in Fig. 1, in mice with inhibited myocardial βARK1 basal R* is presumably less phosphorylated and can proceed to stimulate G_s, producing cAMP and enhancing myocardial function. Thus, signaling is increased when βARK1 is inhibited, which, as demonstrated by the βARK1-inhibitor mice, leads to enhanced cardiac function (13).

In transgenic mice with three- to five fold βARK1 overexpression specifically in the myocardium, there was a significant attenuation of basal adenylyl cyclase activity, which appeared to be mediated by an alteration in the β_1-AR complex, Since less receptors were in the high-affinity "coupled" state (13). In agreement with this biochemical data, in vivo hemodynamic measurements in anesthetized mice revealed significant attenuation of isoproterenol-induced cardiac contractility (13). These data suggest that myocardial β_1-ARs are in vivo substrates for this GRK, and strengthen the hypothesis that myocardial βARK1 activity is critical physiology and that the increased βARK1 levels seen in human heart failure may indeed be contributing to β-AR signaling dysfunction. Therefore these data, coupled with the phenotype of the βARK1-inhibitor mice described above, suggest that βARK1 inhibition may represent a novel therapeutic approach to improving myocardial function in patients with heart failure. Notably in this regard, β-antagonists, which may be effective for chronic therapy for heart failure (29), appear to decrease βARK1 activity (30). This finding, together with that of increased βARK1 expression in a state of chronic β-adrenergic stimulation, such as is seen in heart failure, suggests that βARK1 expression and GRK activity may be coupled very tightly to levels of β-AR signaling.

Recently, transgenic mice have been generated with α-MyHC-targeted overexpression of GRK5 in order to study this myocardially expressed receptor kinase. In a line of transgenic mice with ~30-fold overexpresssion of GRK5, myocardial adenylyl cyclase activity was significantly blunted at baseline and in response to isoproterenol (14). In vivo cardiac inotropy was also severely crippled in response to isoproterenol in GRK5-overexpressing animals compared to nontransgenic littermate controls (14). Thus, GRK5 appears to be capable, when overexpressed in vivo, of desensitizing and uncoupling myocardial β_1- and β_2-ARs, which has also been observed recently in vitro studies (12). This suggests that GRK5, like βARK1, may be critical to normal and compromised heart function.

With the generation of the α-MyHC-GRK5 transgenic mice, it is possible to compare directly responses in these animals to those in the α-MyHC-βARK1 mice. In vivo isoproterenol responses as described above were significantly more attenuated in the GRK5-overexpressing animals *(13, 14)* presumably because of the degree of over expression (30- vs 3-fold).

Since signaling through G-protein-coupled receptors other than β-ARs is also important for myocardial regulation, we have utilized βARK1 and GRK5 transgenic mice to study signaling through cardiac AngII receptors. AngII has been shown to be involved in the regulation of cardiac growth and myocardial inotropy *(14)*. In vivo cardiac responses to AngII were studied in βARK1 and GRK5-overexpressing mice, and interestingly, the data revealed specific differences between these two GRKs. AngII responses were significantly attenuated in βARK1-overexpressing animals, whereas GRK5 overexpressors had normal cardiac responses to AngII, indicating that myocardial AngII receptors are not regulated by GRK5-mediated desensitization, despite the robust expression of this enzyme. Thus, these mice provide powerful model systems to study the in vivo substrate specificity that these GRKs possess. Thus, these GRKs may play distinct roles in the normal regulation of cardiac physiology.

Overexpression of Gα$_s$ Protein

Transgenic manipulation of the myocardial β-AR-G$_s$-adenylyl cyclase signaling system has not been limited to the receptor or receptor kinase (Table 1). Transgenic mice with myocardial overexpression of the α-subunit of G$_s$ were recently described *(31)*. These mice, which had approximately three fold Gα$_s$ overexpression targeted to the myocardium by the rat α-MyHC promoter, demonstrated no change in the steady state maximal cyclase activity as measured by in vitro assays. At a physiological level, as assessed by echocardiography on 10-mo-old animals, there was no change in basal contractility, but infusions of catecholamines led to enhanced contractility and increased heart rate relative to control non transgenic animals *(32)*. Thus, it appears that overexpression enhances the efficacy of the β-AR-G$_s$-adenylyl cyclase signaling pathway.

SUMMARY AND FUTURE DIRECTIONS

Understanding cardiac contractility is essential for advances in the treatment of cardiac disease, particularly heart failure. The availability of cDNA clones encoding adrenergic receptors and GRKs, coupled with transgenic animal technology myocardial-specific promoters, has made it possible to study the consequences of specific alterations in the myocardial adrenergic receptor systems in vivo. These transgenic mice have advanced the understanding of signaling through adrenergic receptors in the heart, both under normal and pathophysiological conditions, and represent important experimental models to test hypotheses about receptor theory, myocardial hypertrophy, and therapeutics. Future research will combine transgenic and gene targeting technologies, which allow for the targeted and selective manipulation of candidate molecules, with models of clinically important diseases, such as hypertrophy and heart failure. Monitoring the physiological phenotype in these models will provide an extremely powerful approach to the understanding of disease processes where normal regulatory mechanisms have failed. Furthermore, transgenic mice overexpressing β$_2$-ARs and a βARK1 inhibitor suggest that gene transfer may represent an exciting novel therapeutic approach for cardiovascular disease.

REFERENCES

1. Field LJ. Transgenic mice in cardiovascular research. Annu Rev Physiol 1993;55:97–114
2. Koch WJ, Milano CA, Lefkowitz RJ. Transgenic Manipulation of myocardial G-protein-coupled receptors and receptor kinases. Circ Res 1996;78:511–516.
3. Cohn JN. Plasma norepinephrine and mortality. Clin Cardiol 1995;18(Suppl):I-9–12.
4. Brodde O. Beta-adrenoceptors in cardiac disease. Pharmac of Ther 1993;60:405–430.
5. Xiao R-P, Lakatta EG. β_1-adrenoceptor stimulation and β_2-adrenoceptor stimulation differ in their effects on contraction, cytosolic Ca^{2+}, and Ca^{2+} current in single rat Ventricular cells. Cir Res 1993;73:286–300.
6. Atschuld RA, Starling RC, Hamlin RL, Billman GE, Hensley J, Castillo L, Fertel RH, Hohl CM, Robitaille P-ML, Jones LR, Xiao R-P, Lakatta EG. Response of failing canine and human heart cells to β_2-adrenergic stimulation. Circulation 1995;92:1612–1618.
7. Bristow MR, Minobe W, Rasmussen R, Hersberger RE, Hoffman BB. Alpha-1 adrenergic receptors in the nonfailing and failing human heart. J Pharmacol Exp Ther 1988;247:1039–1045.
8. Terzic A, Puceat M, Vassort G, Vogel SM. Cardiac α_1-adrenoceptors: An overview. Pharmacol Rev 1993;45:147–175.
9. Kariya K, Karns LR, Simpson PC. expression of a constitutively activated mutant of the β-isozyme of protein kinase C in cardiac myocytes stimulated the promoter of the β-myosin heavy chain isogene. J Biol Chem 1991;266:10,023–10,026.
10. Hausdorff WP, Caron MG, Lefkowitz RJ. Turning off the signal: Desensitization of β-Adrenergic receptor function. FASEB 1990;4:2881–2889.
11. Inglese J, Freedman NJ, Koch WJ, Lefkowitz RJ. Structure and mechanism of the G-protein-coupled receptor kinases. J Biol Chem 1993;268:23,735–23,738.
12. Freedman NJ, Liggett SB, Drachman DE, Pie G, Caron MG, Lefkowitz RJ. Phosphorylation and desensitization of the human β_1-adrenergic receptor: Involvement of G-protein-coupled receptor kinases and cAMP-dependent protein kinase. J Biol Chem 1995;270:17,953–17,961.
13. Koch WJ, Rockman HA, Samama P, Hamilton R, Bond RA, Milano CA, Lefkowitz RJ. Reciprocally altered cardiac function in transgenic mice overexpressing the β-adrenergic receptor kinase or a βARK1 inhibitor. Science 1995;268:1350–1353.
14. Rockman HA, Choi D-J, Rahman NU, Akhter SA, Lefkowitz RJ, Koch WJ. Receptor specific in vivo desensitization by the G-protein-coupled receptor kinase-5 in transgenic mice. Proc Natl Acad Sci USA 1996;93:9954–9959.
15. Pitcher JA, Inglese J, Higgins JB, Arriza JL, Casey PJ, Kim C, Benovic JL, Kwatra MM, Caron MG, Lefkowitz RJ. Role of $\beta\gamma$-subunits of G proteins in targeting the β-adrenergic receptor kinase to membrane-bound receptors. Science 1993;257:1264–1267.
16. Koch WJ, Inglese J, Stone WC, Lefkowitz RJ. The binding site for the $\beta\gamma$-subunits of heterotrimeric G proteins on the β-adrenergic receptor kinase. J Biol Chem 1993;268:8256–8260.
17. Premont RT, Koch WJ, Inglese J, Lefkowitz RJ. Identification, purification and characterization of GRK5, a member of the family of G-protein-receptor kinases. J Biol Chem 1994;269:6832–6841.
18. Pitcher JA, Fredericks ZL, Stone WC, Premont RT, Stoffel RH, Koch WJ, Lefkowitz RJ. Phosphatidylinositol-4,5-bisphosphate (PIP_2)-enhanced G-protein-coupled receptor kinase (GRK) activity: Location, structure, and regulation of the PIP_2 binding site distinguishes the GRK subfamilies. J Biol Chem 1996;271:24,907–24,913.
19. Pitcher JA, Touhara K, Payne ES, Lefkowitz RJ. Pleckstrin homology domain-dedicated membrane association and activation of the beta-adrenergic receptor kinase requires coordinate interaction with $G_{\beta\gamma}$ subunits and lipids. J Biol Chem 1995;270:11,709,11,710.
20. Bristow MR, Minobe WA, Reynolds MV, Port JD, Rasmussen R, Ray PE, Feldman AM. Reduced β_1 receptor messenger RNA abundance in the failing human heart. J Clin Invest 1993;92:2737–2745.
21. Lohse MJ. G-protein-coupled receptor kinases and the heart. Trends Cardiovasc Med 1995;5:63–68.
22. Feldman AM. Experimental issues in assessment of G protein function in cardiac disease. Circulation 1991;84:1852–1861.
23. Bohm M. Alteration of β-adrenoreceptor-G-protein-regulated adenylyl cyclase in heart failure. Mol Cell Biochem 1995;147:147–160.
24. Milano CA, Allen LF, Rockman HA, Dolber PC, McMinn TR, Chien KR, Johnson TD, Bond RA, Lefkowitz RJ. Enhanced myocardial function in transgenic mice overexpression the $\beta2$-adrenergic receptor. Science 1994;264:582–586.

25. Bond RA, Johnson TD, Milano CA, Rockman HA, McMinn TR Apparsunndaram S, Kenakin TP, Allen LF, Lefkowitz RJ. Physiologic effects of inverse agonists in transgenic mice with myocardial overexpression of the β2-adrenoceptor. Nature 1995;374:272–275.

26. Rockman HA, Hamilton R, Milano CA, Mao L, Jones LR, Lefkowitz RJ. Enhanced myocardial relaxation in vivo in transgenic mice overexpression the β_2-adrenergic receptor is associated with reduced phospholamban protein. J Clin Invest 1996;97:1–6.

27. Lefkowitz RJ, Cotecchia S, Samama P, Costa T. Constitutive activity of receptors coupled to guanine nucleotide proteins. Trends Pharmacol Sci 1993;14:303–307.

28. Milano CA, Dolber PC, Rockman HA, Bond RA, Venable ME, Allen LF, Lefkowitz RJ. Myocardial expression of a constitutively active α_{1B}-adrenergic receptor in transgenic mice induces cardiac hypertrophy. Proc Natl Acad Sci USA, 1994;91:10,109–10,113.

29. Bristow MR, O'Connel JB, Gilbert EM, French WJ, Leatherman G, Kantrowitz NE, Orie J, Smucker ML, Marshall G, Kelly P, Deitchman D, Anderson JL. Dose-response of chronic β-blocker treatment in heart failure from either idiopathic dilated or ischemic cardiomyopathy. Bucindolol Investigators. Circulation 1994;89:1632–1642.

30. Ping P, Gelzer-Bell R, Roth DA, Kiel D, Insel PA, Hammond HK. Reduced β-adrenergic receptor activation decrease G protein expression and β-adrenergic receptor kinase activity in porcine heart. J Clin Invest 1995;95:1271–1280.

31. Gaudin C, Ishikawa Y, Wight DC, Mahdavi V, Nadal-Ginard B, Wagner TE, Vatner DE, Homcy CJ. Overexpression of G_{sa} protein in the hearts of transgenic mice. J Clin Invest 1995;95:1676–1683.

32. Iwase M, Bishop SP, Uechi M, Vatner DE, Shannon RP, Kudej RK, Wight DC, Wagner TE, Ishikawa Y, Homcy CJ, Vatner SF. Adverse effects of chronic endogenous sympathetic drive induced by cardiac G_{sa} overexpression. Circ Res 1996;78:517–524.

33. Rockman HA, Koch WJ, Milano CA, Lefkowitz RJ. Myocardial β-adrenergic receptor signaling in vivo: Insights from transgenic mice. J Mol Med 1996;74:489–495.

17

Dopamine Receptors in Human Disease
Lessons from Targeted Mouse Mutants

Domenico Accili, MD, John Drago, MD, PhD, and Sara Fuchs, PhD

CONTENTS

The neurotransmitter dopamine exerts a broad array of effects on the central nervous system, the cardiovascular, endocrine, and the genito-urinary systems *(1,2)*. In the central nervous system, dopamine affects locomotion and behavior. In the cardiovascular system, dopamine affects heart rate and myocardial contractility. Dopamine effects on blood pressure and blood volume have been postulated to involve both brainstem and direct renal mechanisms, as well as peripheral blood flow and fluid balance *(3)*. In the endocrine system, dopamine is a potent modulator of hypothalamic and pituitary functions. To elicit its effects, dopamine binds to specific receptors on the surface of target cells. In recent years, a spate of contributions have led to the identification of five subtypes of dopamine receptors. The five receptors are subdivided into two classes, referred to as D1-like, and D2-like *(4,5)*. It is generally held that each class mediates different effects. However, the specific role of each individual subtype has thus far been unclear. In this chapter, we analyze the role of mouse models of dopamine receptor defects in furthering our understanding of this complex system and its implications for the function of dopamine receptors in human disease.

From: *Contemporary Endocrinology: G Proteins, Receptors, and Disease*
Edited by: A. M. Spiegel, Humana Press Inc., Totowa, NJ

CLASSIFICATION AND STRUCTURAL ANALYSIS
OF DOPAMINE RECEPTORS

It has been known for almost three decades that dopamine can modulate adenylyl cyclase activity in specific areas of the brain. The observation of the opposing actions of dopamine on adenylyl cyclase in different tissues *(6,7)* suggested the presence of two distinct subclasses of dopamine receptors long before molecular cloning techniques came of age. The D2 receptor was the first dopamine receptor to be cloned, using a homology screening approach with a hamster β_2-adrenergic receptor as a probe *(8)*. Steady progress throughout the 1980s led to the discovery of more dopamine receptor genes and the determination of the putative amino acid sequence of their protein products *(9–14)*. Five different subtypes of dopamine receptors have been identified. They have been referred to as D1–D5, or D1-like (D1 and D5, also known as D1A and D1B in the rodent literature) and D2-like (D2, D3, and D4). Despite this remarkable diversity, the pharmacological and functional properties of the five receptor subtypes have confirmed the initial hypothesis that dopamine receptors can either stimulate (D1 and D5) or inhibit (D2, D3, and D4) adenylyl cyclase activity through binding to specific G proteins *(15–19)*. The notion that dopamine receptors have evolved from two main ancestral genes is also supported by the observation that D1-like receptors are encoded by intronless genes, whereas D2-like receptor genes are divided by intron sequences, the positions of which are conserved in all members of the family, and in some opsin genes *(20–22)*.

Sequence alignment of the five dopamine receptor cDNAs reveals a typical structure for G-protein-coupled receptors with seven membrane-spanning domains, three extracellular, and three intracellular loops. Sequence homology is highest in the membrane-spanning domains, where it ranges from 52% among D2-like to 75% between the two D1-like receptors. The third intracellular loop is highly divergent even within members of the same class. It has been suggested that specificity of signaling may reside within this domain. All receptors contain a putative palmitoylation site at the carboxy-terminal end, as well as potential sites of N-linked glycosylation at the amino-terminal end.

Alternative splicing of mRNA sequences results in the generation of two isoforms of D2 receptors in humans, rat, and mouse. The two isoforms differ by the presence or absence of a 29 amino acid stretch in the third intracellular loop *(23,24)*. Because of the critical role of this region in coupling to G proteins, the two isoforms have been the object of intense scrutiny. Evidence for binding of specific α-subunits to the two receptor isoforms is, however, conflicting *(25–28)*. The two isoforms are mostly coexpressed by the same cell types. A similar splicing pattern has been reported for the mouse D3 receptor, but not for the human homolog *(21,29)*.

In addition to the identification of internally spliced D2 receptor isoforms, several truncated mRNAs encoding D3 receptors have been reported, the physiologic significance of which is uncertain *(21,30,31)*.

The D4 receptor contains a unique repeat sequence of 48-bp in the third intracellular loop. This repeat sequence is highly polymorphic, being reiterated 2–10 times in normal individuals *(11,32)*. Unlike the simple repeat sequences identified in the product of the myotonic dystrophy gene, or in the androgen receptor gene in patients with the fragile X syndrome, no instability has been demonstrated for this sequence. The presence of this highly polymorphic marker has greatly simplified the genetic analysis of the D4 locus in psychiatric disorders. Although no evidence for linkage of D4 receptor poly-morphisms to major psychiatric diseases has thus far been found *(33–38)*, two reports have rekindled the hypothesis that there might exist an association between genetic variations at the D4 locus and specific personality traits *(39,40)*.

ANATOMICAL LOCALIZATION AND PHARMACOLOGICAL CHARACTERIZATION OF DOPAMINE RECEPTORS

In the central nervous system, most dopaminergic neurons arise from the midbrain and project to the forebrain and other areas. Dopaminergic neurons are found in the nigrostriatal, mesocorticolimbic, and tuberoinfundibular pathways *(41)*. The first path-way is mainly involved in motor control. Degeneration of the dopaminergic neurons of the substantia nigra pars compacta is the pathological hallmark of Parkinson's disease.

The role of the mesocorticolimbic pathway has proven to be more elusive. Although it has been associated with emotional stability and behavioral control, evidence linking dopamine receptor dysfunction to disorders like psychoses and schizophrenia is largely indirect, being substantially based on the fact that dopamine levels are elevated in schizo-phrenic patients and that neuroleptic drugs are D2-like receptor antagonists *(42,43)*. Furthermore, a substantial body of evidence indicates that dopamine receptors may be involved in regulating the response to drugs of addiction *(44,47)*. Although in Parkinson's disease loss of dopaminergic innervation to the putamen is most evident, pathological studies have shown some loss in corticolimbic targets *(48)*.

The implication of dopaminergic neurons of the tuberoinfundibular pathway in repro-duction and lactation through their effects on prolactin, gonadotropins, and thyroid hor-mone secretion is firmly established. Dopamine is a potent inhibitor of prolactin secretion, and galactorrhea is a common side effect of neuroleptic treatment. Thyroid-stimulating hormone (TSH), gonadotropin, and growth hormone (GH) secretion are also negatively regulated by dopamine *(49)*.

Marked differences exist in the anatomical distribution of dopamine receptors in the central nervous system. D1 and D2 receptors are the most abundant. It has been esti-mated that they represent more than 90% of all dopamine receptors. D3, D4, and D5 receptors are two orders of magnitude less abundant. Such figures are, however, mis-leading, since the local distribution of individual receptor subtypes varies substantially. In the ventral region of the striatum known as the islands of Calleja, for example, D3 receptors are the most abundant form of D2-like dopamine receptors *(50,51)*.

D1 and D2 receptors, being the most abundant subtypes, are highly expressed in the striatum *(4)*. D1 receptors are predominant in the basal ganglia (nucleus accumbens, caudate-putamen, and olfactory tubercles), but they are also found in the cortex *(52)*. D1 receptors are mainly expressed in the striatonigral neurons, whereas D2 receptors are found in striatopallidal projection neurons *(53)*. D5 receptor mRNA is found in areas that do not contain D1 receptors, such as the hippocampus, lateral mammillary bodies, and thalamus *(54)*. In contrast, D2 receptors are most abundant in the dopaminergic neu-rons of the substantia nigra, where no D1 receptors are found, and are also present in the cortex, thalamus, and mesencephalon *(55–57)*. It has long been debated whether D1 and D2 receptors colocalize to the same cell type. It appears that most striatal projection neu-rons only express D1 or D2 receptors; however, a body of evidence suggests that the two receptors colocalize in a subpopulation of neurons *(58)*. In addition, D1 and D3 receptors colocalize in the islands of Calleja, whereas different D1-like and D2-like receptors do not *(56,57,59)*.

Other subtypes of dopamine receptors are found in the mesocorticolimbic pathway. The D3 receptor is expressed in the shell of the nucleus accumbens by neurotensin-containing neurons, as well as the islands of Calleja and the hypothalamus *(50,51)*. D4 receptors are found in cortical and limbic areas, whereas they are not present in the basal ganglia *(59)*.

Dopamine receptors are also found outside the central nervous system. D1 receptors are found in various tissues; most notably the kidney and the parathyroid glands *(60,61)*. Their role appears to be related to fluid balance and Ca^{++} homeostasis through stimulation of parathyroid hormone (PTH) secretion. D2 receptors are found in atria, vascular smooth muscle, kidney, and pituitary, and are thought to control heart rate, blood pressure, and hormone secretion. D4 receptors are also found in heart. Through its action on the pituitary D2 receptor, dopamine inhibits secretion of prolactin, gonadotropins, TSH, and GH *(56)*. D2 receptors are found on pancreatic β-cell tumors, but their physiologic role in insulin secretion is unclear. D3 receptors are found in kidney, where they may be involved in blood pressure control by regulating the response to a saline load *(62)*.

D1 and D2 receptors are found in the adrenal cortex and medulla, with D2 receptors being the predominant type. D2 receptors are particularly enriched in the zona glomerulosa, where they may contribute to aldosterone regulation *(63)*.

Another important feature of dopamine receptors is their different affinity for dopamine and other dopaminergic compounds. D5 and D3 receptors appear to have the highest affinity for dopamine, leading to the suggestion that they may function as autoreceptors *(64)*. This function is also consistent with their localization to dopamine-secreting neurons, and with the observation that pharmacological lesions of dopaminergic neurons with the dopamine analog 7-OH-dopamine are associated with a marked decrease in D3 receptor expression *(65)*.

Although ligands that can discriminate between D1-like and D2-like subtypes are available, there are no agents known to be selective for any given molecular species of receptor. Initially, the D3 receptor had been thought to be a specific receptor for some neuroleptics *(12)*. Pharmacological studies, it should be noted, have largely been conducted in cells transfected with various receptor cDNAs and may, therefore, not represent faithfully the situation in vivo, where the bioavailability of the drug, the concentration of target receptors, and their affinity for the ligand may be influenced by factors that are absent in cultured cells. Studies of the "atypical" neuroleptic clozapine have provided the impetus for the development of novel agonists and antagonists specific for individual subtypes of dopamine receptors. Clozapine has been shown to control behavioral symptoms in schizophrenic patients without the disabling parkinsonian side effects and tardive dyskinesia. Clozapine binds to D4 receptors with a 10-fold higher affinity than D2 receptors *(66)*. Thus, clozapine is considered to be relatively D4-specific. Likewise, D3-specific agonists and antagonists are now being evaluated in preliminary clinical studies. For example, the D3-selective antagonist UH232 has behavior-stimulating effects in rodents, whereas the D3 "specific" agonist 7-OHDPAT has inhibitory effects on locomotion *(67)*.

The ability of the various subtypes of dopamine receptors to mediate second messenger generation has been studied in a variety of in vitro systems, mostly using cells transfected with the various subtypes. The current paradigm is that D1-like receptors stimulate cAMP formation through coupling with G_s, whereas D2-like receptors decrease cAMP formation through coupling with $G_{i/o}$. The specific α-subunits responsible for mediating these effects have not been isolated. In addition, dopamine receptors in specific tissues have been shown to elicit arachidonate release and modulate ion channels, such as in lactotroph cells, where stimulation of K^+-channels leads to a drop of intracellular Ca^{2+} levels and inhibition of prolactin release (27,68–71).

The search for mediators of dopamine receptor effects has led to the identification of a dopamine-regulated phosphoprotein (DARPP), an M_r 32,000 protein that colocalizes with D1 receptors at various sites, including the striatum and the kidney. DARPP-32 is phosphorylated in response to dopamine; the phosphorylated DARPP-32 is an inhibitor of protein phosphatase-1, and has been shown to inhibit the NA/K-dependent ATPase in renal tubules (60,72).

MICE LACKING D1 RECEPTORS

Mutant mice have been generated by two groups (73,74). Drago et al. showed that a nonsense mutation of the D1 receptor caused growth retardation and increased mortality in homozygous mice. Interestingly, the apparent cause of death in D1-deficient mice appears to be a generalized failure to thrive after weaning, with selective impairment of motivated behavior, such as drinking and eating, which could be partially avoided by isolating the animals and making food readily available on the cage floor. This behavior is wholly consistent with known effects of dopamine, which plays a critical role in motivation and reward mechanisms. Growth retardation could not be explained by hypocalcemia, renal failure, or growth hormone deficiency.

The D1-mutant mice generated by Xu et al. are somewhat different from those described by Drago et al. For example, there is no mention of increased mortality in the report of Xu et al. Such differences are common in the knockout literature and should not befuddle the reader. The effects of any given mutation can be modulated by the complex of genes required to elicit a biological response. It is becoming increasingly clear that all targeted alleles exhibit some extent of variation in their phenotype. These differences are referred to as "penetrance" in the geneticist's parlance. Penetrance is influenced by many factors, including the presence of strain-specific "modifier" genes, i.e., genes that interact with the main disease gene to determine the phenotype (75). The influence of the genetic background on the phenotypic expression has been the subject of intense discussion (76–78).

The same preamble should be kept in mind to interpret behavioral studies of the D1 mutant mice. In the study of Xu et al., mice lacking D1 receptors are hyperactive in an activity cage test, in which the locomotor activity of the animals is monitored automatically by way of photon beams. The only behavioral abnormality reported by Drago et al. is a selective impairment of rearing, which is considered a normal exploratory behavior in rodents. Pharmacological studies have shown that rearing can be affected by dopaminergic drugs. It should be further emphasized that the studies of Drago et al. were conducted using a different technique, in which investigators observed the animals and scored their behavior over a 15-min period in an open field.

Lack of dopamine D1 receptors does not interfere with the development of dopaminergic neurons, but it does decrease overall brain size (74,79). Expression of specific mRNAs that colocalize with D1 receptor neurons in the striatum is reduced in D1-

deficient mice. Specifically, dynorphin and substance P are expressed at considerably lower levels than in normal mice. In contrast, enkephalin, a neuropeptide that is expressed in D2-positive striatopallidal projection neurons remains unchanged. The specificity of the changes in the neuropeptide expression profile is consistent with 6-hydroxydopamine lesioning studies in rat, in which downregulated substance P and dynorphin expression is reversed by D1 agonist administration *(53)*, whereas correction of enkephalin overexpression requires a D2 agonist. The degree to which modulation of neuropeptide gene expression in mice lacking functional D1 dopamine receptors from early development mirrors the changes seen in mature rats treated with 6-hydroxydopamine is reassuring and certainly authenticates the use of these mice as a valid model for human studies.

D1 receptor-deficient mice have also strikingly confirmed the importance of this receptor subtype in drug addiction and reward mechanisms. Cocaine has been shown to inhibit dopamine reuptake by the dopamine transporter, and thus to sensitize the body to the effects of dopamine *(44,47)*. The relative role of D1 and D2 receptors in this response, however, has long been debated. Animals lacking D1 receptors are insensitive to the locomotor-activating effects of cocaine. However, mutant mice given high doses display increased sniffing and grooming as well as behavior suggestive of serotonin receptor overstimulation *(79,80)*. The place preference experimental paradigm was used to address the issue of cocaine addiction. In this experiment, normal mice given repeated small doses of cocaine are seen to change their behavior in a way that correlates with anticipated cocaine administration. In contrast to the effect of cocaine on locomotion, this drug was seen to have a positive rewarding effect and result in a change in place preference to an equal degree in wild-type, heterozygous, and D1 homozygous mice *(81)*. These results cannot be generalized to the claim that there are normal reward mechanisms operating in D1 mutants. Cocaine is a highly reinforcing drug, and experiments need to be repeated with less reinforcing substances before such conclusions can be drawn. With respect to the peripheral actions of dopamine, it should be noted that mice lacking D1 receptors are hypertensive *(2)*.

MICE LACKING D2 RECEPTORS

Mice devoid of D2 receptors present with the most easily discernible phenotype among dopamine receptor-mutant mice *(82)*. Their growth is slightly impaired, and their motor behavior is blunted, with akinesia, postural abnormalities, abnormal gait, and bradykinesia. Autoradiographic studies with iodo-sulpride confirmed the complete ablation of D2 receptors, with residual binding sites in the islands of Calleja, presumably corresponding to D3 receptors. The absence of D2 receptors was accompanied by alterations of gene expression in D2 neurons. Enkephalin mRNA was increased, but tyrosine hydroxylase was unchanged, suggesting that the dopamine synthetic pathway was unaffected by the absence of D2 receptors. The increased enkephalin expression parallels the changes seen in 6-hydroxydopamine-treated rats.

Reproductive function is severely impaired in mice lacking D2 receptors. Their gonads are considerably reduced in size. Lack of inhibition of prolactin secretion is an important factor to be considered in the pathogenesis of the endocrine abnormalities of D2-deficient mice. However, it is possible that more subtle abnormalities in gonadotropin production may also play a role. Reproductive endocrinologists are being called to task to unravel these complex mechanisms.

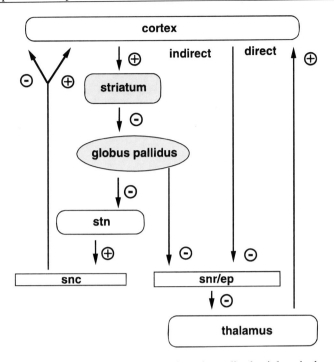

Fig. 1. Basal ganglia physiology. The basic circuitry of basal ganglia physiology is shown. Dopaminergic transmission occurs through two pathways, a direct output from D1 neurons to the substantia nigra pars reticulata/entopeduncular nucleus (SNR/EP), and an indirect pathway from D2 neurons to the same outflow nucleus via the external segment of the globus pallidus and subthalamic nucleus (STN). In Parkinson's disease, there is an underactivity of the direct pathway and an overactivity of the final limb of the indirect pathway (i.e., glutamatergic output from the STN to the outflow nucleus), the overall result is an upregulation of inhibitory discharge from SNR/EP nucleus and clinical bradykinesia. The (+) or stimulatory transmitter is glutamate (from cortex to striatum and from subthalamic nucleus to the outflow nucleus), and the (−) or inhibitory transmitter is γ-amino-butyric acid.

DOPAMINE RECEPTOR KNOCKOUTS AND PARKINSON'S DISEASE

A dissection of the roles of the two main dopamine receptor subtypes is essential to understanding the pathogenesis of Parkinson's disease. Dopaminergic transmission in the basal ganglia has been hotly debated for decades *(83)*. The prevailing view is that dopaminergic transmission occurs through two paths, a direct output pathway from D1 neurons to the substantia nigra pars reticularis/entopeduncular nucleus complex outflow nucleus, and an indirect output from D2 neurons through the external segment of the globus pallidus and subthalamic nucleus to the same outflow nucleus. The outflow nucleus is tonically active and influences thalamic activity, which in turn influences body movement through cortical activity. According to this model, death of dopaminergic neurons in Parkinson's disease results in understimulation of both D1 and D2 dopamine receptors. The effect of this is an overactivity of the final limb of the indirect pathway mediated by uninhibited glutamatergic subthalamic neurons acting on the outflow nucleus and an underactivity of the D1-mediated direct pathway again acting on the outflow nucleus (Fig. 1). Parkinsonian bradykinesia is the predicted outcome in this model of basal ganglia circuitry. There are many complicating issues that surface in a discussion of basal ganglia physiology. Among these issues is the role played by striatal interneurons *(84)*, some of which have dopamine and substance P receptors, the influence of the proposed synergy between D1 and D2 receptors, and finally the controversy concerning receptor coexpression on single projection neurons.

Clearly, dopamine receptors other than D1 and D2 are involved in mediating the clinical features of Parkinson's disease. Mood and anxiety changes occur commonly in patients with Parkinson's disease with frequent motor fluctuations. Patients in whom levodopa levels are controlled by infusion were found to have onset of bradykinesia, heightened anxiety levels, and depressive mood swings following the cessation of infusion *(85)*. In addition, cognitive slowing is also thought to occur in association with the motor "off" state. Significant cognitive differences were particularly noted in the delayed recall of complex verbal material *(86)*. Psychological accompaniments of severe bradykinesia may be florid and almost psychotic in extent. Off-phase screaming is a good example of this phenomenon *(87)*.

The combined lessons of the D1 and D2 receptor knockouts are quite interesting. The findings confirm the paramount role of D2 receptor understimulation in the bradykinesia of Parkinson's disease, and of D1 subtype in drug addiction and motivated behavior. Bradykinesia seen in D2-deficient mice is consistent with the pivotal role of indirect pathway neurons in the pathophysiology of Parkinson's disease. It is somewhat surprising that one of the two strains of D1-deficient mice shows signs of increased locomotor activity, since the prediction would have been that in the absence of D1 receptor stimulation, the animals may develop a hypoactive state, as is observed following administration of D1 antagonists. In this respect, the behavior of the mutant strain described by Drago et al. *(73)* is most consistent with the expected role of D1 receptors. However, the jury is still out on this point. Clarification awaits the results of experiments conducted on knockout mice generated from multiple back-crosses.

MICE LACKING D3 RECEPTORS

The role of D3 receptors has been a difficult one to tackle owing to the low abundance and the restricted tissue distribution of this gene. The development of a mouse strain with a targeted mutation of the D3 receptor gene is a first step toward understanding the function of this subpopulation of dopamine receptors *(88)*. Lack of dopamine D3 receptors has been well documented in this study. Autoradiographic studies show that D3-specific binding is absent in the islands of Calleja, the only brain structure in which D3 receptors are very abundant (Fig. 2) *(50,51)*. This study demonstrates that mice lacking D3 dopamine receptors are hyperactive in a test for exploratory behavior, with increased locomotor activity and rearing. Data derived from genetic ablation of the D3 gene in mice are thus consistent with pharmacological studies in which 7-OH-DPAT, a dopaminergic agonist that binds preferentially to D3 receptors, inhibits locomotor activity *(67)*, whereas UH232, a D3-preferring antagonist, causes hyperactivity. Although the selectivity of these drugs remains controversial, these studies support the conclusion that hyperactivity in D3 receptor mutant mice is the result of ablation of D3 receptors rather than the effect of compensatory changes.

This study provides evidence for a specific role of the D3 receptor subtype to regulate behavior. Its most immediate implication is that alterations of D3 receptor function may be responsible for behavioral disorders associated with hyperactivity. This work bears also on the treatment of behavioral disorders. It has been known for several years that

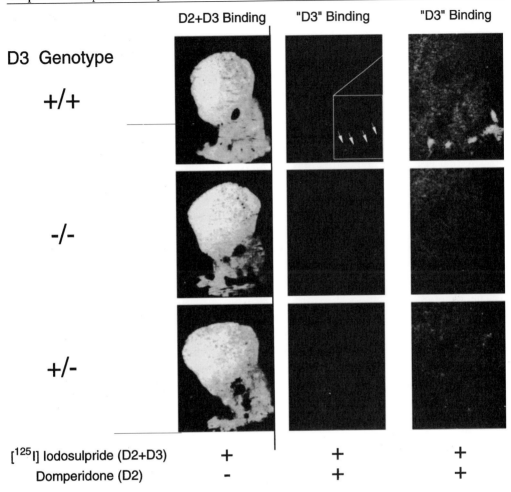

Fig. 2. Autoradiographic studies in D3 receptor-deficient mice. Visualization of D3 and D2 receptors was obtained using ^{125}I-iodosulpride autoradiography. Coronal brain sections through the striatum, nucleus accumbens, olfactory tubercles, and islands of Calleja from +/+, +/–, and –/– mice were incubated with ^{125}I-iodosulpride in the absence (left column) or in the presence (middle column) of the D2-preferring ligand domperidone (100 nM) to compete ^{125}I-iodosulpride binding to D2 receptors and selectively visualize D3 receptors. The right hand column shows an enlargement (3×) of the D3 receptor binding panels in order to better visualize the islands of Calleja, which can be seen, marked with arrows, at the bottom of the +/+ D3 binding panels.

D3 dopamine receptors possess high affinity for neuroleptic drugs commonly employed in the treatment of manic-depressive illness and schizophrenia *(12)*. The effect of these drugs to control the patient's behavioral symptoms may be related to their ability to specifically bind to D3 receptors. The findings provide a further link between the effect of neuroleptics on D3 receptors and behavioral control.

Of interest in this study is the greater than expected reduction of D3 binding in mice heterozygous for the D3 mutation. The authors surmise that the >50% reduction observed in heterozygous mice may be the result of a dominant negative effect of the mutant allele to inhibit binding to D3 receptors expressed from the wild-type allele. The mutant allele encodes a truncated receptor lacking sequences downstream of the second intracellular loop. It is noteworthy that a D3 receptor mRNA deleted at the carboxy-terminus has been detected in brains of normal human subjects as well as schizophrenic patients. Further data on this point should provide insight into possible mechanisms of dominant negative inhibition of G-protein-coupled receptors.

DOPAMINE RECEPTORS AND SCHIZOPHRENIA

The pathogenesis of schizophrenia and other psychotic disorders has been linked to an overactive dopamine system. Furthermore, it has been suggested, but never definitely proven, that D3 and D4 receptors may play a role in the pathogenesis of behavioral disorders and schizophrenia *(66,89)*. These disorders have a strong genetic component. They are commonly referred to as complex traits, i.e., traits with non-Mendelian inheritance. Genetic studies of behavioral disorders in humans are rather unwieldy, because the gene pool of human populations is exceedingly complex. Laboratory mice present distinct advantages for genetic studies. First, they are genetically homogeneous ("inbred"), and second, the function of specific genes in the disease process can be addressed by means of genetic manipulations, such as gene "knockouts."

The genetics of behavioral disorders, like those of other common complex traits, such as diabetes, hypertension, and cancer pose a formidable challenge to currently available methods of disease detection. Genetic heterogeneity, polygenic inheritance, incomplete penetrance, and phenocopies contribute to the complexity of this endeavor. Although the availability of a dense linkage map of the human and mouse genome will contribute to simplifying the daunting task of sifting through millions of base pairs to detect susceptibility loci, it is likely that other methods will have to be employed in order to home in on the genes identified through genome-wide scans. Mouse genetics, through gene knockouts and analysis of quantitative traits and modifier genes, has an important role to play, as do molecular and biochemical studies of candidate genes.

A number of studies have addressed whether sequence variations at various dopamine receptor loci could be implicated in the pathogenesis of schizophrenia *(33–37,90–93)*. Although the majority of these studies have ruled out a role for dopamine receptors in major psychoses and schizophrenia, it should be emphasized that the complex genetics of neuropsychiatric illness can hardly lend itself to association studies and linkage analysis. Thus, these negative reports speak more to the inadequacy of current detection techniques than to a true exclusion of a role of dopamine receptors in these disorders.

CONCLUSIONS AND PERSPECTIVES

Considerable progress has been made in the identification of specific roles for individual subtypes of dopamine receptors. Gene knockouts have been extremely valuable to dissect the contributions of various components of the dopamine system. In addition to the dopamine receptor mutants reviewed here, mice with a mutant dopamine transporter gene have been derived *(94)*, as well as numerous mutant strains in the monoamine synthetic pathway *(95–97)* and their receptor family. Obviously, the derivation of mutant mice is only a stepping stone in the analysis of gene function. Pharmacological and behavioral characterization of the mutant mice, as well as genetic crosses with other mutations of the same gene family will gradually fill in the numerous blanks in the emerging picture of dopamine action.

Among the limitations of gene knockouts, we should continue to be aware of the fact that conclusions reached in a knockout mouse may not be applicable to humans. Furthermore, when a given gene exerts a variety of complex functions, it is likely that only those functions required for survival of the mouse will be observed in a knockout experiment, and that more adaptive functions will be overlooked. Conversely, when a gene is a part of a family of genes, compensation by related genes may overshadow the real contribution of the gene of interest to the process under investigation. Finally, it is becoming increasingly clear that genetic diversity among different mouse strains is important to determine the phenotype. The effects of modifier genes can hardly be overlooked; however, their role in human disease remains to be established (98). To begin to address more specific questions, we can now resort to inducible and tissue-specific knockouts (99,100). These techniques have rapidly moved into the realm of possibilities for many investigators. It is likely that substantial progress will be made within the next few years in our understanding of the physiologic role of dopamine receptors.

REFERENCES

1. Hornykiewicz O. Dopamine (3-hydroxytyramine) and brain function. Pharmacol Rev 1966;18:925–964.
2. Albrecht FE, Drago J, Felder RA, Printz MP, Eisner GM, Robillard JE, Sibley DR, Westphal HJ, Jose PA. Role of the D1A dopamine receptor in the pathogenesis of genetic hypertension. J Clin Invest 1996;97:2283–2288.
3. Van der Buuse M, Jones CR, and Wagner J. Brain dopamine D-2 receptor mechanisms in spontaneously hypertensive rats. Brain Res Bull. 1992;28:289–297.
4. Sokoloff P, Schwartz J-C. Novel dopamine receptors half a decade later. Trends Pharmacol Sci 1995;16:270–275.
5. Sibley DR, Monsma FJ. Molecular biology of dopamine receptors. Trends Pharmacol Sci 1992; 13:61–69.
6. Kebabian JW, Calne DB. Multiple receptors for dopamine. Nature 1979;277:93–96.
7. Stoof JO, Kebabian JW. Opposing roles for D-1 and D-2 dopamine receptors in efflux of cyclic AMP from rat neostriatum. Nature 1981;294:366–368
8. Bunzow JR, Van TH, Grandy DK, Albert P, Salon J, Christie M, Machida CA, Neve KA, Civelli O. Cloning and expression of a rat D2 dopamine receptor cDNA. Nature 1988;336:783–787
9. Dearry A, Gingrich JA, Falardeau P, Fremeau RJ, Bates MD, Caron MG. Molecular cloning and expression of the gene for a human D1 dopamine receptor. Nature 1990;347:72–76
10. Sunahara RK, Niznik HB, Weiner DM, Stormann TM, Brann MR, Kennedy JL, Gelernter JE, Rozmahel R, Yang YL, Israel Y, et al. Human dopamine D1 receptor encoded by an intronless gene on chromosome 5. Nature 1990;347:80–83.
11. Van Tol H, Bunzow JR, Guan HC, Sunahara RK, Seeman P, Niznik HB, Civelli O. Cloning of the gene for a human dopamine D4 receptor with high affinity for the antipsychotic clozapine. Nature 1991;350:610–614.
12. Sokoloff P, Giros B, Martres M-P, Bouthenet M-L, Schwartz J-C. Molecular cloning and characterization of a novel dopamine receptor (D_3) as a target for neuroleptics. Nature 1990;347:146–151.
13. Monsma FJ, Mahan LC, McVittie LD, Gerfen CR, Sibley. Molecular cloning and expression of a D1 dopamine receptor to adenylyl cyclase activation. Proc Natl Acad Sci USA 1990;87:6723–6727
14. Sunahara RK, Guan HC, O'Dowd BF, Seeman P, Laurier LG, Ng G, George SR, Torchia J, Van TH, Niznik HB. Cloning of the gene for a human dopamine D5 receptor with higher affinity for dopamine than D1. Nature 1991;350:614–619.
15. Vallar L and Meldolesi J. Mechanisms of signal transduction at the dopamine D2 receptor. Trends Pharmacol Sci 1989;10:74–77.
16. Vallar L, Muca C, Magni M, Albert P, Bunzow J, Meldolesi J, Civelli O. Differential coupling of dopaminergic D2 receptors expressed in different cell types. Stimulation of phosphatidylinositol 4,5-biphosphate hydrolysis in LtK-fibroblasts, hyperpolarization, and cytosolic-free Ca^{2+} concentration decrease in GH4C1 cells. J Biol Chem 1990;265:10,320–10,326.

17. Tiberi M, Jarvie KR, Silvia C, Falardeau P, Gingrich JA, Godinot N, Bertrand L, Yang FT, Fremeau RJ, Caron MG 1991 Cloning, molecular characterization, and chromosomal assignment of a gene encoding a second D1 dopamine receptor subtype: differential expression pattern in rat brain compared with the D1A receptor. Proc Natl Acad Sci USA 88:7491–7495.

18. Memo M, Lovenberg W, Hanbauer I. Agonist-induced subsensitivity of adenylate cyclase coupled with a dopamine receptor in slices from rat corpus striatum. Proc Natl Acad Sci USA 1982;79: 4456–4460.

19. Neve KA, Henningsen RA, Bunzow JR, Civelli O. Functional characterization of a rat dopamine D-2 receptor cDNA expressed in a mammalian cell line. Mol Pharmacol 1989;36:446–451.

20. Minowa MT, Minowa T, Monsma FJ, Sibley DR, Mouradian MM. Characterization of the 5' flanking region of the human D1A dopamine receptor gene. Proc Natl Acad Sci USA 1992;89:3045–3049.

21. Giros B, Martres MP, Pilon C, Sokoloff P, Schwartz JC. Shorter variants of the D3 dopamine receptor produced through various patterns of alternative splicing. Biochem Biophys Res Commun 1991;176:1584–1592.

22. Fryxell KJ, Meyerowitz EM. The evolution of rhodopsins and neurotransmitter receptors. J Mol Evol 1991;33:367–378.

23. Giros B, Sokoloff P, Martres MP, Riou JF, Emorine LJ, Schwartz JC. Alternative splicing directs the expression of two D2 dopamine receptor isoforms. Nature 1989;342:923–926.

24. Monsma FJ, McVittie LD, Gerfen CR, Mahan LC, Sibley DR. Multiple D2 dopamine receptors produced by alternative RNA splicing. Nature 1989;342:926–929.

25. Montmayeur JP, Guiramand J, Borrelli E. Preferential coupling between dopamine D2 receptors and G-proteins. Mol Endocrinol 1993;7:161–170.

26. Senogles SE. The D2 dopamine receptor isoforms signal through distinct Gi alpha proteins to inhibit adenylyl cyclase. A study with site-directed mutant Gi alpha proteins. J Biol Chem 1994;269:23, 120–23,127.

27. Liu YF, Civelli O, Grandy DK, Albert PR. Differential sensitivity of the short and long human dopamine D2 receptor subtypes to protein kinase C. J Neurochem 1992;59:2311–2317.

28. Fishburn CS, Elazar Z, Fuchs S. Differential glycosylation and intracellular trafficking for the long and short isoforms of the D2 dopamine receptor. J Biol Chem 1995;270:29,819–29,824.

29. Fishburn CS, Belleli D, David C, Carmon S, Fuchs S. A novel short isoform of the D3 dopamine receptor generated by alternative splicing in the third cytoplasmic loop. J Biol Chem 1993;268: 5872–5878.

30. Schmauss C, Haroutunian V, Davis KL, Davidson M. Selective loss of dopamine D3-type receptor mRNA expression in parietal and motor cortices of patients with chronic schizophrenia. Proc Natl Acad Sci USA 1993;90:8942–8946.

31. Snyder LA, Roberts JL, Sealfon SC. Alternative transcripts of the rat and human dopamine D3 receptor. Biochem Biophys Res Commun 1991;180:1031–1035.

32. Lichter JB, Barr CL, Kennedy JL, Van TH, Kidd KK, Livak KJ. A hypervariable segment in the human dopamine receptor D4 (DRD4) gene. Hum Mol Genet 1993;2:767–773.

33. Petronis A, Macciardi F, Athanassiades A, Paterson AD, Verga M, Meltzer HY, Cola P, Buchanan JA, Van TH, Kennedy JL. Association study between the dopamine D4 receptor gene and schizophrenia. Am J Med Genet 1995;60:452–455.

34. Macciardi F, Petronis A, Van TH, Marino C, Cavallini MC, Smeraldi E, Kennedy JL. Analysis of the D4 dopamine receptor gene variant in an Italian schizophrenia kindred. Arch Gen Psychiatry 1994;51:288–293.

35. Macciardi F, Verga M, Kennedy JL, Petronis A, Bersani G, Pancheri P, Smeraldi E. An association study between schizophrenia and the dopamine receptor genes DRD3 and DRD4 using haplotype relative risk. Hum Heredity 1994;44:328–336.

36. Barr CL, Kennedy JL, Lichter JB, Van TH, Wetterberg L, Livak KJ, Kidd KK. Alleles at the dopamine D4 receptor locus do not contribute to the genetic susceptibility to schizophrenia in a large Swedish kindred. Am J Med Genet 1993;48:218–222.

37. Coon H, Byerley W, Holik J, Hoff M, Myles WM, Lannfelt L, Sokoloff P, Schwartz JC, Waldo M, Freedman R, et al. Linkage analysis of schizophrenia with five dopamine receptor genes in nine pedigrees. Am J Hum Genet 1993;52:327–334.

38. Gelernter J, Pakstis AJ, Pauls DL, Kurlan R, Gancher ST, Civelli O, Grandy D, Kidd KK. Gilles de la Tourette syndrome is not linked to D2-dopamine receptor. Arch Gen Psychiatry 1990;47: 1073–1077.

39. Benjamin J, Li L, Patterson C, Greenberg B, Murphy D, Hamer D. Population and familial association between the D4 dopamine receptor gene and measures of novelty seeking. Nature Genet 1996;12:81–84.

40. Ebstein R, Novick O, Umansky R, Priel B, Osher Y, Blaine D, Bennett E, Nemanov L, Katz M, Belmaker R. Dopamine D4 receptor (D4DR) exon III polymorphism associated with the human personality trait of novelty seeking. Nature Genet 1996;12:78–80.

41. Civelli O, Bunzow JR, Grandy DK. Molecular diversity of the dopamine receptors. Annu Rev Pharmacol Toxicol 1993;33:281–307.

42. Karobath M, Leitich H. Antipsychotic drugs and dopamine-stimulated adenylate cyclase prepared from corpus striatum of rat brain. Proc Natl Acad Sci USA 1974;71:2915–2918.

43. Sokoloff P, Andrieux M, Besancon R, Pilon C, Martres MP, Giros B, Schwartz JC. Pharmacology of human dopamine D3 receptor expressed in a mammalian cell line: comparison with D2 receptor. Eur J Pharmacol 1992;225:331–337.

44. Caine SB, Koob GF. Modulation of cocaine self-administration in the rat through D3 dopamine receptors. Science 1993;260:1814–1816.

45. Self DW, Nestler EJ. Molecular mechanisms of drug reinforcement and addiction. Annu Rev Neurosci 1995;18:463–495.

46. Self DW, Stein L. Pertussis toxin attenuates intracranial morphine self-administration. Pharmacol Biochem Behav 1993;46:689–695.

47. Steiner H, Gerfen CR. Dynorphin opioid inhibition of cocaine-induced, D1 dopamine receptor-mediated immediate-early gene expression in the striatum. J Comp Neurol 1995;353:200–212.

48. Agid Y, Javoy-Agid F, Ruberg M. Biochemistry of neurotransmitters in Parkinson's Disease. Butterworth, London, 1987.

49. Reichlin S. Neuroendocrinology. In: Wilson JD, Foster DW, eds. Williams Textbook of Endocrinology. Saunders, Philadelphia, 1994, pp. 135–219.

50. Landwehrmeyer B, Mengod G, Palacios JM. Differential visualization of dopamine D2 and D3 receptor sites in rat brain. A comparative study using in situ hybridization histochemistry and ligand binding autoradiography. Eur J Neurosci 1993;5:145–153.

51. Landwehrmeyer B, Mengod G, Palacios JM. Dopamine D_3 receptor mRNA and binding sites in human brain. Mol Brain Res 1993;18:187–192.

52. Besson MJ, Graybiel AM, Nastuk MA. [3H]SCH 23390 binding to D1 dopamine receptors in the basal ganglia of the cat and primate: delineation of striosomal compartments and pallidal and nigral subdivisions. Neuroscience 1988;26:101–119.

53. Gerfen CR, Engber TM, Mahan LC. D1 and D2 dopamine receptor-regulated gene expression of striatonigral and striatopallidal neurons. Science 1990;250:1429–1432.

54. Meador-Woodruff JH, Mansour A, Grandy DK, Damask SP, Civelli O, Watson SJJ. Distribution of D5 dopamine receptor mRNA in rat brain. Neurosci Lett 1992;145:209–212.

55. Joyce JN, Janowsky A, Neve KA. Characterization and distribution of [125I]epidepride binding to dopamine D2 receptors in basal ganglia and cortex of human brain. J Pharmacol Exp Ther 1991; 257:1253–1263.

56. Murray AM, Ryoo HL, Gurevich E, Joyce JN. Localization of dopamine D3 receptors to mesolimbic and D2 receptors to mesostriatal regions of human forebrain. Proc Natl Acad Sci USA 1994;91: 11,271–11,275.

57. Diaz J, Levesque D, Lammers CH, Griffon N, Martres MP, Schwartz JC, Sokoloff P. Phenotypical characterization of neurons expressing the dopamine D3 receptor in the rat brain. Neuroscience 1995; 65:731–745.

58. Surmeier DJ, Eberwine J, Wilson CJ, Cao Y, Stefani A, Kitai ST. Dopamine receptor subtypes colocalize in rat striatonigral neurons. Proc Natl Acad Sci USA 1992;89:10,178–10,182.

59. Meador-Woodruff JH, Grandy DK, Van TH, Damask SP, Little KY, Civelli O, Watson SJJ. Dopamine receptor gene expression in the human medial temporal lobe. Neuropsychopharmacology 1994;10:239–248.

60. Felder CC, Blecher M, Jose PA. Dopamine-1-mediated stimulation of phospholipase C activity in rat renal cortical membranes. J Biol Chem 1989;264:8739–8745.

61. O'Connell DP, Botkin SJ, Ramos SI, Sibley DR, Ariano MA, Felder RA, Carey RM. Localization of dopamine D1A receptor protein in rat kidneys. Am J Physiol 1995;268:1185–1197.

62. Jose P, Drago J, Accili D, Eisner G, Felder R. Transgenic mice to study the role of dopamine receptors in cardiovascular function. Clin Exp Hyperten 1997;19(1&2):15–25.

63. Amenta F. In: Amenta F, ed. Peripheral Dopamine Receptors. CRC, Boca Raton, 1990 pp. 39–60.

64. Rivet JM, Audinot V, Gobert A, Peglion JL, Millan MJ. Modulation of mesolimbic dopamine release by the selective dopamine D3 receptor antagonist, (+)-S 14297. Eur J Pharmacol 1994;265:175–177.

65. Levesque D, Martres MP, Diaz J, Griffon N, Lammers CH, Sokoloff P, Schwartz JC. A paradoxical regulation of the dopamine D3 receptor expression suggests the involvement of an anterograde factor from dopamine neurons. Proc Natl Acad Sci USA 1995;92:1719–1723.

66. Seeman P and Van TH. Dopamine receptor pharmacology. Trends Pharmacol Sci 1994;15:264–270.

67. Svensson K, Carlsson A, Waters N. Locomotor inhibition by the D3 ligand R-(+)-7-OH-DPAT is independent of changes in dopamine release. J Neural Transm 1994;95:71–74.

68. Mahan LC, Burch RM, Monsma FJ, Sibley DR. Expression of striatal D1 dopamine receptors coupled to inositol phosphate production and Ca^{2+} mobilization in *Xenopus oocytes*. Proc Natl Acad Sci USA 1990;87:2196–2200.

69. Malgaroli A, Vallar L, Elahi FR, Pozzan T, Spada A, Meldolesi J. Dopamine inhibits cytosolic Ca^{2+} increases in rat lactotroph cells. Evidence of a dual mechanism of action. J Biol Chem 1987;262:13,920–13,927.

70. Vallar L, Vicentini LM, Meldolesi J. Inhibition of inositol phosphate production is a late, Ca^{2+} dependent effect of D2 dopaminergic receptor activation in rat lactotroph cells. J Biol Chem 1988;263:10,127–10,134.

71. Kanterman RY, Mahan LC, Briley EM, Monsma FJ, Sibley DR, Axelrod J, Felder CC. Transfected D2 dopamine receptors mediate the potentiation of arachidonic acid release in Chinese hamster ovary cells. Mol Pharmacol 1991;39:364–369.

72. Meister B, Holgert H, Aperia A, Hokfelt T. Dopamine D1 receptor mRNA in rat kidney: localization by in situ hybridization. Acta Physiol Scand 1991;143:447–449.

73. Drago J, Gerfen CR, Lachowicz JE, Steiner H, Hollon TR, Love PE, Ooi GT, Grinberg A, Lee EJ, Huang SP, Bartlett PF, Jose PA, Sibley DR, Westphal H. Altered striatal function in a mutant mouse lacking D1A dopamine receptors. Proc Natl Acad Sci USA 1994;91:12,564–12,568.

74. Xu M, Moratalla R, Gold LH, Hiroi N, Koob GF, Graybiel AM, Tonegawa S. Dopamine D1 receptor mutant mice are deficient in striatal expression of dynorphin and in dopamine-mediated behavioral responses. Cell 1994;79:729–742.

75. Lander ES, Schork NJ. Genetic dissection of complex traits. Science 1994;265:2037–2048.

76. Gerlai R. Gene-targeting studies of mammalian behavior: is it the mutation or the background genotype? Trends Neurosci 1996;19:177–181.

77. Crawley JN. Unusual behavioral phenotypes of inbread mouse strains. Trends Neurosci 1996;19:181,182.

78. Lathe R. Mice, gene targeting and behavior: more than just genetic background. Trends Neurosci 1996;19:183–186.

79. Drago J, Gerfen CR, Westphal H, Steiner H. Differential regulation of Substance P and immediate-early gene expression by cocaine in forebrain of D1 dopamine receptor-deficient mice. Neuroscience, 1996;74:813–823.

80. Xu M, Hu X-T, Cooper DC, Moratalla R, Graybiel AM, White FJ, Tonegawa S. Elimination of cocaine-induced hyperactivity and dopamine-mediated neurophysiological effects in dopamine D1 receptor mutant mice. Cell 1994;79:945–955.

81. Miner LL, Drago J, Chamberlain P M, Donovan D, Uhl GR. Retained cocaine place preference in D1 receptor deficient mice. Neuroreport 1995;6:2314–2316.

82. Baik J-H, Picetti R, Saiardi A, Thiriet G, Dierich A, Depaulis A, Le Meur M, Borrelli E. Parkinsonian-like locomotor impairment in mice lacking dopamine D2 receptors. Nature 1995;377:424–428.

83. Nestler EJ. Hard target: understanding dopaminergic neurotransmission. Cell 1994;79:923–926.

84. Kawaguchi Y, Wilson CJ, Augood SJ, Emson PC. Striatal interneurons: chemical, physiological and morphological characterization. Trends Neurosci 1995;18:527–535.

85. Maricle RA, Nutt JG, Carter JH. Mood and anxiety fluctuations in Parkinson's disease associated with levodopa infusion: Preliminary findings. Movement Disord 1995;10:329–332.

86. Mohr E, Fabbrini G, Williams J. Dopamine and memory function in Parkinson's disease. Movement Disord 1989;4:113–120.

87. Riley DE, Lang AE. The spectrum of levodopa-related fluctuations in Parkinson's disease. Neurology 1993;43:1459–1464.

88. Accili D, Fishburn CS, Drago J, Steiner H, Lachowicz JE, Park B-H, Gauda EB, Lee EJ, Cool MH, Sibley DR, Gerfen CR, Westphal H, Fuchs S. A targeted mutation of the D3 dopamine receptor gene is associated with hyperactivity in mice. Proc Natl Acad Sci USA 1996;93:1945–1949.

89. Seeman P, Ulpian C, Bergeron C, Riederer P, Jellinger K, Gabriel E, Reynolds GP, Tourtellotte WW. Bimodal distribution of dopamine receptor densities in brains of schizophrenics. Science 1984; 225:728–731.

90. Sabate O, Campion D, d'Amato T, Martres MP, Sokoloff P, Giros B, Leboyer M, Jay M, Guedj F, Thibaut F, et al. Failure to find evidence for linkage or association between the dopamine D3 receptor gene and schizophrenia. Am J Psychiatry 1994;151:107–111.

91. Gelemter J, Kennedy JL, Grandy DK, Zhou QY, Civelli O, Pauls DL, Pakstis A, Kurlan R, Sunahara RK, Niznik HB, et al. Exclusion of close linkage of Tourette's syndrome to D1 dopamine receptor. Am J Psychiatry 1993;150:449–453.

92. Barr CL, Kennedy JL, Pakstis AJ, Castiglione CM, Kidd JR, Wetterberg L, Kidd KK. Linkage study of a susceptibility locus for schizophrenia in the pseudoautosomal region. Schizophr Bull 1994;20:277–286.

93. Shaikh S, Collier D, Arranz M, Ball D, Gill M, Kerwin R. DRD2 Ser311/Cys311 polymorphism in schizophrenia. Lancet 1994;343:1045, 1046.

94. Giros B, Jaber M, Jones SR, Wightman RM, Caron MG. Hyperlocomotion and indifference to cocaine and amphetamine in mice lacking the dopamine transporter. Nature 1996;379:606–612.

95. Zhou QY, Quaife CJ, Palmiter RD. Targeted disruption of the tyrosine hydroxylase gene reveals that catecholamines are required for mouse fetal development. Nature 1995;374:640–643.

96. Thomas SA, Matsumoto AM, Palmiter RD. Noradrenaline is essential for mouse fetal development. Nature 1995;374:643–646.

97. Kobayashi K, Morita S, Sawada H, Mizuguchi T, Yamada K, Nagatsu I, Hata T, Watanabe Y, Fujita K, Nagatsu T. Targeted disruption of the tyrosine hydroxylase locus results in severe catecholamine depletion and perinatal lethality in mice. J Biol Chem 1995;270:27,235–27,243.

98. Dietrich WF, Lander ES, Smith JS, Moser AR, Gould KA, Luongo C, Borenstein N, Dove W. Genetic identification of Mom-1, a major modifier locus affecting Min-induced intestinal neoplasia in the mouse. Cell 1993;75:631–639.

99. Gu H, Zou YR, Rajewsky K. Independent control of immunoglobulin switch recombination at individual switch regions evidenced through Cre-loxP-mediated gene targeting. Cell 1993;73:1155–1164.

100. Kuhn R, Schwenk F, Aguet M, Rajewsky K. Inducible gene targeting in mice. Science 1995; 269:1427–1429.

The β₃-Adrenergic Receptor and Susceptibility to Obesity, the Insulin Resistance Syndrome, and Noninsulin-Dependent Diabetes Mellitus

Jeremy Walston, MD, Kristi Silver, MD, and Alan R. Shuldiner, MD

CONTENTS

INTRODUCTION

Genetics of Noninsulin-Dependent Diabetes Mellitus (NIDDM) and Obesity

Although most forms of NIDDM in humans do not exhibit simple Mendelian inheritance, the large contribution of heredity is well recognized *(1–5)*. Progress toward an understanding of the genetic basis of NIDDM has been largely restricted to a few distinct monogenic syndromes with predictable modes of inheritance. For example, one form of autosomal-dominant maturity-onset diabetes of the young (MODY) is caused by mutations in the glucokinase (MODY2) gene *(6,7)* autosomal-recessive syndromes of extreme insulin resistance are the result of mutations in the insulin receptor gene *(8)* and maternally inherited diabetes and deafness (MIDD) is the result of mutations in mitochondrial DNA *(9)*. These rare subphenotypes of diabetes are examples in which single gene defects have a major influence on the phenotype and for which environmental influences on expression of the phenotype are negligible.

By contrast, the common forms of NIDDM are likely to be caused by a pool of variant genes (polygenic inheritance) *(3–5)*. The effect of each variant gene will be modest, and thus, several will be required in an individual for expression of the diabetic phenotype. These NIDDM "susceptibility" genes are likely to be common and to differ between

From: *Contemporary Endocrinology: G Proteins, Receptors, and Disease*
Edited by: A. M. Spiegel Humana Press Inc., Totowa, NJ

populations (genetic heterogeneity). In addition to genetic predisposition, environmental provocations (i.e., caloric excess and sedentary lifestyle) and time are required for the development of diabetes (late-onset/incomplete penetrance).

Obesity is a major risk factor for the development of insulin resistance and NIDDM *(10–16)*. Both degree *(12–17)* and duration *(18)* of obesity, as well as the distribution of adipose tissue *(14,17,19–22)* influence this risk. A central (upper) body distribution of adipose tissue, which is a prominent feature of the insulin resistance syndrome (central obesity, hyperinsulinemia/insulin resistance, glucose intolerance, hypertension, and dyslipidemia), confers a greater risk for the development of NIDDM than a lower-body distribution of adipose tissue. Similar to NIDDM, obesity in humans is a complex disorder with both genetic and environmental components *(23,24)*. Although substantial progress has been made in defining the genetic basis of obesity in several monogenic rodent models e.g., *ob/ob* mouse—leptin gene *(25)*; *db/db* mouse and Zucker *[fa/fa]* rat—leptin receptor gene *(26,27)*, *fa/fa* mouse—carboxypeptidase E gene *(28)*, tubby mouse—tubby gene *(29)* AyAy yellow mouse—agoutigene *(30)*. Although rare individuals with extreme obesity have mutations in the leptin gene, it is unclear whether any of these genes are determinants of genetic susceptibility to typical obesity in humans *(31,32)*.

In times of nutrient scarcity, gene variants that increased caloric efficiency may have had a selective advantage in evolution *(33)*. These "thrifty" gene variants are likely to be the same genes that confer susceptibility to obesity and NIDDM during times of nutrient excess. The selective pressures of famine may have been very potent, and may in part account for the high prevalence of obesity in countries where high-fat and high caloric diets are typical. It is likely that obesity susceptibility genes will be prevalent in many populations.

Regulation of Energy Expenditure by the Sympathetic Nervous System and Its Relationship to Obesity

Several studies have linked decreases in energy expenditure (thermogenesis) with increased susceptibility to obesity *(34–38)*. Energy expenditure is regulated by the sympathetic nervous system, which mediates increases in thermogenesis induced by cold exposure or feeding through its effects on brown adipose tissue (BAT) (nonshivering thermogenesis) *(39–45)*. Norepinephrine released from sympathetic nerve terminals binds to β-adrenergic receptors on BAT. These seven membrane-spanning receptors couple to regulatory G proteins, which mediate the activation of adenylyl cyclase and the increase in intracellular cAMP concentrations. This pathway accelerates lipolysis, and the liberated fatty acids serve as substrates for oxidation in mitochondria. Since BAT expresses uncoupling protein-1, oxidative phosphorylation is uncoupled from the generation of ATP, and heat is generated *(39–45)*.

Except for neonates and adults with pheochromocytomas, humans do not have discrete anatomic regions of BAT. However, molecular markers specific for BAT (e.g., uncoupling protein-1) exist in visceral adipose tissue of humans of all ages *(46,47)*. Current evidence supports an important role of the sympathetic nervous system as a regulator of energy expenditure in humans, in part through its modulation of thermogenesis in BAT-related tissues *(43,44,48–51)*.

Leptin, a protein secreted by adipocytes, and its receptor also play a role in the sympathetic nervous system-mediated control of adipocyte metabolism *(25,45,52)*. As

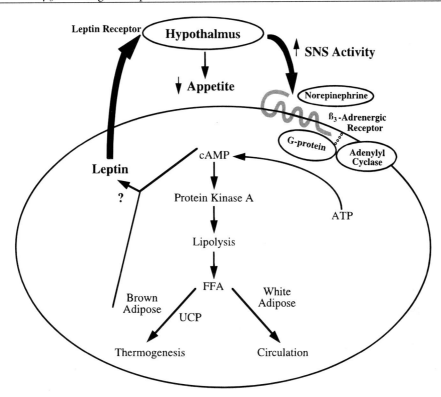

Fig. 1. Schematic of the leptin-β₃AR axis. Leptin is produced by adipocytes and released into the circulation. Leptin travels to the hypothalamus where it binds to leptin receptors. Stimulation of the leptin receptor results in a decrease in appetite and an increase in sympathetic nervous system activity. Release of norepinephrine at the sympathetic nerve terminals in adipose tissue activates β₃-AR. In turn, the G-protein second messenger cascade is stimulated producing an increase in adenylyl cyclase activity, an increase in cAMP levels, activation of protein kinase A, and an increase in lipolysis. In white adipose tissue, the liberated free fatty acids enter the circulation and are used elsewhere in the body. In brown adipose tissue, the uncoupling protein uncouples oxidative phosphorylation from ATP production. As a result, free fatty acids are used for thermogenesis or heat production. Additionally, activation of the β₃AR results in a decrease in leptin levels, which closes the negative feedback loop. The exact mechanism whereby β₃AR activation decreases leptin production is not known.

adipose tissue mass enlarges, leptin is secreted into the circulation in increasing quantities. Leptin crosses the blood–brain barrier and binds to receptors in the hypothalamus, which in turn leads to a decrease in appetite and an increase in energy expenditure *(45,52–57)*. This increase in metabolic rate is likely mediated by increased sympathetic nervous system activity, which stimulates β-adrenergic receptors on adipocytes *(55,58)* (Fig. 1).

The β₃-Adrenergic Receptor (β₃AR) and Energy Expenditure: Potential Role in Obesity in Rodents

The β₃AR is homologous to the β₁- and β₂-adrenergic receptors *(59)*. It is expressed in adipose tissue and has distinct pharmacologic properties. Some studies indicate that the β₃AR is the predominant mediator of norepinephrine-induced lipolysis in rodent adipose tissue, and that molecular defects in the regulation and/or function of the β₃AR may be a common pathway that contributes to obesity. For example, even though defects in the $\beta_3 AR$ gene are not the cause of obesity in the *ob/ob* (leptin-deficient) mouse and Zucker *fa/fa* (leptin receptor-deficient) rat, both display markedly decreased expression of $\beta_3 AR$ mRNA in adipose tissue *(60,61)*. In the *ob/ob* mouse, $\beta_3 AR$ mRNA levels in adipose tissue are reduced by approx 300-fold compared to lean mice *(61)*. Further, stimulation of adenylyl cyclase by the $\beta_3 AR$ selective agonist BRL37344 is severely blunted *(61)*. Thus, the defective thermogenesis previously demonstrated in the *ob/ob* mouse may be owing in part to decreased $\beta_3 AR$ expression *(62,63)*. Decreased $\beta_3 AR$ expression in obesity also may be mediated by transcriptional downregulation of the $\beta_3 AR$ by hyperinsulinemia *(64)*.

Lowell and coworkers recently created a mouse devoid of functional $\beta_3 AR$ by targeted disruption of the $\beta_3 AR$ gene *(65,66)*. These mice have a marked decrease in catecholamine-stimulated lipolysis providing support for a role of the $\beta_3 AR$ in the regulation of adipocyte metabolism. At 15 wk of age (early adulthood), female $\beta_3 AR$ knockout mice have two fold greater fat mass than female controls with an intact $\beta_3 AR$ gene.

Pharmacologic studies provide additional evidence for a role for the $\beta_3 AR$ in obesity. $\beta_3 AR$ agonists increase the number of mitochondria and expression of uncoupling protein in BAT *(67,68)*. Administration of $\beta_3 AR$-specific agonists to obese mice results in an increase in resting metabolic rate (thermogenesis), a reduction in weight, an increase in sensitivity to insulin, and an improvement in islet β-cell responsiveness *(69–71)*.

The $\beta_3 AR$ in Humans

Although early reports of expression of the $\beta_3 AR$ in human tissues were inconsistent *(72,73)*, recent studies using more sensitive and specific approaches (e.g., reverse transcription-PCR) have shown that the $\beta_3 AR$ is expressed in perinephric and visceral adipose tissue, and is much less abundant in subcutaneous adipose tissue *(74)*. Expression of the $\beta_3 AR$ in human adipose tissue parallels that of uncoupling protein, a marker widely regarded as being specific for BAT, suggesting that small amounts of BAT (or a BAT homolog) may be admixed with white adipose tissue in visceral adipose tissue in humans, and that these cells may be the primary site of $\beta_3 AR$ expression *(74)*.

The human $\beta_3 AR$ is also expressed in gallbladder, ileum, colon, and myocardial tissue, and is absent or negligible in skeletal muscle, liver, lung, kidney, thyroid, and lymphocytes *(74,75)*. Studies of function of the $\beta_3 AR$ in the gastrointestinal tract are in progress. The $\beta_3 AR$-specific agonist CL316,243 inhibits smooth muscle contraction in the sphincter of Oddi in a prairie dog model, suggesting that the $\beta_3 AR$ may be involved in the regulation of bile acid secretion into the gastrointestinal tract *(76)*. In the myocardium, $\beta_3 AR$ agonists act as negative inotrops via alternative coupling to G_i *(73)*. In vitro studies also indicate that the $\beta_3 AR$ may couple to G_i in some cell types *(77)*.

Although the $\beta_3 AR$ is a major mediator of catecholamine-stimulated lipolysis in rodent BAT, functional studies of the $\beta_3 AR$ in human (and monkey) adipose tissue remain controversial *(72,73,78,79)*. Inconsistencies between studies may be owing in part to the fact that the rodent $\beta_3 AR$ and human $\beta_3 AR$ have different pharmacological properties, and that specific human $\beta_3 AR$ agonists are not yet available. In addition, differences in the site(s) of adipose tissue studied (e.g., subcutaneous vs visceral) and other methodological details may be responsible for inconsistencies among studies. Some have found little or negligible $\beta_3 AR$-stimulated lipolysis, suggesting that the $\beta_1 AR$ may be the major mediator of catecholamine-mediated lipolysis in human and monkey adipose tissue *(72,73,79)*. By contrast, Lonqvist and coworkers demonstrated β₃AR mediated lipolysis in human visceral adipose tissue *(80)*. Further, omental adipose tissue from subjects who are obese showed significantly greater β₃AR-mediated lipolysis than adipose tissue from nonobese individuals *(80)*. Increased β₃AR-mediated lipolysis may be one mechanism whereby obese individuals have elevated circulating free fatty acids, which may be responsible in part for insulin resistance in obese individuals *(81,82)*. Alternatively, decreased sympathetic activity, which is a feature of obesity in some humans *(51,83–86)*, may lead to reduced β₃AR expression/stimulation, thereby resulting in altered energy balance.

Pharmacological studies of β₃AR agonists in humans are also controversial. Some studies have shown beneficial effects with increased resting metabolic rate (RMR), weight loss, and improved glucose tolerance, whereas other studies have been less convincing *(87–91)*. Differences among studies may be owing to differing pharmacological properties of the agonists used. Beneficial effects of some agonists may have been the result of cross-reactivity with the β₁AR, since tremor and increased heart rate were side effects in some studies *(90)*. Since the pharmacological properties of the rodent and human β₃AR differ, some agonists designed to activate the rodent receptor may not be effective in humans. Alternatively, β₃AR expression may be too low in adipose tissue of humans to be an effective target for therapeutic intervention.

GENETICS OF THE β₃ AR IN HUMANS

Given the role of the sympathetic nervous system in regulating energy expenditure and the observation that small daily differences in resting metabolic rate can lead to weight gain *(91)*, molecular defects in the regulation and/or function of the β₃AR may result in a predisposition to obesity and the metabolic abnormalities associated with obesity, such as NIDDM or the insulin resistance syndrome. The human β₃AR gene is located on chromosome 8p11–8p12, and encodes a 408 amino acid protein within two exons *(59,92,93)*. Exon 1 encodes the 5′-untranslated region and the first 402 amino acids, whereas exon 2 encodes the last six amino acids and the 3′-untranslated region. In addition to TATA and CAAT sequences, the proximal 5′-regulatory region contains four putative cAMP response elements (CREs), one glucocorticoid response element (GRE), and an AP1 binding site *(67,68,93)*. Unlike other adrenergic receptors, chronic stimulation of the β₃AR results in transcriptional upregulation through the generation of cAMP *(67,94)*.

The Trp64Arg β₃ AR Variant: Worldwide in Distribution

Using molecular scanning methods, we identified a missense mutation (Trp64Arg) in the first intracellular loop of the human β₃AR gene (Fig. 2) *(95,96)*. This variant was first identified in Pima Indians, a population with a very high prevalence of both obesity and NIDDM. The Trp64Arg β₃AR variant is common in this population, with an allele frequency of 0.31 (genotype frequency: 46% normal homozygotes [NN], 45% Trp64Arg heterozygotes [NM], 9% Trp64Arg homozygotes [MM]). Subsequent studies of diverse ethnic populations show that the Trp64Arg β₃AR variant is worldwide in distribution, but with varying frequency among populations *(97)* (Table 1). To date, the only population in which this variant has not been detected is the Nauruans of the South Pacific, a genetically isolated population with a very high prevalence of obesity and NIDDM *(97)*.

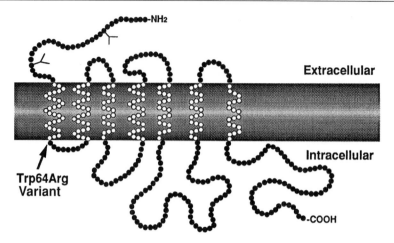

Fig. 2. Schematic of the β_3AR. Each circle represents an amino acid. The Trp64Arg missense mutation is at the junction between the first transmembrane domain and the first intracellular loop.

Evidence for Clinical Importance of the Trp64Arg β_3AR Variant

Given the preferential expression of the β_3AR in visceral adipocytes and the potential role this receptor plays in regulating energy expenditure, it is hypothesized that the variant receptor leads to a lower metabolic rate and a predisposition to the development of visceral obesity. Central obesity may in turn influence the development of several features of the insulin resistance syndrome and may accelerate the onset of NIDDM. Support for this hypothesis comes from a number of studies (Table 2).

PIMA INDIANS OF ARIZONA

Association studies in 642 unrelated Pima Indians (390 with NIDDM and 252 without NIDDM) showed that the prevalence of NIDDM was slightly, but not significantly higher in Pima subjects who were homozygous for the Trp64Arg β_3AR variant *(95)*. The average age of onset of NIDDM was significantly earlier in Trp64Arg β_3AR homozygotes than in heterozygotes or normal homozygotes (36 ± 1.6 yr in MM, 40 ± 0.8 yr in NM, and 41 ± 0.8 yr in NN; $p = 0.02$). Early onset NIDDM, defined as diabetes onset prior to age 25, was three-fold more frequent in Trp64Arg β_3AR homozygotes than normal homozygotes or heterozygotes. Since type I diabetes is rare or nonexistent in Pima Indians *(98)*, these individuals most likely represent an early onset form of NIDDM.

Association studies in 210 nondiabetic Pima subjects showed a trend toward a lower resting metabolic rate in subjects with the Trp64Arg β_3AR variant. After adjustment for fat-free mass, fat mass, and gender (known covariates of RMR), Trp64Arg homozygotes expended an average of 82 kcal/d less than normal homozygotes ($p = 0.06$); heterozygotes were intermediate with an average RMR that was 36 kcal/d less than normal homozygotes ($p = 0.19$) (overall significance for analysis of covariance [ANCOVA], $p = 0.14$). Body mass index (BMI) tended to be higher in nondiabetic subjects with the Trp64Arg β_3AR variant (35.2 ± 2.0 kg/m^2 in MM, 34.1 ± 0.7 kg/m^2 in NM, and 33.9 ± 0.7 kg/m^2 in NN) *(95)*. No significant associations or trends were found in this Pima cohort with insulin sensitivity as measured by fasting and 2-h insulin values after an oral glucose challenge, or by euglycemic hyperinsulinemic clamp. Similarly, no differences

Table 1
Allele Frequencies and Predicted Genotype of Trp64Arg β₃AR

Population	Allele frequency, alleles typed	Frequencies (%)		
		Trp64Arg homozygotes MM	Trp64Arg heterozygotes NM	Normal homozygotes NN
Pima Indians *(95)*	0.31 (1284)	9.6	42.8	47.6
Japanese *(102)*	0.20 (700)	4.0	32.0	64.0
Mexican Americans *(107)*	0.13 (124)	1.7	22.6	75.7
African Americans *(95)*	0.12 (98)	1.4	21.2	77.4
Chinese *(97)*	0.12 (104)	1.4	21.2	77.4
Chinese American *(97)*	0.12 (60)	1.4	21.2	77.4
Indian (subcontinent) *(97)*	0.09 (88)	0.8	16.4	82.8
Caucasians				
Finland *(99)*	0.11 (770)	1.2	19.6	79.2
France *(108)*	0.10 (370)	1.0	18.0	81.0
Baltimore *(95)*	0.08 (96)	0.6	14.8	84.6
Samoans *(97)*	0.06 (84)	0.4	11.2	88.8
Nauruans *(97)*	0.00 (78)	0	0	100

were found in cholesterol or triglyceride levels, waist-to-hip ratio, or blood pressure among β₃AR genotypes.

FINNISH CAUCASIANS

In a study of 335 Finnish Caucasian subjects (128 with NIDDM and 207 without NIDDM), the prevalence of NIDDM was no higher in Finnish subjects with the Trp64Arg variant than those without the variant *(99)*. However, similar to Pimas homozygous for the variant, Finnish Caucasians heterozygous for the Trp64Arg variant had a significantly earlier age of onset of NIDDM (56 ± 1 yr in NM and 61 ± 1 yr in NN; $p = 0.04$). Although there was no statistical difference in BMI, nondiabetic subjects with the variant had significantly higher glucose levels 2 h after an oral glucose challenge (5.8 ± 0.2 mmol/L in NM and 5.3 ± 0.1 mmol/L in NN; $p = 0.006$), higher 2-h insulin levels (59.1 ± 7.9 μU/mL in NM and 41.0 ± 2.9 μU/mL in NN; $p = 0.005$), lower glucose disposal rates during a euglycemic hyperinsulinemic clamp (5.3 ± 0.6 mg/kgin NM and 6.5 ± 0.4 mg/kg in NN; $p = 0.04$), higher waist-to-hip ratios (0.92 ± 0.01 in NM and 0.89 ± 0.01 in NN; $p = 0.02$), and higher diastolic blood pressures (82 ± 1 mmHg in NM and 78 ± 1 mmHg in NN; $p < 0.01$) than those without the variant. Further, quantitative trait linkage analysis in sibling pairs confirmed that the Trp64Arg variant is linked to increased waist-to-hip ratio, as well as increased area under the curve during an oral 2-h glucose tolerance test for both plasma glucose and insulin. These findings suggest that the Trp64Arg β₃AR variant, even in its heterozygous state, is likely to contribute to several features of the insulin resistance syndrome (central fat distribution, hyperinsulinemia, and increased blood pressure), as well as an earlier onset of diabetes in Finnish Caucasians *(99)*.

In another study of 170 Finnish Caucasians, the allele frequency of the Trp64Arg variant was no different between obese and nonobese subjects, nor was there an associa-

Table 2
Summary of Genetic Studies for the Trp64Arg β₃AR Variant

Study	Population	Central obesity	Hyperinsulinemia	↑ Diastolic BP	Earlier Onset NIDDM	↑ BMI	Other[a]
Walston et al. (95)	Pima[a,b]	*	*	*	***	**	↓ older male Trp64Arg homozygotes; trend for ↓ RMR
Kadowaki et al. (102)	Japanese[b]		*		**	*	↑ SBP in heterozygotes only
Yoshida et al. (106)	Japanese[c,d]	*				*	↓ Weight loss, ↓ RMR
Fujiwasa et al. (103)	Japanese[c]					*	Meta-analysis positive for association with NIDDM
Sakane et al. (105)	Japanese[c]				*	*	↑ Maximal BMI
Awata et al. (114)	Japanese[c]				*	*	Maximal BMI, FH NIDDM
Odawara et al. (115)	Japanese[c]						Meta-analysis in Japanese no association with NIDDM
Silver et al. (107)	Mexican Am.[e]	*	*	*	*	**	– TG, LDL, HDL
Wider et al. (99)	Finns[e]	*	*	*	*	*	Linkage with ↑ WHR, ↑ insulin in sib pairs; ↑ glucose during 2-hr OGTT

Reference	Population					Other associations
Urhammer et al. (111)	Danish[b]	*				TG, ↑ LDL, ↓ S, trend ↓ S_G
Gagnon et al. (112)	Swedish[e] Canadian[e]	**			**	trend for insulin AUC, ↑ RMR by linkage analysis, ↑ maximal weight in Canadians only
Kurabayashi et al. (109)	Australian[e]	*			*	Earlier menarche, ↑ gravidity, ↑ parity
Elbein et al. (113)	Utah Morman[e]	*		*	*	No linkage in families
Zhang et al. (110)	British[e]	*	*		*	↓ RMR
Clement et al. (108)	French[e]				*	↑ Weight gain

[a] Abbreviations: AUC, are under the curve; BMI, body mass index; OGTT, oral glucose tolerance test; RMR, resting metabolic rate; SBP, systolic blood pressure; S_G, glucose effectiveness; S_I, insulin sensitivity index; WHR, waist-to-hip ratio.
[b] Associations in Trp64Arg homozygotes only.
[c] Associations in Trp64Arg homozygotes and heterozygotes.
[d] Associations in females only.
[e] Associations in Trp64Arg heterozygotes only (too few Trp64Arg homozygotes to study separately).
[f] Associations in females <70 yr old only.
*$p > 0.1$; **$p = 0.06 - 0.1$; ***$p \leq 0.05$.

tion of the variant with waist-to-hip ratio, lean body mass, fat mass, or glucose or insulin values during an oral glucose tolerance test *(100)*. However, obese subjects with the Trp64Arg variant had significantly lower resting metabolic rates than those without the variant (1569 ± 73 kcal/d in NM and 1635 ± 142 kcal/d in NN; $p = 0.004$) *(100)*. In a third study of Finns, subjects with the Trp64Arg variant had significantly increased rate of weight gain from age 20 and decreased insulin sensitivity *(101)*.

JAPANESE

The effects of the Trp64Arg β_3AR variant have been the subject of intensive investigation in Japanese subjects. In a study by Kadowaki and coworkers, in a study of 350 Japanese subjects (159 with NIDDM and 191 without NIDDM), there was no association of the Trp64Arg variant with NIDDM, although there was a trend toward an earlier onset of NIDDM in those with the variant *(102)*. The Trp64Arg variant was significantly associated with increased BMI (24.7 ± 1.4 kg/m^2 in MM, 22.9 ± 0.3 kg/m^2 in NM, and 22.1 ± 0.2 kg/m^2 in NN; $p = 0.009$). Japanese subjects homozygous for the Trp64Arg variant had significantly higher fasting and 2-h insulin levels during an oral glucose tolerance test compared with normal homozygotes, again suggesting greater insulin resistance in those homo-zygous for the variant allele. Systolic and diastolic blood pressure also tended to be higher in Japanese subjects with the Trp64Arg β_3AR variant *(102)*.

In a study by Fujisawa and coworkers of 295 Japanese subjects, homozygotes for the Trp64Arg variant had significantly higher BMI than heterozygotes or those homozygous for the normal β_3AR (25.5 ± 3.9 kg/m^2 in MM and 22.6 ± 4.1 kg/m^2 in NM; $p < 0.05$, and 22.8 ± 3.8 in NN; $p < 0.05$) *(103)*. Those homozygous for the variant tended to have an earlier age of onset of NIDDM, but this trend did not achieve statistical significance. The allele frequency of the Trp64Arg variant was slightly, but not significantly higher in NIDDM subjects than in control subjects. However, when these data were combined with all other studies that had been published at that time into a meta-analysis (Pima Indians and Finnish Caucasians), homozygosity for the Trp64Arg variant was significantly associated with NIDDM (relative risk 1.72, 95% Cl = 1.00–2.95, $p < 0.05$) *(104)*.

In another group of 368 Japanese subjects, the Trp64Arg β_3AR variant significantly associated with an earlier onset of NIDDM (36.9 ± 7.5 yr in MM, 40.3 ± 9.6 yr in NM, and 43.0 ± 9.4 yr in NN; $p < 0.01$) *(105)*. Like earlier studies, there was no association with NIDDM *per se*. Although the Trp64Arg variant did not associate with current BMI, NIDDM subjects homozygous for the variant had significantly greater maximal lifetime BMI (27.6 ± 2.7 kg/m^2 in MM and 25.1 ± 1.3 kg/m^2 in NN; $p < 0.05$) *(105)*.

Yoshida and coworkers studied 88 Japanese women self-referred to a weight management program for obesity and 100 nonobese women *(106)*. There was no association of the Trp64Arg variant with obesity. However, within the obese group, those with the Trp64Arg variant had significantly greater waist-to-hip ratios and visceral to subcutaneous adipose tissue ratios as measured by computed tomography (CT) scan, suggesting a central pattern of fat distribution. Further, obese subjects with one or two copies of the Trp64Arg variant had significantly lower adjusted resting metabolic rates, and lost significantly less weight during 3 mo of intensive diet and exercise therapy (–5.2 ± 2.8 kg in MM, –5.5 ± 3.8 kg in NM, and –8.3 ± 4.9 kg in NN; $p < 0.05$). These findings suggest for the first time that the Trp64Arg genotype has prognostic value, and may be a useful clinical marker to identify individuals who will have greater difficulty losing weight *(106)*.

MEXICAN AMERICANS OF SAN ANTONIO, TEXAS

Silver and coworkers performed genotype analysis for the Trp64Arg β_3AR variant in 61 unrelated Mexican Americans *(107)*. The Trp64Arg variant significantly associated with earlier age of onset of NIDDM (41.3 ± 4.6 yr in NM and 55.6 ± 2.6 yr in NN; $p < 0.02$), and in nondiabetics with elevated 2-h insulin levels during an oral glucose tolerance test (810 ± 120 pmol/L in NM and 384 ± 6 pmol/L in NN; $p < 0.005$). Mexican American subjects with the variant allele also tended to have higher BMI, waist-to-hip ratios, and diastolic blood pressures. Four hundred twenty-one (421) related subjects from 31 families in the San Antonio Family Diabetes Study were also studied. Using measured genotype analysis to estimate genotype-specific means for each trait, those who were homozygous for the Trp64Arg variant had significantly higher 2-h insulin levels ($P = 0.04$), and trends toward higher BMI compared to the other two groups. No associations of these traits were apparent in Trp64Arg β_3AR heterozygotes in this analysis *(107)*.

MORBIDLY OBESE FRENCH CAUCASIANS

In a cohort of 185 morbidly obese French Caucasians *(108)*, the Trp64Arg variant significantly associated with increased weight (140 ± 8 kg in NM and 126 ± 2 kg in NN; $p = 0.03$) and increased capacity to gain weight over a 25-yr period (67 ± 6 kg in NM and 51 ± 2 kg NN; $p = 0.007$). These findings suggest that the Trp64Arg β_3AR variant is likely to predispose to weight gain and obesity in Caucasians *(108)*.

OTHER STUDIES

Recent findings in elderly Australian Caucasians further support a potential role of the Trp64Arg β_3AR variant as a determinant of obesity and features of the insulin resistance syndrome, and extend these findings to include reproductive history in women *(109)*. In this study, 686 elderly subjects from a cross-section of the normal Australian population were studied. In women, the Trp64Arg variant (heterozygotes) significantly associated with obesity as well as increased diastolic blood pressure (even after adjustment for age and BMI). In women under 70 yr of age, there was also significant association of the Trp64Arg variant with increased central adiposity as measured by spinal dual X-ray absorptiometry (DEXA) scan. No such associations were observed in men. Interestingly, women with the Trp64Arg variant had significantly earlier ages of menarche (12.8 ± 1.3 yr in NM and 13.4 ± 1.5 yr in NN; $p = 0.006$) and greater parity (3.8 ± 2.0 offspring in NM and 3.0 ± 1.9 offspring in NN; $p = 0.005$) *(109)*. These findings suggest that women with the Trp64Arg β_3AR variant may have had increased fat mass even during adolescence, since fat mass is known to influence the age of menarche.

In 227 British Caucasians, Zhang and coworkers showed that the Trp64Arg variant significantly associates with BMI (35.6 ± 3.5 kg/m^2 in MM, 31.1 ± 1.0 kg/m^2 in NM, 29.7 ± 0.4 kg/m^2 in NN; $p = 0.029$), but not with insulin resistance or NIDDM *(110)*. In this same cohort, a commonly occurring variant in the insulin receptor substrate-1 gene (Gly972Ala IRS-1) was associated with insulin resistance and NIDDM, but not obesity. The authors suggested that these two commonly occurring variants contribute separately to traits related to obesity and NIDDM, and are examples of polygenic inheritance of a heterogeneous disorder *(110)*.

Urhammer and coworkers studied 380 Danish Caucasians *(111)*. Although there were no differences in any traits related to the insulin resistance syndrome or NIDDM in heterozygotes, Trp64Arg homozygotes had significantly greater BMI and insulin resistance. One weakness of this study is that the number of homozygotes was small ($n = 3$).

Importantly, some well-performed studies failed to show any associations of the Trp64Arg variant with obesity, age of onset of diabetes, or other related traits *(112–114)*. Gagnon and coworkers studied 242 men and women from the Quebec Family Study, and 385 women from the Swedish Obese Subjects. In neither cohort was there evidence for association of the Trp64Arg variant with BMI, fat mass, central obesity, insulin or glucose levels, blood pressure, resting metabolic rate, or changes in weight over time. Quantitative trait linkage analysis of these same characteristics in the Quebec Family Study were also negative with the exception of resting metabolic rate in which those with the Trp64Arg variant had significantly lower values ($p = 0.04$) *(112)*. Similarly, there was no evidence of association or linkage of the Trp64Arg β_3AR or polymorphic markers near the β_3AR locus with NIDDM, age of onset of diabetes, BMI, waist-to-hip ratio, glucose, or insulin levels in 617 Utah Mormon subjects from 42 families *(113)*. Finally, association studies by Awata and Kaayama revealed no evidence of association of the Trp64Arg variant with NIDDM, age of onset of NIDDM, maximal, or current BMI in Japanese subjects *(114)*, and a meta-analysis by Odawara and coworkers of a combined Japanese cohort failed to show association of the variant with NIDDM *(115)*

Current Controversy over the Relevance of the Trp64Arg β_3AR Variant: Phenotypic Expression May Depend on Multiple Factors

Comparisons among the study populations reveal distinct differences in the phenotypic expression of the Trp64Arg variant both quantitatively (i.e., gene dose) and qualitatively. For example, in Pima Indians, homozygosity for the Trp64Arg variant is associated with an earlier onset of NIDDM, whereas heterozygotes are minimally, if at all affected *(95)*. By contrast, in Mexican Americans *(107)* and Finns *(99)*, heterozygotes have significantly earlier onsets of NIDDM. Furthermore, in Japanese *(106)*, Finns *(99)*, Australian women under the age of 70 *(109)*, and possibly in Mexican American women *(107)*, there is association of the Trp64Arg variant with central obesity (increased waist-to-hip ratio), but there is no such association of the variant with central obesity in Pima Indians *(95)*. The difference in insulin resistance/hyperinsulinemia among β_3AR genotypes is most marked in Finnish Caucasians *(99)* and Mexican Americans *(107)* (heterozygotes affected), less prominent in Danes *(111)* and Japanese *(102)* (only homozygotes affected), and absent in Pima Indians *(95)*. Finally, some studies fail to show any associations of the Trp64Arg variant with obesity, age of onset of diabetes, or other related traits *(112–114)*. We suggest that given the complex nature of obesity and NIDDM in humans, these apparent differences in phenotypic expression of the Trp64Arg β_3AR variant among study populations are expected. There are several possible explanations for apparent differences among study populations *(116)*.

First, ethnic (genetic) background is likely to have a marked effect on the phenotypic expression of the Trp64Arg variant both quantitatively (gene dose) and qualitatively. The Trp64Arg variant may influence more than one trait related to the insulin resistance syndrome (epistasis), but which one(s) may depend on other yet-to-be-identified genetic factors that may be distinct in a given ethnic population or cohort. Further, the presence of other common NIDDM and obesity susceptibility genes in a population may modify the effect of the Trp64Arg variant, or even mask its effect on a given phenotype altogether. Well-described examples of these genetic mechanisms include (1) the marked variation in phenotypic expression of the *ob* gene mutation on penetrance of diabetes and the degree of obesity in different inbred mouse strains *(117)*, and (2) the differences in phenotypic expression of the Δ-Phe^{508} cystic fibrosis transmembrane conductance regulator (CFTR) between races or families *(118)*.

Second, environmental provocations are likely to be required for phenotypic expression of the Trp64Arg β₃AR variant. Differences in the degree of type(s) of environmental provocations among study populations may account for some of the variation. Sakane and coworkers *(105)* have suggested that environmental factors may explain in part why studies of two Japanese populations were positive for association of the Trp64Arg β₃AR variant with an earlier onset of NIDDM and traits related to the insulin resistance syndrome, whereas a third Japanese study was not *(114)*.

Third, gender may be an important determinant of phenotypic expression of the Trp64Arg β₃AR variant. In some studies, women with the Trp64Arg variant have higher BMI and waist-to-hip ratios than women without the variant, but men with the variant are less (if at all) affected *(106,107,109)*. These data in humans are consistent with those of Susulic and coworkers *(65)*, who demonstrated that female β₃AR knockout mice have approximately twofold greater fat mass than wild-type female controls, whereas males are less affected.

Fourth, differences among studies may be owing to subtleties in study design, subject ascertainment, phenotypic characterization, or statistical analyses. For example, in our studies of Mexican Americans *(107)*, when subjects were unrelated, there were significant associations in Trp64Arg heterozygotes for an earlier onset of NIDDM and hyperinsulinemia. When this cohort was expanded to include all available family members, associations in heterozygotes were no longer apparent, but associations in Trp64Arg homozygotes for hyperinsulinemia persisted. Further, variability in the relative sensitivities of different statistical genetic analytic approaches may account in part for discrepancies among studies. Recently, Risch and Merikangas *(119)* suggested that for complex disorders caused by several genes, each with a modest effect, linkage analysis is much less sensitive than association studies. Thus, it is not surprising that with study designs based on family collections and linkage analysis, evidence for involvement of the Trp64Arg variant in some populations is lacking *(112,113)*.

Finally, it is possible that associations are spurious owing to stratification bias, multiple comparisons, or other factors *(120,121)*. However, since associations with traits related to obesity and NIDDM cluster together and have been documented in many independent studies, it is unlikely that they are all spurious. Rather, the inability of some studies to show association is more likely owing to the modest effect of the Trp64Arg β³AR variant combined with the other caveats described above.

Function of the Trp64Arg β₃AR Variant

Early studies of the functional characteristics of the Trp64Arg β₃AR are inconclusive. Recently, Candelore and coworkers *(122)* expressed the normal and Trp64Arg β₃AR variant in Chinese hamster ovary (CHO) cells. Studies of ligand binding, adenylyl cyclase activation, and desensitization failed to show any differences between the normal β₃AR and the Trp64Arg variant. However, in a similar study, the Trp64Arg β₃AR variant had decreased maximal activation of adenylyl cyclase *(123)*. In a study of omental adipose tissue, there were no differences in rates of lipolysis between those homozygous for the normal β_3AR and those heterozygous for the Trp64Arg variant *(124)*. Since omental adipose tissue from Trp64Arg homozygotes was unavailable, these studies do not rule out the possibility that there may be a subtle functional defect, particularly in Trp64Arg homozygotes. In vivo studies of appearance rates of free fatty acids and free fatty acid turnover in Pima Indians failed to detect difference among the three β_3AR genotypes *(125)*. However, since β_3AR-mediated lipo-lysis in omental adipose tissue is likely to constitute only a small proportion of the total, measures of whole-body turnover may not be a sensitive enough approach to tease out potential defects in β_3AR function. Additional in vitro and in vivo studies of function will be required, including provocation with specific β_3AR agonists, which are active in humans.

CONCLUSIONS

There is strong evidence that the Trp64Arg β_3AR variant associates with obesity, several features of insulin resistance syndrome, and an earlier onset of NIDDM. The effect of the variant is modest and may be similar to the ApoE4 allele in Alzheimer's disease; it is neither necessary nor sufficient to cause the disease, but when pres-ent, leads to a significantly earlier onset *(126)*. Factors, such as ethnic (genetic) background, subject selection/ascertainment (e.g., lifestyle, gender, relatedness), and statistical analyses, may influence phenotypic expression both quantitatively (gene dose) and qualitatively. It is likely that this paradigm will be relevant for other common complex genetic disorders in humans.

REFERENCES

1. Harris MI, Hadden WC, Knowler WC, et al. Prevalence of diabetes and impaired glucose tolerance and plasma levels in U.S. populations aged 20–74 yr. Diabetes 1987;36:523–534.
2. Rich SS. Mapping genes in diabetes. Genetic epidemiological perspective. Diabetes 1990; 39:1315–1319.
3. Rotter JL, Vadheim CM, Rimoin DL. Genetics of diabetes mellitus. In: Rifkin H, Porte D Jr, eds. Diabetes Mellitus: Theory and Practice. Elsevier, Amsterdam, 1990, pp. 378–413.
4. Elbein SC, Hoffman MD, Bragg KL, Mayorga RA. The genetics of NIDDM. Diabetes Care 1994;17:1523–1533.
5. Shuldiner AR, Silver K. Candidate genes for type II diabetes mellitus. In: LeRoith D, Olefsky JM, Taylor SI, eds. Diabetes Mellitus: A Fundamental and Clinical Text. Lippincott, Philadelphia, 1996, pp. 565–574.
6. Vionnet N, Stoffel M, Takeda J, et al. Nonsense mutation in the glucokinase gene causes early-onset non-insulin-dependent diabetes mellitus. Nature 1992;356:721, 722.
7. Froguel P, Zouali H, Vionnet N, et al. Familial hyperglycemia due to mutations in glucokinase. Definition of a subtype of diabetes mellitus. N Engl J Med 1993;328:697–702.
8. Taylor SI, Cama A, Accili D, et al. Mutations in the insulin receptor gene. Endoc Rev 1992;13: 566–595.
9. Kadowaki T, Kadowaki H, Mori Y, et al. A subtype of diabetes mellitus associated with a mutation of mitochondrial DNA. N Engl J Med 1994;330:962–968.
10. Bennett PH, Knowler WC, Rushforth NB, et al. The role of obesity in the development of diabetes in the Pima Indians. In: Vague PH, ed. Excerpta Medica, Diabetes and Obesity. Oxford, Amsterdam, 1979, pp. 117.
11. Modan M, Karasik A, Halkin H, et al. Effect of past and concurrent body mass index on prevalence of glucose intolerance and type 2 (non-insulin-dependent) diabetes and on insulin response. The Israel study of glucose intolerance, obesity and hypertension. Diabetologia 1986;29:82.

12. Barrett-Connor E. Epidemiology, obesity, and non-insulin-dependent diabetes mellitus. Epidemiol Rev 1989;11:172–181.

13. Papoz L, Eschwege E, Warnet J, et al. Incidence and risk factors of diabetes in the Paris prospective study (G.R.E.A.). In: Eschwege E, ed. Advances in Diabetes Epidemiology. Elsevier Amsterdam, 1982, pp. 113–122.

14. Hartz A, Rupley D, Kalkhoff R, et al. Relationship of obesity to diabetes: influence of obesity level and body fat distribution. Prev Med 1983;12:351–357.

15. Knowler W, Pettitt D, Saad M, et al. Obesity in the Pima Indians: its magnitude and relationship with diabetes. Am J Clin Nutr 1991;53:1543–1551.

16. Morris R, Rimm D, Hartz A, et al. Obesity and heredity in the etiology of non-insulin-dependent diabetes mellitus in 32,662 adult white women. Am J Epidemiol 1989;130:112–121.

17. Reaven GM. Role of insulin resistance in human disease. Banting Lecture. Diabetes 1988;37:1595–1607.

18. Everhart J, Pettitt D, Bennett P, et al. Duration of obesity increases the incidence of NIDDM. Diabetes 1992;41:235–240.

19. Marin P, Anderson B, Ottosson M, et al. The morphology and metabolism of intra abdominal adipose tissue in men. Metabolism 1992;41:1242.

20. Haffner S, Stern M, Hazuda H, et al. Do upper-body and centralized adiposity measure different aspects of regional body-fat distribution? Relationship to non-insulin-dependent diabetes mellitus, lipids, and lipoproteins. Diabetes 1987;36:43–51.

21. Kissebah A, Pelris A. Biology of regional body fat distribution: relationship to non-insulin-dependent diabetes mellitus. Diabetes Metab Rev 1989;5:83–109.

22. Stern MP. Diabetes and cardiovascular disease. The "common soil" hypothesis. Diabetes 1995;44:369–374.

23. Stunkard A, Sorensen T, Hanis C, et al. An adoption study of human obesity. N Engl J Med 1986;314:193–197.

24. Bouchard C, Despres J, Tremblay A. Genetics of obesity and human energy metabolism. Proc Nutr Soc 1991;50:139–147.

25. Zhang Y, Proenca R, Maffei M, et al. Positional cloning of the mouse obese gene and its human homologue. Nature 1994;372:425–432.

26. Chen H, Charlat O, Tartaglia LA, et al. Evidence that the diabetes gene encodes the leptin receptor: Identification of a mutation in the leptin receptor gene in db/db mice. Cell 1996;84:491–495.

27. Chua SC, Chung WK, Wu-Peng XS, et al. Phenotypes of mouse diabetes and rat fatty due to mutation in the Ob (leptin) receptor. Science 1996;271:994–996.

28. Naggert JK, Fricker LD, Varlamov O, et al. Hyperproinsulinemia in obese fat/fat mice associated with a carboxypeptidase E mutation which reduces enzyme activity. Nature Genet 1995;10:135–142.

29. Kleyn PW, Fan W, Kovats SG, et al. Identification and characterization of the mouse obesity gene *tubby*: A member of a novel gene family. Cell 85; 281–290.

30. Bultman SJ, Michaud EJ, Woychik RP. Molecular characterization of the mouse agouti locus cell 1992;71:1195.

31. Montague CT, Farooql IS, Whitehead JP, et al. Congenital leptin defect is associated with severe early onset of obesity in humans. Nature 1997;387:903–908.

32. Bouchard C. The causes of obesity: advances in molecular biology but stagnation on the genetic front. Diabetologia 1996;39:1532–1533.

33. Neel JV. The thrifty genotype revisited. In: Kobberling J, Tattersall R, eds. The Genetics of Diabetes Mellitus. Proceedings of the Serono Symposium Academic. London, 1982, pp. 283–293.

34. Ravussin E, Bogardus C. A brief overview of human energy metabolism and its relationship to essential obesity. Am J Clin Nutr 1992;55:242–245S.

35. Fontvieille A, Lillioja S, Ferraro R, et al. Twenty-four-hour energy expenditure in Pima Indians with type 2 (non-insulin-dependent) diabetes mellitus. Diabetologia 1992;35:753–759.

36. Bouchard C, Tremblay A, Nadeau A, et al. Genetic effect in resting and exercise metabolic rates. Metabolism 1989;38:364–370.

37. Hewitt J, Stunkard A, Carroll D, et al. A twin study approach towards understanding genetic contributions to body size and metabolic rate. Acta Genet Med Gemellol 1990;40:133–146.

38. Ravussin E, Lillioja M, Knowler W, et al. Reduced rate of energy expenditure as a risk factor for body-weight gain. N Engl J Med 1988;318:467–472.

39. Himms-Hagen J. Brown adipose tissue thermogenesis: interdisciplinary studies. FASEB J 1990; 4:2890–2898.

40. Rothwell NJ, Stock MJ. A role for brown adipose tissue in diet-induced thermogenesis. Nature 1979;281:31–35.

41. Foster DO, Frydman ML. Tissue distribution of cold-induced thermogenesis in conscious warm- or cold-acclimated rats reevaluated from changes in tissue blood flow: the dominant role of brown adipose tissue in the replacement of shivering by nonshivering thermogenesis. Can J Physiol Pharmacol 1979;57:257–270.

42. Davis TRA, Johnston DR, Bell FC, et al. Regulation of shivering and nonshivering heat production during acclimation of rats. Am J Physiol 1960;198:471–475.

43. Saad M, Alger S, Zurlo F, et al. Ethnic differences in sympathetic nervous system-mediated energy expenditure. Am J Physiol 1991;261:E789–E794.

44. Bray GA, York DA, Fisler JS. Experimental obesity: a homeostatic failure due to defective nutrient stimulation of the sympathetic nervous system. Vitam Horm 1989;45:1–124.

45. Flier JS. The adipocyte: storage depot or node on the energy information superhighway? Cell 1995;80:15–18.

46. Emorine L, Blin N, Strosberg AD. The human β3-adrenoceptor: The search for a physiological function. Trends Pharmacol Sci 1994:15:3–7.

47. Lonnqvist F, Krief S, Storsberg AD, Nyberg S, Emorine LJ, Arner P. Evidence for a functional beta-3-receptor in man. Br J Pharmacol 1993;110:929–936.

48. Rowe JW, Young JB, Ninaker KL, et al. Effect of insulin and glucose infusions on sympathetic nervous system activity in normal man. Diabetes 1981;30:219–225.

49. Landsberg L, Young JB. The role of the sympathoadrenal system in modulating energy expenditure. J Clin Endocrinol Metab 1984;13:475–499.

50. Katzeff HL, O'Connell M, Horton ES, et al. Metabolic studies in human obesity during overnutrition and undernutrition: thermogenic and hormonal responses to norepinephrine. Metab Clin Exp 1986;35:166–175.

51. Christin L, O'Connell M, Bogardus C, et al. Norepinephrine turnover and energy expenditure in Pima Indians and white men. Metabolism 1993;42:723–729.

52. Caro JF, Sinha MK, Klaczynski JW, Zhang PL, Considine RV. Leptin: The tale of an obesity gene. Diabetes 1996;45:1455–1462.

53. Halaas JL, Gajiwala KS, Maffei M, et al. Weight reducing effects of the plasma protein encoded by the obese gene. Science 1995;269:543–546.

54. Pelleymounter MA, Cullen MJ, Baker MB, et al. Effects of the obese gene product on body weight regulation in *ob/ob* mice. Science 1995;269:540–543.

55. Campfield LA, Smith FJ, Guisez Y, Devos R, Burn P. Recombinant mouse OB protein: Evidence for a peripheral signal linking adiposity and central neural networks. Science 1995;169:546–549.

56. Tartaglia LA, Dembski M, Weng X, et al. Identification and expression cloning of a leptin receptor, OB-R. Cell 1995;83:1263–1271.

57. Considine RV, Sinha MK, Heiman ML, et al. Serum immunoreactive- leptin concentrations in normal-weight and obese humans. N Engl J Med 1995;334:292–295.

58. Collins S, Kuhn C, Petro A, et al. Role of leptin in fat regulation. Nature 1996;380:677.

59. Emorine LJ, Marullo S, Briend-Sutren M-M, et al. Molecular characterization of the human β3-adrenergic receptor. Science 1989;245:1118–1121.

60. Muzzin P, Revelli JP, Kuhne F, et al. An adipose tissue-specific β-adrenergic receptor. Molecular cloning and down-regulation in obesity. J Biol Chem 1991;266:24,053–24,058.

61. Collins S, Daniel K, Rohlfs E, et al. Impaired expression and functional activity of the β3- and β1-adrenergic receptors in adipose tissue of congenitally obese (C57BL/6J ob/ob) mice. Mol Endocrinol 1994;8:518–527.

62. Trayhurn P, James WPT. Thermoregulation and nonshivering thermogenesis in the genetically obese (*ob/ob*) mouse. Pfluegers Arch Eur J Physiol 1978;373:189–193.

63. Thurbly PL, Trayhurn P. The role of thermoregulatory thermogenesis in the development of obesity in genetically obese (*ob/ob*) mice pair-fed with lean siblings. Br J Nutr 1979;42:377–385.

64. Feve B, Elhadri K, Quignard-Boulange A, Pairault J. Transcriptional down-regulation by insulin of β3-adrenergic receptor expression in 3T3-F442A adipocytes: A mechanism for repressing the cAMP signalling pathway. Proc Natl Acad Sci USA 1994;91:5677–5681.

65. Susulic VS, Frederich RC, Lawitts J, et al. Targeted disruption of the beta 3-adrenergic receptor gene. J Biol Chem 1995;270:29,483–29,492.

66. Ito M, Grujic D, Susulic VS, et al. Generation of mice expressing human but not murine beta-3-adrenergic receptors (abstract). 10th International Conference of Endocrinology, San Francisco, CA, June 1996 vol. 1, 1996, p. 389.

67. Thomas R, Holt B, Schwinn D, et al. Long-term agonist exposure induces upregulation of β3-adrenergic receptor expression via multiple cAMP response elements. Biochemistry 1992; 89:4490–4494.

68. Liggett S, Schwinn D. Multiple potential regulatory elements in the 5′ flanking region of the β-adrenergic receptor. J DNA Sequencing and Mapping 1991;2:61–63.

69. Himms-Hagen J, Cui J, Danforth E Jr. Effect of CL-316,243, a thermogenic β3-agonist, on energy balance and brown and white adipose tissues in rats. Am J Physiol 1994;266:R1371–R1382.

70. Revelli J, Muzzin P, Giacobino J, Muzzin P, Giacobino J. Modulation in vivo of β-adrenergic-receptor subtypes in rat brown adipose tissue by the thermogenic agonist Ro16-8714. Biochem J 1992; 283:743–746.

71. Yoshida T. The antidiabetic β3-adrenoceptor agonist BRL 26830A works by release of endogenous insulin. Am J Nutr 1992;55:237S–241S.

72. Thomas R, Liggett S. Lack of β3-adrenergic receptor mRNA expression in adipose and other metabolic tissues in the adult human. Mol Pharmacol 1992;43:343–348.

73. Rosenbaum M, Malbon C, Hirsch J, et al. Lack of β3-adrenergic effect on lipolysis in human subcutaneous adipose tissue. J Clin Endocrinol Metab 1993;77:352–355.

74. Krief S, Lonnquist F, Raimbault S, et al. Tissue distribution of β3-adrenergic receptor mRNA in man. J Clin Invest 1993;91:344–349.

75. Gauthier C, Travernier G, Charpentier F, Laning D, LeMarec H. Functional β3-adrenoceptor in the human heart. J Clin Invest 1996;98:556–562.

76. Martin SA, Johnston SM, Nakeeb A, et al. Effect of CCK and CL316,243: A novel β3-adrenoceptor agonist on sphincter of ODDI motility in the prairie dog. Annual Meeting of the American College of Surgeons, San Francisco, CA, 1996.

77. Chaudhry A, MacKenzie RG, Georgic LM, Granneman JG. Differential interaction of β₁ and β₃-adrenergic receptors with Gᵢ in rat adipocytes. Cell Signalling 1994;6:457–465.

78. Arbeeny C, Meyers D, Skwish S, Dickinson K. Strategies for the identification of potent beta-3-adrenergic receptor agonists for the clinical treatment of obesity and NIDDM (abstract). International Business Communications Third International Symposium on Obesity, Washington DC, 1996.

79. Viguerie-Bascands N, Bousquiet-Melou A, Galitzky J, et al. Evidence for numerous brown adipocytes lacking functional beta-3-adrenoceptors in fat pads from nonhuman primates. J Clin Endocrinol Metab 1996;81:368–375.

80. Lonnqvist F, Thorne A, Nilsell K, Hoffstedt J, Arner P. A pathogenic role of visceral fat β3-adrenoceptors in obesity. J Clin Invest 1995;95:1109–1116.

81. Randle PJ, Garland PB, Hales CN, Newsholme EA. The glucose fatty-acid cycle: its role in insulin sensitivity and the metabolic disturbances of diabetes mellitus. Lancet 1963;1:785–789.

82. Boden G. Role of fatty acids in the pathogenesis of insulin resistance and NIDDM. Diabetes 1997;46:3–10.

83. Ravussin E, Swinburn BA. In: Stunkard AJ, Wadden TA, eds. Obesity: Theory and Therapy. Raven, New York, 1993, pp. 97–123.

84. Bogardus C, Lillioja S, Mott D, et al. Evidence for reduced thermic effect of insulin and glucose infusions in Pima Indians. J Clin Invest 1985;75:1264–1269.

85. Spraul M, Ravussin E, Fontvieille AM, et al. Reduced sympathetic nervous activity: a potential mechanism predisposing to body weight gain. J Clin Invest 1993;92:1730–1735.

86. Spraul M, Anderson EA, Bogardus C, et al. Muscle sympathetic nerve activity in response to glucose ingestion. Diabetes 1994;43:191–196.

87. Connacher AA, Jung RT, Mitchell PEG. Weight loss in obese subjects on a restricted diet given BRL 26830A, a new atypical β-adrenoceptor agonist. Br Med J 1988;296:1217–1220.

88. Haesler E, et al. Effect of a novel β-adrenoceptor agonist (Ro40-2148) on resting energy expenditure in obese women. Int J Obes 1994;18:313–322.

89. Cawthorne M, Sennitt M, Arch J, et al. BRL 35135, a potent and selective atypical β-adrenoceptor agonist. Am J Clin Nutr 1992;55:252S–257S.

90. Connacher A, Bennet W, Jung R. Clinical studies with the β-adrenoceptor agonist BRL 26830A. Am J Clin Nutr 1992;55:258S–261S.

91. Pietri-Rouxel F, Strosberg AD. Pharmacological characteristics and species-related variations of beta-3-adrenergic receptors. Fund Clin Pharmacol 1995;9:211–218.

92. Granneman J, Lahners K, Chaudhry A. Characterization of the human β3-adrenergic receptor gene. Mol Pharmacol 1993;44:264–270.

93. Spronsen AV, Nahmias C, Krief S, et al. The promotor and intron/exon structure of the human and mouse β3-adrenergic-receptor genes. Eur J Biochem 1993;213:1117–1124.

94. Champigny O, Ricquier D, Blondel O, et al. β3-adrenergic receptor stimulation restores message and expression of brown-fat mitochondrial uncoupling protein in adult dogs. Pharmacology 1991;88:10,774–10,777.

95. Walston J, Silver K, Bogardus C, et al. Time of onset of non-insulin dependent diabetes mellitus and genetic variation in the β_3-adrenergic-receptor gene. N Engl J Med 1995;333:343–347.

96. Arner P. The β_3-adrenergic receptor—a cause and cure of obesity? 1995;333:382, 383.

97. Silver K, Walston W, Wang Y, Dowse G, Zimmet P, Shuldiner AR. Molecular scanning for mutations in the β_3-adrenergic receptor gene in Nauruans with obesity and noninsulin dependent diabetes mellitus. J Clin Endocrinol Metab 1996;81:4155–4158.

98. Knowler WC, Bennett PH, Bottazz GF, Doniach D. Islet cell antibodies and diabetes mellitus in Pima Indians. Diabetologia 1979;17:161–164.

99. Widen E, Lehto M, Kanninen T, et al. Association of a polymorphism in the β_3-adrenergic-receptor gene with features of the insulin resistance syndrome in Finns. N Engl J Med 1995;333:347–351.

100. Sipilainen R, Uusitupa M, Heikkinen S, Rissanen A, Laakso M. Polymorphism of the β_3-adrenergic receptor gene affects basal metabolic rate in obese Finns Diabetes 1997;46:77–80.

101. Ghosh S, Ally D, Hauser E, et al. The beta-3-adrenergic receptor codon 64 variant is not associated with age-at-diagnosis of NIDDM nor with obesity in the FUSION (Finish US Investigation of NIDDM) study (abstract). Diabetes 1996;45(Suppl 2):229A.

102. Kadowaki H, Yasuda K, Iwamoto K, et al. A mutation in the β_3-adrenergic receptor gene is associated with obesity and hyperinsulinemia in Japanese subjects. Biochem Biophys Res Commun 1995;215:55–560.

103. Fujisawa T, Ikegami H, Yamato E, et al. Association of Trp64Arg mutation of the β_3-adrenergic receptor with NIDDM and body weight gain. Diabetologia 1996;39:349–352.

104. Knowler, WC. Association of Trp64Arg mutation of the β_3-adrenergic receptor gene with NIDDM. Diabetologia 1996;39:1411.

105. Sakane N, Yoshida T, Yoshioka K, et al. Genetic variation in the β_3-adrenergic receptor in Japanese NIDDM patients. Diabetes Care, 1996;19:34–35.

106. Yoshida T, Sakane N, Umedawa T, et al. Mutation of the β_3-adrenergic receptor gene and response to treatment of obesity. Lancet 1996;346:1433–1434.

107. Silver K, Mitchell BD, Walston J, Sorkin JD, Stern MP, Roth J, Shuldiner AR. Trp64Arg beta-3-adrenergic receptor and obesity in Mexican Americans, Am Journal of Human Genetics 1997; in press.

108. Clement K, Vaisse C, Manning B. St. J, et al. Genetic variation in the β_3-adrenergic receptor and an increased capacity to gain weight in patients with morbid obesity. N Engl J Med 1995;333:351–354.

109. Kurabayashi T, Carey DGP, Morrison NA. The β_3-adrenergic receptor gene Trp64Arg mutation is overrepresented in obese women. Effects on weight, BMI, abdominal fat, blood pressure, and reproductive history in an elderly Australian population. Diabetes 1996;45:1358–1363.

110. Zhang Y, Wat N, Stratton IM, et al. UKPDS 19: heterogeneity in NIDDM: separate contributions of IRS-1 and β3-adrenergic-receptor mutations to insulin resistance and obesity respectively with no evidence for glycogen synthase gene mutations. Diabetologia 1996;39:1505–1511.

111. Urhammer SO, Clausen JO, Hansen T, Pedersen O. Insulin sensitivity and body weight changes in young white carriers of the codon 64 amino acid polymorphism of the β_3-adrenergic receptor gene. Diabetes 1996;45:1115–1120.

112. Gagnon J, Mauriege P, Roy S, et al. The Trp64Arg mutation of the β_3-adrenergic receptor gene has no effect on obesity phenotypes in the Quebec family study and Swedish obese subjects cohorts. J Clin Invest 1996;98:2086–2093.

113. Elbein S, Hoffman M, Barrett K, et al. Role of the beta-3-adrenergic receptor locus in obesity and noninsulin-dependent diabetes among members of Caucasian families with a diabetic sibling pair. J Clin Endocrinol Metab 1996;81:4422–4427.

114. Awata T, Kaayama S. Genetic variation in the β_3-adrenergic receptor in Japanese NIDDM patients. Diabetes Care 1996;19:271,272.

115. Odawara M, Sasaki K, Yamashita K. β_3-Adrenergic receptor gene variant and Japanese NIDDM: A pitfall in meta-analysis. Lancet 1996;348:896–897

116. Shuldiner AR, Silver K, Roth J, Walston J. Beta-3-adrenergic receptor gene variant in obesity and insulin resistance. Lancet 1996;348:1584,1585.

117. Shafrir E. Frontiers in Diabetes Research: Lessons from Animal Diabetes IV. Shafir E, ed. Smith-Gordon, London.

118. The Cystic Fibrosis Genotype-Phenotype Consortium Correlation between genotype and phenotype in patients with cystic fibrosis. N Engl J Med 1993;329:1308–1313.

119. Risch N, Merlkangas K. The future of genetic studies of complex human diseases. Science 1996;273:1516,1517.

120. Cox NJ, Bell GI. Disease associations. Chance, artifact, or susceptibility genes? Diabetes 1989;38:947–950.

121. Maurieg P, Bouchard C. Trp64Arg mutation in β_3-adrenoceptor gene of doubtful significance for obesity and insulin resistance. Lancet 1996;348:699,700.

122. Candelore MR, Deng L, Tota LM, Kelly LJ, Cascieri MA, Strader CD. Pharmacological characterization of a recently described human β_3-adrenergic receptor mutant. Endocrinology 1996; 137:2638–2641.

123. Strosberg AD. Structure and function of the human β_3-adrenergic receptor. 10th International Congress of Endocrinology, Washington, D.C. 1996;1:28.

124. Li LS, Lonnqvist F, Luthman H, Arner P. Phenotypic characterization of the Trp64Arg polymorphism in the β_3-adrenergic receptor gene in normal weight and obese subjects. Diabetologia 1996;39:857–860.

125. Snitker S, Odeleye OE, Hellmer, J, et al. No effect of the Trp64Arg β_3-adrenoceptor variant on *in vivo* lipolysis in subcutaneous adipose tissue. Diabetologia 1997;40:838–842.

126. Saunders AM, Strittmatter WJ, Schmechel D, et al. Association of apolipoprotein E allele E4 with late-onset familial and sporadic Alzheimer's disease. Neurology 1993;43:1467–1471.

INDEX